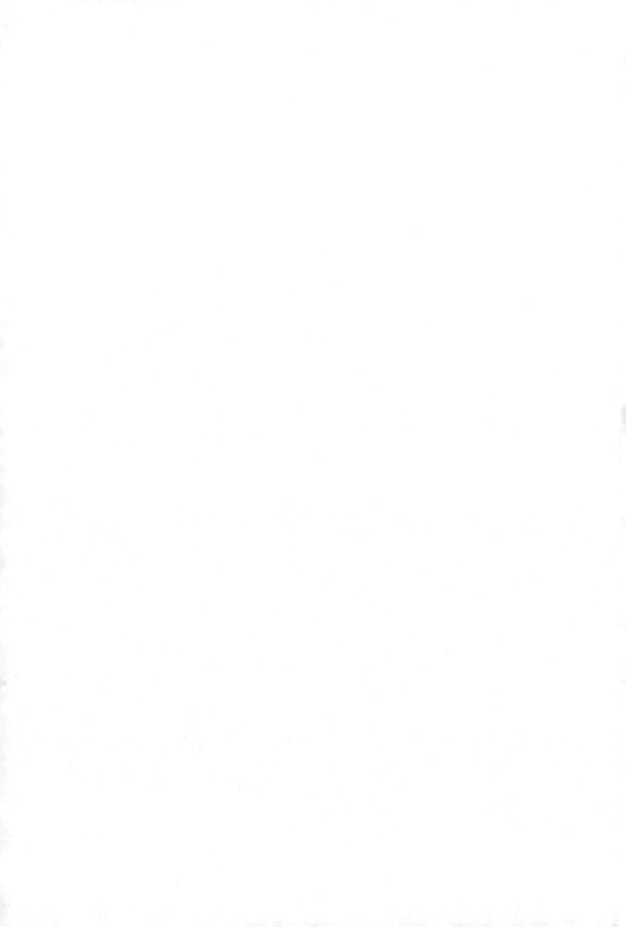

Implementation Science

This accessible textbook introduces a wide spectrum of ideas, approaches, and examples that make up the emerging field of implementation science, including implementation theory, processes and methods, data collection and analysis, brokering interest on the ground, and sustainable implementation.

Containing over 60 concise essays, each addressing the thorny problem of how we can make care more evidence-informed, this book looks at how implementation science should be defined, how it can be conducted, and how it is assessed. It offers vital insight into how research findings that are derived from healthcare contexts can help make sense of service delivery and patient encounters. Each entry concentrates on an important concept and examines the idea's evidence base, root causes and effects, ideas and applications, and methodologies and methods. Revealing a very human side to caregiving, but also tackling its more complex and technological aspects, the contributors draw on real-life healthcare examples to look both at why things go right in introducing a new intervention and at what can go wrong. *Implementation Science: The Key Concepts* provides a toolbox of rich, contemporary thought from leading international thinkers, clearly and succinctly delivered.

This comprehensive and enlightening range of ideas and examples brought together in one place is essential reading for all students, researchers, and practitioners with an interest in translating knowledge into practice in healthcare.

Frances Rapport is Professor of Health Implementation Science at Macquarie University's Centre for Healthcare Resilience and Implementation Science, Sydney, Australia, is Academic Lead, MD Research, Macquarie University, and holds an Honorary Chair as Professor of Qualitative Health Research at Swansea University's Medical School, UK. She currently leads a team of implementation scientists examining new models of implementation to support the translation of research outcomes into practical solutions for healthcare delivery and improvement. Rapport has a visiting professorship in Bournemouth University, UK, and was previously a visiting professor at Harvard University (Psychiatry), Texas University, Galveston (Medical Board), and the University of Tromsø (Medical Humanities) in Norway.

Robyn Clay-Williams is Associate Professor of Human Factors and Resilience and an internationally regarded health services researcher, who leads a research stream at the Australian Institute of Health and Innovation (AIHI), Macquarie University, Sydney, Australia. Her expertise is in creating health systems that can function effectively in the presence of complexity and uncertainty. Dr Clay-Williams' research bridges the gap between theory and practice by developing products and processes that are usable and ready for implementation. She has a background in aviation and, prior to her academic career, was a military test pilot with the Royal Australian Air Force.

Jeffrey Braithwaite is Founding Director of the AIHI, Director of the Centre for Healthcare Resilience and Implementation Science, and Professor of Health Systems Research, Faculty of Medicine, Health and Human Sciences, Macquarie University, Sydney, Australia. He has appointments at six other universities internationally, and he is a board member and President of the International Society for Quality in Health Care (ISQua) and consultant to the World Health Organization (WHO). Working with 152 countries on their reform initiatives, his research on safer, higher quality, and more resilient care examines health systems and their capacity to implement change and improvement, attracting funding of more than AUD 171 million. He is particularly interested in healthcare as a Complex Adaptive System and applying complexity science to healthcare problems.

Implementation Science

The Key Concepts

**Edited by Frances Rapport,
Robyn Clay-Williams, and
Jeffrey Braithwaite**

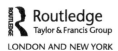

Routledge
Taylor & Francis Group

LONDON AND NEW YORK

Cover image credit: © Getty Images

First published 2022
by Routledge
4 Park Square, Milton Park, Abingdon, Oxon OX14 4RN

and by Routledge
605 Third Avenue, New York, NY 10158

Routledge is an imprint of the Taylor & Francis Group, an informa business

British Library Cataloguing-in-Publication Data
A catalogue record for this book is available from the British Library

Library of Congress Cataloging-in-Publication Data
Names: Rapport, Frances, 1960– editor. | Clay-Williams, Robyn, editor. |
     Braithwaite, Jeffrey, 1954– editor.
Title: Key concepts in implementation science : translation and improvement
     in medicine and healthcare / edited by Frances Rapport, Robyn Clay-Williams
     and Jeffrey Braithwaite.
Description: Abingdon, Oxon ; New York, NY : Routledge, 2022. | Includes
     bibliographical references and index.
Identifiers: LCCN 2021056873 (print) | LCCN 2021056874 (ebook) |
     ISBN 9780367626136 (hardback) | ISBN 9780367626112 (paperback) |
     ISBN 9781003109945 (ebook)
Subjects: LCSH: Evidence-based medicine—Textbooks. | Medical
     care—Textbooks.
Classification: LCC R723.7 .K48 2022 (print) | LCC R723.7 (ebook) |
     DDC 610—dc23/eng/20220330
LC record available at https://lccn.loc.gov/2021056873
LC ebook record available at https://lccn.loc.gov/2021056874

ISBN: 978-0-367-62613-6 (hbk)
ISBN: 978-0-367-62611-2 (pbk)
ISBN: 978-1-003-10994-5 (ebk)

DOI: 10.4324/9781003109945

Typeset in Times New Roman
by Apex CoVantage, LLC

Contents

Figures

Tables

Boxes

Contributors

Gregory A. Aarons is a clinical and organizational psychologist, Professor in the Department of Psychiatry at the University of California San Diego (UCSD), Co-director of the UCSD Dissemination and Implementation Science Center (UCSD-DISC), and Director of the Child and Adolescent Services Research Center (CASRC). He is co-developer of the Exploration, Preparation, Implementation, Sustainment (EPIS) framework (https://episframework.com) and developer of the Leadership and Organizational Change for Implementation strategy (https://implementationleadership.com). He focuses on leadership and organization support strategies and evidence-based practice implementation and sustainment in behavioural health. His implementation and scale-up strategies are being used in behavioural health, schools, child welfare, HIV prevention, and trauma care in the United States, Norway, and West Africa.

David C. Aron is Director of Clinical Program Research and Education at the Cleveland VA Medical Center. He is a clinical endocrinologist, health services researcher, and leader of the VA Quality Scholars Fellowship Program, a training program in quality improvement. He is Professor of Medicine and Epidemiology and Biostatistics at the School of Medicine, Case Western Reserve University. He is also Adjunct Professor of Organizational Behaviour at the Weatherhead School of Management, where he teaches a class on Managing Complex Systems. He is the author of a recent book titled *Complex Systems in Medicine: A Hedgehog's Tale of Complexity in Clinical Practice, Research, Education and Management*.

David W. Bates is an internationally renowned expert in health information technology, patient safety, and quality. His work has focused on improving clinical decision-making, patient safety, quality of care, and cost-effectiveness. He is Chief of the Division of General Internal Medicine at Brigham and Women's Hospital in Boston, Professor of Medicine at Harvard Medical School, and Professor of Health Policy and Management at the Harvard School of Public Health, where he co-directs the Program in Clinical Effectiveness. He has been elected to the Institute of Medicine, is a past president of the International Society of Quality in Health Care, and is past chairman of the Board of the American Medical Informatics Association.

Sarah A. Birken is Associate Professor in the Department of Implementation Science in the School of Medicine and Member of Wake Forest Baptist Health's Comprehensive Cancer Center at Wake Forest University, North Carolina, United States. Her research focuses on translating evidence into practice. Specifically, she studies middle managers' role in implementing evidence-based practices, the implementation of innovations in cancer care, and the selection and application of implementation theories. Birken also co-hosts AcaDames, a podcast about women in academia. She is an avid runner and loves nesting at home and in her garden with friends and family.

Jackie Bridges runs a research program at the University of Southampton, UK, focusing on the organization and delivery of healthcare to older people with complex needs. Dr Bridges is interested in organizational change and professional work, drawing on the methods and theoretical perspectives of the social sciences. Her research focuses on healthcare systems and workforce, particularly nursing, examining organizational conditions in which health workers are able to deliver responsive, high-quality care to older people with complex needs. She leads the Ageing and Dementia Research Group in the School of Health Sciences and is an investigator for the National Institute for Health Research Applied (NIHR) Research Collaborative (ARC) Wessex.

Pascale Carayon is the Leon and Elizabeth Janssen Professor in Engineering, Director of the Center for Quality and Productivity Improvement, Founding Director of the Wisconsin Institute for Healthcare Systems Engineering, and leader of the interdisciplinary Systems Engineering Initiative for Patient Safety (SEIPS) at the University of Wisconsin–Madison, United States. She received her engineer diploma from the Ecole Centrale de Paris, France, and her PhD in industrial engineering from the University of Wisconsin–Madison. She has research experience analysing, designing, and improving complex work systems such as those in healthcare and focuses on patient safety and healthcare issues such as design of health information technologies.

David Chambers is Deputy Director for Implementation Science in the Division of Cancer Control and Population Sciences (DCCPS) at the National Cancer Institute (NCI). Dr Chambers focuses on advancing the field of implementation science through funding opportunity announcements, training programs, research activities, dissemination platforms, and enhancement of partnerships and networks to integrate research, practice, and policy. He publishes on strategic research directions in implementation science and serves as a plenary speaker at numerous scientific conferences. He received his AB degree (with Honours) in economics from Brown University (1997) and MSc and DPhil in management studies (1998 and 2001, respectively) from Oxford University, UK.

Huey T. Chen is Professor in the Department of Public Health and Director of the Center for Applied Research and Evaluation in the College of Health Professions at Mercer University. He previously served as branch chief and senior evaluation scientist at the Centers for Disease Control and Prevention (CDC), as well as Professor at the University of Alabama at Birmingham, United States. Dr Chen has worked with community organizations, health-related agencies, government agencies, and educational institutions. He has conducted both large-scale and small-scale evaluations in the United States and internationally and has written extensively on program theory, theory-driven evaluation, the bottom-up evaluation approach, and the integrated evaluation perspective.

Mark Clark is Associate Professor of Medical Humanities at the University of the Incarnate Word School of Osteopathic Medicine, San Antonio, Texas, United States. As a member of the founding faculty, Dr Clark helped establish a new medical school curriculum that integrates the medical humanities and promotes professional identity formation. He has published work related to narrative issues in medicine, the doctor–patient relationship, literature and medicine, and professional identity formation. Previously, he served as Director of the Graduate Program for the Institute of the Medical Humanities at the University of Texas Medical Branch and as a faculty member, Department of English, Saint Louis University.

Jenelle Clarke is a postdoctoral research fellow at the School of Social Policy, Health Services Management Centre, University of Birmingham, UK. Her current research project, "The Rituals of Integrated Working", funded by The Healthcare Improvement Studies (THIS) Institute, explores improvement initiatives within integrated mental health and social teams, specifically children and adolescent and older people services. Previously, Clarke has been a co-collaborator and research fellow on a NIHR-funded grant, "Healthcare Leadership with Political Astuteness (HeLPA): A Qualitative Study of How Service Leaders Understand and Mediate the 'Politics and Power' of Major Health System Change", looking at the organizational politics involved in major health system change.

Ellen Coeckelberghs is a postdoctoral researcher at the Leuven Institute for Healthcare Policy at KU Leuven, Belgium, and deputy coordinator of the Belgian-Dutch clinical pathway network. This is a social capital network of more than 50 healthcare organizations sharing knowledge, data, experiences, and expertise on the development, implementation, evaluation, and continuous follow-up of care pathways. She is also membership manager of the European Pathway Association and is involved in national and international research about care pathways. She co-authored the national care pathway for low back pain. Internationally, she has undertaken projects on care pathways for nutrition problems in gastrointestinal cancer and geriatric hip fractures.

Laura Damschroder is an implementation researcher with the Veterans Affairs Center for Clinical Management Research in Ann Arbor, Michigan, United States, and a principal investigator for the Maintaining Implementation through Dynamic Adaptations (MIDAS) Center. She is also Adjunct Associate Professor at Queensland University of Technology in Brisbane, Australia. Laura Damschroder is lead developer of the Consolidated Framework for Implementation Research (CFIR), one of the most widely used frameworks in implementation science. She has been a visiting scholar at many international institutions, leads national workshops, and mentors early career implementation researchers. She focuses on applying theory in implementation research and developing pragmatic approaches for understanding context and tailoring strategies for implementation success.

Ellen S. Deutsch practised as a paediatric otolaryngology surgeon for 20 years before taking a full-time position in simulation and completing a master's degree in healthcare quality and patient safety. She has served in leadership roles in national otolaryngology and international simulation organizations. Most recently, she served as a senior scientist at the Children's Hospital of Philadelphia (CHOP) and adjunct associate professor at the University of Pennsylvania. She has expertise in patient safety data analysis and display. Her goals include implementing human factors principles and enhancing the resilience of healthcare delivery systems to empower clinicians to improve patient safety and provider satisfaction.

Ivana Durcinoska was, until recently, a researcher at the Ingham Institute for Applied Research and the University of New South Wales, Sydney, Australia. Her research traverses cancer, Social Network Analysis, and health services, including a passion for patient-centred approaches to care. Her work on the Patient-Reported Outcome Measures for Personalized Treatment and Care (PROMPT-Care) system is particularly well regarded.

She has contributed to studies using multiple research methods, including randomized trials, the development of decision algorithms, and population-based surveys of patients.

Mark G. Ehrhart is Professor of Industrial and Organizational Psychology at the University of Central Florida. His research interests include organizational climate and culture, organizational citizenship behaviour, and leadership and the application of these topics across levels of analysis and in behavioural and mental health settings. His recent work focuses on organizational context in the implementation of evidence-based practice in mental health, child welfare, substance abuse treatment, and nursing settings. He is lead author (with Dr Benjamin Schneider and Dr William Macey) of the 2014 book *Organizational Climate and Culture: An Introduction to Theory, Research, and Practice*.

Moriah E. Ellen is Senior Lecturer in the Department of Health Systems Management, Guilford Glazer Faculty of Business and Management, Ben-Gurion University of the Negev, Israel. She is also Assistant Professor at the Institute of Health Policy, Management and Evaluation at the University of Toronto, Canada, and Investigator at the McMaster Health Forum, Canada. Dr Ellen's primary research interests are health systems and policy, knowledge transfer and exchange, and addressing the use of unnecessary healthcare services. Specifically, she has addressed infrastructures needed for evidence-informed policymaking and health system initiatives to reduce the overuse of tests, treatments, and procedures.

Per-Erik Ellström is Senior Professor of Education at Linköping University, Sweden. He is also the founder and former director of the Centre for Studies of Humans, Technology, and Organization (1994–2005) and the HELIX Excellence Centre (2006–2012) at the same university. HELIX is a multidisciplinary research centre with a focus on learning, innovation, change, and development in organizations. Ellström's research interests include professional learning, practice-based innovation, organizational change and development, leadership, and interactive research. He has published several books and a large number of articles and other publications. In addition, 20 PhD students have finished their exams under his supervision.

Glyn Elwyn is Professor at the Dartmouth Institute for Health Policy and Clinical Practice, United States, and at the Scientific Institute for Quality of Healthcare at Radboud University Nijmegen Medical Centre in the Netherlands. He holds visiting professor positions in Switzerland and the UK. Glyn Elwyn studies coproduction, shared decision-making, and the application of machine learning to digital recordings of clinical encounters. He leads an international interdisciplinary team examining the implementation of shared decision-making in clinical settings. He developed Option Grid™ patient decision aids and evidence-based tools. He is the lead editor of *Shared Decision Making: Evidence-Based Patient Choice*, Oxford University Press, 3rd edition, 2016.

Benjamin Gardner is Senior Lecturer at King's College London, UK. His main research interest lies in understanding the concept of habit, identifying the precise role(s) of "habit" in real-world behaviours, and how insights from habit theory can be used to explain and change behaviour. He has published more than 70 papers on habit, variously covering theory development, measurement, behaviour prediction, intervention design and evaluation, and state-of-the-art theoretical and empirical reviews. He is a chartered member of the British Psychological Society and co-leads the European Health Psychology Society Habit Special Interest Group.

Emily R. Haines is a postdoctoral fellow in Wake Forest School of Medicine's Cancer Prevention and Control Training Program, North Carolina, United States. Her doctorate is from the University of North Carolina at Chapel Hill Gillings School of Global Public Health where she studied implementation and organization science. Dr Haines' research focuses on the implementation of evidence-based practices in cancer care organizations with a particular interest in applied novel methods in implementation research (e.g., ethnography; user-centred design) to assess implementation context to improve implementation. Her other research interests include adolescent and young adult cancer care and the application of organizational theory in implementation science.

Henna Hasson is Professor of Implementation Science and Director of the Medical Management Centre at Karolinska Institutet, Sweden. Her research focus is on the implementation of innovative work practices and de-implementation of low value care. She has a great interest in the practical impact of her research as a Head of Unit for Implementation, Center for Epidemiology and Community Medicine at Stockholm Region, Sweden. She is a project leader for several ongoing research projects investigating implementation of interventions. The results of these projects can be used to analyse how, when, and in what context the interventions might work.

Carolyn J. Hill joined the Manpower Demonstration Research Corporation (MDRC) from Georgetown University, where she was Associate Professor of Public Policy. She is working on the Mother and Infant Home Visiting Program Evaluation, the Families Forward Demonstration, the Understanding Poverty: Childhood and Family Experiences Study, the Get Ready Guilford Initiative, and a technical assistance project on the coordination between welfare-to-work programs under Temporary Assistance for Needy Families (TANF) and workforce development services funded by the Workforce Innovation and Opportunity Act (WIOA). She also co-curates MDRC's Implementation Research Incubator and helps lead MDRC's Implementation Research Group, supporting innovative implementation research methods across the organization's policy areas and studies.

Erik Hollnagel is an internationally recognized specialist in the fields of resilience engineering, system safety, human reliability analysis, cognitive systems engineering, and intelligent human-machine systems. He is presently Senior Professor of Patient Safety at the University of Jönköping, Sweden. Hollnagel is also Visiting Professorial Fellow, Faculty of Medicine and Health Sciences at Macquarie University (Australia); Visiting Fellow of the Institute for Advanced Study of the Technische Universitat München (Germany); and Professor Emeritus at the Department of Computer and Information Science (IDA) at Linköping University (LIU), Sweden. Erik Hollnagel has been president of the European Association of Cognitive Ergonomics (1994–2000) and member of the Swedish Reactor Safety Council (1996–2002).

Louise Hull is Deputy Director of the Centre for Implementation Science at King's College London, UK, and leads the methodology theme of the centre. She is also Deputy Co-lead of the NIHR ARC South London Implementation Research theme. Hull trained as a psychologist and holds a BSc in psychology and an MSc in research methods in psychology. She completed her PhD in patient safety at Imperial College London. Her research interests fall within the areas of patient safety, improvement science, and implementation science, and she has led the development and validation of non-technical and teamwork assessment tools for use in healthcare.

Karen Hutchinson is a postdoctoral research fellow with the AIHI, Macquarie University, Sydney, Australia. She completed a PhD at the University of Sydney in 2018 taking a social model perspective to research younger onset dementia. Her current research examines the experiences of families living with parental refractory (uncontrolled) epilepsy and roles and responsibilities of epilepsy nurses in Australia. Dr Hutchinson is a physiotherapist working with adults living with complex and chronic neurological conditions. She is on the NHMRC Younger Onset Dementia Special Interest Group, Young Carers Research Advisory Group with Carers NSW, and Chair of the AIHI Implementation Science Interest Group.

Amy M. Kilbourne is Director of the US Department of Veterans Affairs Quality Enhancement Research Initiative (QUERI) and Professor of Learning Health Sciences at the University of Michigan. With over 40 centres across the United States, QUERI's mission is to improve patient health outcomes by accelerating the implementation of research findings into real-world practice. As QUERI director, Dr Kilbourne established the first national network of training programs focused on implementation strategies, supporting provider-based tools or methods used to facilitate the spread of effective clinical practices. She has worked tirelessly to improve outcomes and reduce health disparities through implementation science methods' applications across different communities and healthcare settings.

Roman Kislov is a reader in organization studies at Manchester Metropolitan University, UK; an honorary senior research fellow at The University of Manchester; and a deputy lead for Implementation Science in the NIHR ARC, Greater Manchester. He conducts qualitative research on the processes and practices of knowledge mobilization, with a particular interest in knowledge brokering, co-production of research, and application and development of theory in implementation science. His work crosses disciplinary boundaries between organization studies, public administration, and health services research.

Virginia Knox is President of the MDRC, United States, prior to which she served as vice president and leader of the organization's Families and Children Policy Area. Over 25 years she has brought leadership to developing, evaluating, and improving social programs and strengthening evidence-based policymaking. She has designed evaluations of central interest to policymakers and practitioners and provided them with actionable conclusions. She has focused on how increased access to assistance for low-income parents can improve lives, and she has led or co-led MDRC's evaluation of many programs, including the Get Ready Guilford Initiative and the Building Bridges and Bonds evaluation.

Klay Lamprell is a health systems researcher with the AIHI, Macquarie University, Sydney, Australia. Dr Lamprell's work examines patients' experiences of healthcare and investigates systemic challenges to the delivery of safe, effective, individualized care. She has a background and extensive expertise in journalism and an interest in narrative methodologies. Most recently, she has written about how to narrativize patient-centred care, arguing that patient-centred approaches must begin with caring for clinicians. Recent research interests include patients' longitudinal experience of cancer, in particular melanoma, and how to collect personal accounts of young onset colorectal cancer.

Kate Laver is a past National Health Medical Research Council-Australian Research Council (NHMRC-ARC) Dementia Research Development Fellow and currently an ARC Discovery Early Career Research Fellow. She is both an experienced occupational therapist and a researcher. She has also established herself as a researcher with a reputation for genuine collaboration with patients and members of the public. Dr Laver has expertise in designing and conducting translational research studies that improve the quality of care of community-dwelling older people, particularly those with cognitive frailty. Her research experience also includes testing rehabilitation interventions (fields of dementia and stroke) and other non-pharmacological therapy approaches and use of innovative technologies in rehabilitation.

Luci K. Leykum is the Centre Lead for the Elizabeth Dole Center of Excellence for Veteran and Caregiver Research in the Department of Veterans Affairs, United States. She is also Professor of Medicine and Vice-Chair of the Department of Medicine at Dell Medical School, part of the University of Texas at Austin. Dr Leykum's work has used the lens of complexity science to understand and improve clinical systems, focusing on improving how patients, families, and clinicians relate to each other and make sense of what is happening. Much of her work has been partnered with patients, families, caregivers, and other stakeholders.

Janet C. Long is a health systems researcher with interests and expertise in social and professional networks, knowledge translation, and implementation science. She has a clinical background as a registered nurse and a science background in ecology. This unique combination of clinical, science, and health services research has enabled her to be a powerful connector across the translational gap between research and practice. Her passion is studying social interactions and influences within healthcare using social network theory and methodology. Dr Long's systematic review on brokerage roles in collaborative networks, among other extensive publications in this area, has been highly cited.

Fabiana Lorencatto is the Research Lead and Principal Research Fellow at the University College London's Centre for Behaviour Change. Lorencatto's research focuses on health behaviour change and implementation science – in particular, applying theories and frameworks from the behavioural sciences to understand what factors are driving behaviour as a basis for designing and evaluating theory – and evidence-based interventions to change the behaviour of healthcare professionals, patients, and the public. Her current research focuses on infection prevention control and maternal health. She also has a methodological interest in process evaluations and the assessment of implementation outcomes, particularly intervention fidelity. Lorencatto is an associate editor of *Implementation Science Communications*.

Kristiana Ludlow is a postdoctoral research fellow at the AIHI, Macquarie University, Australia. She is passionate about collaborating with consumers, service users, family members, and workforces to improve the delivery of healthcare, particularly in the aged care sector. Her research interests include care priorities and prioritization, unfinished and missed care, patient- and family-centred care, and the co-design of digital health tools to support information sharing and decision-making.

Russell Mannion has held the Chair in Health Systems at the University of Birmingham, England, since 2010, is an honorary professor at the AIHI, Macquarie University, Sydney, Australia, and is a fellow of Bocconi University, Milan, Italy. Dr Mannion provides consultancy and advice to a range of national and international agencies, including the World Health Organization (WHO), the Organization for Economic Co-operation and Development (OECD), the European Union (EU), and Her Majesty's (HM) Treasury, London.

Carl May is Professor of Medical Sociology at the London School of Hygiene and Tropical Medicine and leads the Innovation and Implementation Science Research Theme in the NIHR North Thames Applied Research Collaborative. His work has focused on professional knowledge and practice in complex healthcare problems, the role of innovative health technologies in managing long-term conditions, and patient and caregiver experiences of care. He is the lead architect of Normalization Process Theory (NPT) (with Dr Tracy Finch and international researchers and practitioners). NPT provides a widely used conceptual framework for understanding the dynamics of implementing treatment modalities and new ways of organizing and delivering care through collective action and collaborative work.

Joanna C. Moullin is an implementation scientist in the Faculty of Health Sciences at Curtin University, Perth, Australia. Dr Moullin completed her PhD applying and advancing the field of implementation science in community pharmacy. She subsequently completed a postdoctoral fellowship at the UCSD, testing leadership and organizational change for implementation intervention in substance use treatment centres. Dr Moullin has extensive knowledge of implementation frameworks, models, and theories and has designed and tested pragmatic implementation measures for use in implementation research and practice. Her research has been published, presented, and applied around the world.

Kazue Nakajima is Executive Director, Japan Organization of Occupational Health and Safety and Professor of the Faculty of Medicine, Osaka University. She is a co-founder of the Department of Clinical Quality Management, Osaka University Hospital. As a Fulbright scholar, she studied health policy and management at the Harvard School of Public Health, completed an internship at the Harvard Risk Management Foundation, and worked for 20 years on patient safety and quality improvement. In 2019, she held the 14th Congress of Japanese Society for Quality and Safety in Health Care as President of the Congress and also hosted the 8th Resilient Health Care Network Meeting in Japan.

Kyota Nakamura is Board Certified in Emergency Medicine and Intensive Care. He is currently Professor of the Department of Clinical Quality Management at Osaka University Hospital in Japan. He has committed himself to education for medical students and healthcare professionals for about 20 years. He is one of the founding members of the simulation centre at Yokohama City University. He has directed and developed many simulation training programs, including in situ simulation, especially on crisis resource management. His specific interests include resuscitation, airway and ventilator management, trauma system, disaster medicine, dynamic team performance, and medical simulation training.

Margit Neher is Associate Professor in the School of Health and Welfare, Jönköping University, Sweden. Dr Neher is engaged in implementation research and teaches implementation science classes. She has interest and extensive expertise in learning processes during clinical change and how learning environments in healthcare contexts may be developed to support effective practices. Her research interests include practice roles and task shifting, as well as workplace learning and behaviour change, in connection with the transition to digital technology use in healthcare. She also researches fidelity and adaptations in evidence-based practice and likes to use a range of qualitative analysis methods and mixed methods.

Per Nilsen is Professor at the Department of Health, Medicine and Caring Sciences, Linköping University, Sweden, with a particular focus on implementation science. He was responsible for building a research program and establishing an international doctoral-level course in implementation science, which has run annually since 2011. Dr Nilsen takes particular interest in issues concerning practice change and the use of theory for understanding implementation challenges. Nilsen is also engaged in health services research and public health studies, where interdisciplinarity, theory use, and behaviour change are common threads.

Terje Ogden is a senior researcher at the Norwegian Center for Child Behavioral Development (NCCBD) and professor at the Norwegian Centre for Learning Environment and Behavioural Research in Education, University of Stavanger, Norway. He is a former research director at NCCBD (2003–2018) and professor at the Institute of Psychology, University of Oslo (2005–2018), Norway. His research interests include the development, implementation, and evaluation of interventions targeting children and youth with mental health and conduct problems. He is also a board member of the Global Implementation Society (GIS) and assistant editor of the US-based journal *Implementation Research and Practice*.

John Øvretveit is Research and Development Officer for Stockholm healthcare system and Professor of Improvement, Implementation and Evaluation at the Karolinska Institute medical university, Stockholm, Sweden. Previously, he was at the Nordic School of Public Health, establishing and running the quality improvement program at Bergen Medical School. He served 12 years as a board director of the US Joint Commission International and currently serves as a board director of the global implementation society leading their COVID-19 implementation response group. Over his career he has published over 400 scientific peer-reviewed articles and 12 books.

Lawrence A. Palinkas is the Albert G and Frances Lomas Feldman Professor of Social Policy and Health in the Suzanne Dworak-Peck School of Social Work at the University of Southern California (USC), United States. He also holds secondary appointments as Professor in the Departments of Anthropology and Preventive Medicine at USC. A medical anthropologist, his primary areas of expertise lie within health services research, preventive medicine, and cross-cultural medicine. Dr Palinkas is particularly interested in behavioural health, global health and health disparities, implementation science, community-based participatory research, and the sociocultural and environmental determinants of health and health-related behaviour with a focus on disease prevention and health promotion.

Mary D. Patterson is a paediatric emergency medicine physician and the associate dean of experiential learning and the Lou Oberndorf Professor of Healthcare Technology at the University of Florida where she directs the Center for Experiential Learning and Simulation. She is past president of the Society for Simulation in Healthcare and has served on the Board of Directors for the Society of Simulation in Healthcare and the International Pediatric Simulation Society. Mary completed her Master of Education at the University of Cincinnati and a Patient Safety Fellowship at Virginia Commonwealth University. She researches simulation, team performance, and patient safety and publishes in patient safety, team performance, and human factors.

Saritte Perlman obtained her undergraduate degree in biological science and theatre studies from the University of Guelph in Canada and subsequently completed her Master of Public Health at Tel Aviv University, Israel. Her research interests include epidemiology of communicable diseases, healthcare quality, public engagement, health policy, and health policy issues where the individual and systems approach cross paths. Perlman currently works at Tel Aviv University School of Public Health as a program coordinator and the Department of Health Systems Management, Faculty of Health Sciences, Ben-Gurion University, conducting research under Prof Moriah E. Ellen.

Michael F. Rayo is Assistant Professor of Cognitive Systems Engineering at the Translational Data Analytics Institute, The Ohio State University. He is also the director of the Cognitive Systems Engineering Laboratory, Symbiotic Healthcare Design Laboratory, and the new Proactive Safety Consortium. His work focuses on building pragmatic tools, practices, and knowledge to help organizations proactively target and mitigate areas of brittleness and protect areas of resilience. His work has been funded by the National Patient Safety Foundation, the Agency for Healthcare Research and Quality, the National Institutes of Health, the Air Force Research Laboratory, and Eurocontrol. He has published on resilience engineering, patient safety, human–machine teaming, and human factors engineering.

Jo Rycroft-Malone trained as a nurse and completed undergraduate and postgraduate degrees in psychology. She has a reputation in mixed methods applied health research, particularly organization and service delivery improvement, and implementation. Her research has been funded through the EU's FP7 Programme, NIHR, Economic and Social Research Council, Medical Research Council, and Canadian Institutes for Health Research. She is Program Director and Chair of the NIHR Health Services and Delivery Research (HS&DR) Programme, Emeritus Senior Research Leader for Health and Care Research Wales, and Chair of the National Institute for Care and Health Excellence (NICE) Implementation Strategy Group.

Tarcisio A. Saurin is Associate Professor at the Industrial Engineering Department of the Federal University of Rio Grande do Sul, Brazil. He has a BSc in civil engineering, an MSc in civil engineering/construction management, and a PhD in industrial engineering. In recent years, he has been a visiting scholar at the University of Salford (England, UK) and Macquarie University (Sydney, Australia). His main research interests are related to the modelling and management of complex socio-technical systems, resilience engineering, and lean production. He has carried out research and consulting projects on these topics in healthcare, manufacturing, construction, and electricity distribution.

Gordon D. Schiff is a general internist and Associate Director of Brigham and Women's Center for Patient Safety Research and Practice, Quality and Safety; Director for the Harvard Medical School (HMS) Center for Primary Care; and Associate Professor of Medicine at HMS. Dr Schiff publishes in medication and diagnosis safety and has contributed to the 2015 National Academy of Medicine report, "Improving Diagnosis in Health Care". He received an award from the Arnold P. Gold Foundation for Medical Humanism to study professional-patient boundaries and relationships, the 2019 Mark Graber Diagnosis Safety Award by the Society for Improving Diagnosis in Medicine, and the John Eisenberg Award (2020) by the National Quality Forum and Joint Commission.

Ulrica von Thiele Schwarz is a registered psychologist and professor of psychology at the School of Health, Care and Social Welfare at Mälardalen University and the Procome research group at the Medical Management Centre, Karolinska Institutet, Sweden. Her research examines how to design, implement, and evaluate interventions in organizations so that the value for service users, staff, organizations, and the system is optimized. This covers a broad range of initiatives such as parental programs, reduction of low value care, and leadership across settings. Her current research includes studies on fidelity and adaptation from a professional perspective, including how decisions are made and how fidelity and adaptation affect professionals' psychosocial work environments.

Nick Sevdalis is a psychologist by training, is a professor and director of the Centre for Implementation Science at King's College London, UK (2015–), and has held academic appointments in the Department of Surgery and Cancer at Imperial College London, UK (2004–2015). Sevdalis's research is in implementation science, improvement science, and applied psychology, focusing on systematically analysing implementation gaps in the delivery of improvement interventions (including checklists, team skills development, and clinical pathway redesign) and public health interventions (including vaccination programs) and developing practical methods to address them. Most recently, he has been developing methodologies that support the design and delivery of implementation studies in the field of healthcare.

Marisa Sklar is a project scientist, licensed clinical psychologist, and program evaluator at UC San Diego's Department of Psychiatry. She led multiple evaluation contracts to use mixed quantitative and qualitative methodologies to assess the impacts of healthcare models and systems on patient, provider, organization, and system-level outcomes. She has an extensive knowledge base in measurement, psychometric theory, statistical methods, mixed methods, evaluation, dissemination, and implementation. Dr Sklar has co-authored numerous publications that present issues with traditional methods for justifying external validity and generalizability in real-world settings and proposed frameworks for overcoming implementation challenges, including the "scaling-out" approach.

Andrea Smith is a Daffodil Fellow at the Daffodil Centre, a partnership between the Cancer Council and the University of Sydney, and until recently was a postdoctoral research fellow at the AIHI, Macquarie University, Sydney, Australia. She also works as an implementation scientist within the Centre of Research Excellence in Melanoma, a collaboration of clinicians and researchers from across New South Wales and Victoria. Dr Smith is involved in collaborative, multidisciplinary research in health promotion and disease prevention, with a current focus on the application of implementation science and practice across the cancer continuum, specifically melanoma and breast cancer.

Ben Smith is Co-deputy Director (Policy and Practice) at the Centre for Oncology Education and Research Translation (CONCERT), Ingham Institute, and the University of New South Wales. His research aims to ensure equitable access to evidence-based psychosocial cancer care for all people living with cancer. He works to build implementation science capacity and collaboration for better cancer outcomes through the Cancer Implementation Science Community of Practice, with a particular interest in the assessment of fear of cancer recurrence, evaluation, and implementation of digital health interventions and clinical trial participation by culturally and linguistically diverse cancer patients. He works with testicular cancer survivors and men with prostate cancer.

James Smith was recently a research fellow at the AIHI, Macquarie University, Sydney, Australia, working on developing a rapid implementation and evaluation strategy for the ZERO Childhood Cancer program, the first personalized medicine program for children with high-risk cancer. Previously, he worked on NIHR-funded projects in the UK. At the University of London, he researched behaviour change in healthcare professionals. At the University of Oxford, he worked on the NIHR-HTA-funded Arthroplasty Candidacy Help Engine (ACHE) project with the Knee Research Group at the Botnar Research Centre. He has researched Patient Reported Outcome Measures (PROMs) and the Musculoskeletal Health questionnaire (Arthritis Research, UK).

Sharon E. Straus is a geriatrician and clinical epidemiologist who trained at the University of Toronto and the University of Oxford. She is Director of the Knowledge Translation Program and Physician-in-Chief, St. Michael's Hospital, and Professor in the Department of Medicine, University of Toronto, Canada. She holds a Tier 1 Canada Research Chair in Knowledge Translation and Quality of Care and has authored more than 450 peer-reviewed publications and three textbooks in evidence-based medicine, knowledge translation, and mentorship. Since 2015, she has consistently been in the top 1 per cent of highly cited clinical researchers with an H-index of 91. She holds more than $57 million in research grants as a principal investigator.

Lawrence Susskind is Ford Professor of Urban and Environmental Planning at the Massachusetts Institute of Technology (MIT), co-founder and Vice-Chair of the Program on Negotiation at Harvard Law School, and founder and Chief Knowledge Officer of the Consensus Building Institute (a not-for-profit that provides neutral services in complex multiparty negotiations around the world). At MIT, he offers a four-week online course through MITxPRO, titled Healthcare Negotiations: Better Outcomes for Sales Professionals. He is the author or co-author of 20 books, including *Good for You, Great for Me*; *The Consensus Building Handbook*; *Multiparty Negotiation*; and *Breaking Robert's Rules*.

Kris Vanhaecht is Associate Professor of Quality and Patient Safety at the KU Leuven Institute for Healthcare Policy in Belgium. He started his work on care pathways in 1998 and is now the secretary general of the European Pathway Association. He leads national and international implementation and evaluation studies on standardization of care processes, next to his academic work on safety and "mangomoments" (patient-centred care). He is involved in research and teaching in Quality in Healthcare, is policy advisor on Quality Management at the University Hospitals Leuven & Flemish Hospital Network, and is an expert on quality for the International Society for Quality in Healthcare (ISQUA).

Justin Waring is Professor of Medical Sociology and Healthcare Organization at the Health Services Management Centre, University of Birmingham, UK. His research investigates the changing organization and governance of health and care services, focusing in particular on the way practices, cultures, and identities can facilitate or stymie the implementation of change. He is interested in the application of social theory to different social, cultural, and organizational contexts as a means of both explaining social phenomena and extending theoretical rigour. Much of his research is ethnographic in character, involving immersive fieldwork and observations with health and care organizations.

Michel Wensing is Professor of Health Services Research and Implementation Science at Heidelberg University Hospital, Germany. He is Head of the MSc Program, Health

Services Research and Implementation Science, and Adjunct Head, Department of General Practice and Health Services Research, Heidelberg University Hospital. Previously, he was Professor at the Radboud University Medical Centre, Nijmegen, the Netherlands, where he continues to hold an affiliation. He has academic degrees in medical sociology (1991), medical sciences (1997), health economics (2007), and health services research (2010). His work focuses on the organization, delivery, and outcomes of primary and ambulatory healthcare. Key themes are the implementation of evidence-based practice, organization of primary care, and alignment with patient preferences.

Johanna Westbrook is Professor and Director of the Centre for Health Systems and Safety Research, AIHI, Macquarie University, Sydney, Australia. She is internationally recognized for her research evaluating the effects of information and communication technology in healthcare, which has led to significant advances in our understanding of how clinical information systems deliver (or fail to deliver) expected benefits. Her highly applied research has supported translation of this evidence into policy, practice, and IT system design changes. In 2014, she was named Australian ICT professional of the year and, in 2019, the national research leader in the field of medical informatics.

Iestyn Williams is Professor of Health Policy and Management and Director of Research at the Health Services Management Centre (HSMC), University of Birmingham, UK. He has led research into the dynamics of service removal and replacement in healthcare and is the author of multiple peer-reviewed papers on this topic. He has specific expertise in priority setting, strategic planning and decision-making, implementation studies, and qualitative evidence synthesis and reporting. He regularly works with healthcare leaders and decision-makers, especially in the National Health Service (NHS) in England, to address the challenges of de-implementation of obsolete or ineffective treatments and services.

Paul Wilson is Senior Lecturer in Implementation Science at the Centre for Primary Care and Health Services Research, The University of Manchester, UK, and Lead for Implementation Science in the NIHR ARC, Greater Manchester. His research interests are focused on evidence-informed decision-making in health policy and practice and the development and evaluation of methods to increase the uptake of research-based knowledge in health systems. He is the co-editor-in-chief of *Implementation Science*, the leading international journal for implementation research.

David D. Woods is Professor in the Department of Integrated Systems Engineering at the Ohio State University and has worked extensively to improve systems safety in high-risk complex settings. He has developed resilience engineering, writing about the dangers of brittle systems and the need to invest in sustaining sources of resilience as part of the response to several NASA accidents. He developed the first comprehensive theory on how systems can build the potential for resilient performance despite complexity. Recently, he started the SNAFU Catchers Consortium, an industry–university partnership to build resilience in critical digital services. He is past president of the Human Factors and Ergonomics Society and of the Resilience Engineering Association.

Ping Yu is Associate Professor at the Centre for Digital Transformation, University of Wollongong, Australia. She is a leader in collaborative, industry-based research that advocates and supports the digital transformative agenda of health and aged care sectors in Australia and overseas. Taking a socio-technical approach to joint problem-solving, she has successfully planned and executed complex, multi-method research on the design, adoption, use, and impact of digital technology in health and aged care for 18 years. Her passion and contribution have been recognized by the Don Walker Award from the Health Informatics Society of Australia for improving access to digital technology by the under-developed economy.

Yvonne Zurynski is Associate Professor of Health System Sustainability at the AIHI, Macquarie University, Sydney, Australia, and leads the Coordinating Centre of the NHMRC Partnership Centre in Health Systems Sustainability. She is Adjunct Associate Professor, University of Tasmania, and Honorary Associate Professor, University of Sydney and Curtin University, in Perth, Western Australia. She is an expert in health services and systems research. As a mixed methods researcher, implementation scientist, epidemiologist, program evaluator, and policy analyst, she consolidates broad knowledge of complex systems from different viewpoints. She has led national epidemiological studies, clinical research studies, service model and policy evaluations, and complex systematic reviews.

Foreword

This new book brings together scholars, researchers, and other leading figures from the field of implementation science who are seeking to promote the use of its concepts and methods much more comprehensively than hitherto to achieve better care for patients. It happened because the editors and many of the authors realized that there is no platform for people to communicate and make available their expertise in implementation science outside formal articles in journals or other academic sources.

The rich collection of essays is pluralist, tackling the topic from numerous theoretical, conceptual, and empirical standpoints. The book is not only aimed at fellow scholars. The scope is broader than what would be pitched to a typical implementation science readership. The writing style is more relaxed, and as a result, the subject is much more accessible to new audiences. It is a book for policymakers, managers and leaders, quality and patient safety specialists, clinicians, students, and patient groups offering explanation and practical advice.

There are 60 essays arranged in three sections covering different domains of implementation science: principles and concepts, methodology and methods, and evidence and evaluation.

In the essay on complexity science, Braithwaite reminds us that the paradigm underpinning activities to get evidence into clinical practice or healthcare delivery is erroneously considered to be a linear proposition. Moreover, if that evidence is derived from high-quality, randomized clinical trial data, the advocate for implementation has the equivalent of a backstage pass for the concert of a major rock star. All doors open, and the doormen bow in deference.

The assumption that the improvement achieved by an intervention in one population of patients can be reliably scaled up to bring national or even global benefits across health systems does not apply in the way that the trial of a therapy might.

In her essay, Damschroder emphasizes that randomized controlled trials produce knowledge of *what* works in highly controlled settings but fail in the task of guiding on *where*, *how*, and *why* the innovation will work in a real-world healthcare context.

Back to complexity again. A clinical therapy is usually something that can be seen, touched, or held in the hands: a tablet, a package of fluid, a metallic object, or a machine. The relationship of the intervention with time is usually clear and easy to describe; for example, applied once, given at regular defined intervals, or used when symptoms recur or laboratory data suggest. An intervention for improvement is something much less tangible; for example, a series of interlocking processes of care, a set of human behaviours directed so as to occur in a particular sequence, or an organizational cultural change tool. Time relates in a different way too: when does it start? When is it finished? What elements need to be sustained, and what can be left behind?

Amongst the most talked about improvement science initiatives with global reach – and there have not been many – in the first two decades of the twenty-first century were those led by Peter Pronovost (then head of the Armstrong Institute for Patient Safety and Quality at Johns Hopkins University, Baltimore, and intensive care physician) and Don Berwick (then president of the Institute of Health Improvement in Boston, Massachusetts).

Pronovost and his team devised a "bundle" of evidence-based clinical interventions aimed at reducing catheter-associated bloodstream infections and implemented it in intensive care units across the state of Michigan, United States, saving an estimated 1,500 lives and $100 million annually. The initiative was implemented in other states and in other countries. *The New Yorker* magazine credited Peter Pronovost with carrying out "work [that] has already saved more lives than that of any laboratory scientist in the past decade".

Soon after his research study in Michigan, I invited Peter Pronovost to join with myself and the World Health Organization (WHO) patient safety team in introducing the care bundle into Europe and Latin America on a pilot basis. The striking early finding was that it did not work very well. This was because the hospitals involved did not put much effort into the change process itself (referred to at the time as "organizational development"), particularly in getting clinical buy-in. This had been a key part of the work in Michigan but was not recognized as mission-critical until it was lacking. Once that had been remedied, the impact was fully realized.

Many of the essays deal with these issues. Put simply, an intervention and its implementation are two different things. It is not enough to "follow the science". As much attention must be given to how an evidence-based intervention will fare in a complex social system like a hospital or a country's entire health system.

The questions posed by Berwick's hugely high-profile 100,000 lives program lay in the evaluation domain of implementation science. He was immediately challenged by his peers to "prove" how many lives had been saved from the huge engagement of hospitals across the United States. The doubts cast by some did not stop calculation of numbers attributed to this complex intervention nor its widespread rollout in similar campaigns in other countries.

The essays, particularly in the third section of the book, deal with the complexities of evaluating in implementation science. Part of this is related to an older scientific prejudice about drawing firm conclusions from observational data. The second section of the book addresses some of the novel methods for resolving the long-standing doubts about "proving", not merely "claiming", impact from improvement programs.

Taking in the deeply impressive breadth and depth of expert content in this book left me reflecting on what I often hear stated as the greatest benefit of improvement science: that it engages frontline healthcare staff in the quality of their services. There is no doubt that the existence of hundreds of thousands of curiosity-driven, granular, quality improvement projects around the world will be benefitting patients and, at times, saving lives. Does it matter that we don't know how much? Or that all this activity is largely uncoordinated at a higher level?

The difficulty with taking a too *laissez-faire* approach is that it ultimately weakens implementation science. It is already too often regarded as a "soft" science. The risks of making it seem even softer are too great.

This book pitches a potentially winning formula of rigour in thought and deed with the simplification of complexity.

Sir Liam Donaldson
Professor of Public Health, London School of Hygiene and Tropical Medicine
Former Chief Medical Officer for England
World Health Organization Patient Safety Envoy

Acknowledgements

The editors would like to acknowledge the contribution of a number of people, without whom this book would not have come to fruition. Firstly, we are incredibly grateful to our international colleagues who authored the essays, bestowing their significant expertise, creativity, and unique insights to assist us in delivering what we hope will be an interesting and novel contribution to the field of implementation science. Our heartfelt thanks also go to the editorial team at the Australian Institute of Health Innovation (AIHI), Macquarie University, Australia, for their considerable effort in coordinating submissions with the authors and producing this compendium. Our research and support team – Mai-Tram Nguyen, Diana Fajardo Pulido, Tayhla Ryder, Kelly Nguyen, and Lieke van Baar – completed the extensive task of formatting the book, creating an index and supporting figures, sourcing biographies and copyright approvals, and editing and proofing the essays. We would also like to thank colleagues at Routledge for their interest in our vision and belief in the initial proposal. Finally, our earnest appreciation goes to four of our AIHI colleagues (Denise Tsiros, K-lynn Smith, Genevieve Dammery, and Jackie Mullins), who kindly undertook the proofreading and copy-editing tasks, providing feedback on the complete manuscript. Any errors that remain are the editors' responsibility. We hope, and trust, you enjoy the result of all these efforts.

Abbreviations

AGHA	Australian Genomics Health Alliance
CAS	Complex Adaptive System
CB	Consensus building
CDS	Clinical decision support
CFIR	Consolidated Framework for Implementation Research
CICI	Context and Implementation of Complex Interventions
COM-B	Capability, Opportunity, Motivation, Behaviour model
da	Data Analysis
dc	Data Collection
EBI	Evidence-based intervention
EBP	Evidence-based practice
ED	Emergency department
EIS	Emergency Implementation Science
EPIS	Exploration, Preparation, Implementation, Sustainment framework
FEFL	Formative Evaluation Feedback Loop
FRAM	The Functional Resonance Analysis Method
FsQCA	Fuzzy-set Qualitative Comparative Analysis
GP	General practitioner
HFE	Human factors engineering
HRQOL	Health-related quality of life
ICU	Intensive care unit
ImpRes	Implementation Science Research Development tool
IN	Intervention
IS	Implementation science
IS	Implementation strategies
KTA	Knowledge-to-Action
LEAP	Learn. Engage. Act. Process.
MRC	Medical Research Council
MST	Multisystemic Therapy
NLP	Natural Language Processing
NPT	Normalization Process Theory
OODA	Observe, Orient, Decide, Act loop
PARIHS	Promoting Action on Research Implementation in Health Services
PDSA	Plan, Do, Study, Act
PMTO	Parent Management Training, the Oregon model

PRECEDE-PROCEED	Predisposing, Reinforcing, and Enabling Constructs in Educational Diagnosis and Evaluation-Policy, Regulatory, and Organizational Constructs in Educational and Environmental Development
PRISM	PReclSion Medicine for Children with Cancer
PRO	Patient Reported Outcome
PROM	Patient Reported Outcome Measure
QUAL	Qualitative
QUAN	Quantitative
QUERI	Quality Enhancement Research Initiative
RCT	Randomized controlled trial
RE-AIM	Reach, Effectiveness, Adoption, Implementation, Maintenance
SEIPS	Systems Engineering Initiative for Patient Safety
TAM-R	Therapist Adherence Measure-Revised
TCRN	Translational Cancer Research Network
TDE	Theory-driven evaluation
TDF	Theoretical Domains Framework
TMF	Theories, models, and frameworks
US	United States
V	Value
VA	Veterans Affairs
WAD	Work-as-Done
WAI	Work-as-Imagined

Models, Theories, Frameworks, and Tools

	Essay/s
2 × 2 framework	19
Action model/Change model schema	43
BARRIERS Scale	8
Behaviour Change Technique Taxonomy framework	26
Behaviour Change Wheel framework	26
Biopsychosocial model	16
Capability, Opportunity, Motivation, Behaviour (COM-B) model	35
Consensus building model	37
Consolidated Framework for Implementation Research (CFIR)	8, 9, 15, 25, 36
Context and Implementation of Complex Interventions	2
Diffusion of Innovation	14, 30
Dynamic Sustainability Framework	59
Exploration, Preparation, Implementation and Sustainment (EPIS) framework	12, 36, 41
Formative Evaluation Feedback Loop (FEFL)	21
Functional Resonance Analysis Method (FRAM)	29
Getting to Outcomes Framework	18
Health Belief Model	14
Implementation Climate	8
Knowledge Action Cycle	59
Knowledge-to-Action Framework	8, 36
Learning Health System framework	5
Normalization Process Theory	7, 13, 25
Nudge Theory	38
Observe, Orient, Decide, Act	24
Organizational Readiness	8
Patient Reported Outcome Measures (PROMs)	15
Plan, Do, Study, Act (PDSA) cycle	20, 21, 24
PRECEDE-PROCEED (Predisposing, Reinforcing, and Enabling Constructs in Educational Diagnosis and Evaluation-Policy, Regulatory, and Organizational Constructs in Educational and Environmental Development)	8
Promoting Action on Research Implementation in Health Services (PARIHS)	8, 9
RE-AIM (Reach, Effectiveness, Adoption, Implementation, Maintenance)	8, 36
Sense, Respond, Probe of the Cynefin process	24
Social Network Analysis	1, 30
Structure-process-outcome triad Model	57
Theoretical Domains Framework	2, 8, 10, 26, 36
Theories of change	44
Three-talk model	16
Systems Engineering Initiative for Patient Safety (SEIPS) model	22

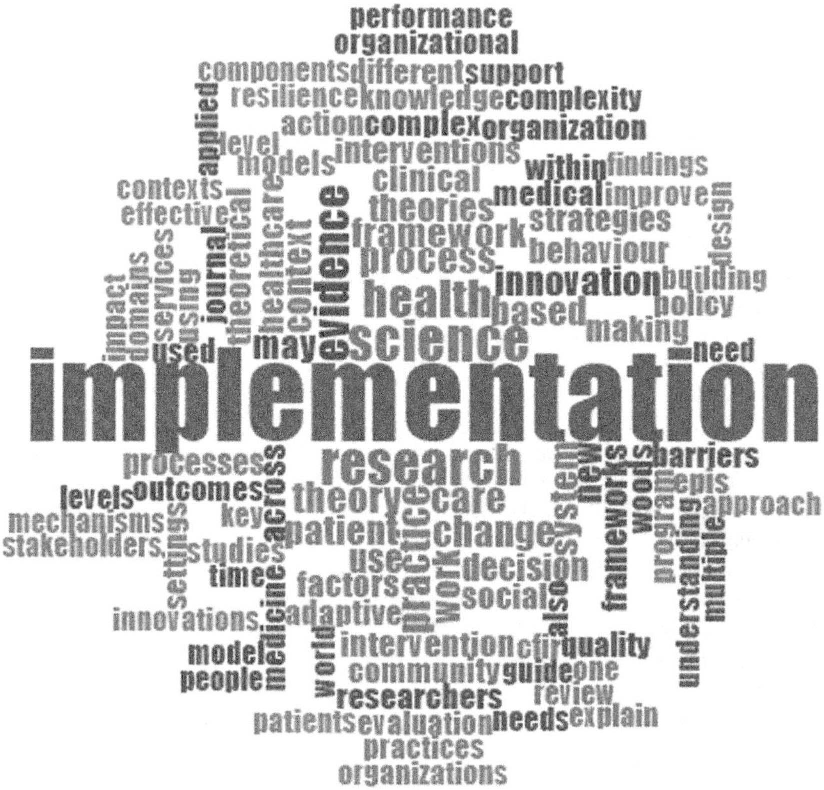
performance
organizational
components
different
support
resilience
knowledge
complexity
applied
action
complex
organization
level
interventions
models
within
findings
contexts
clinical
medical
improve
effective
theories
strategies
design
theoretical
evidence
framework
behaviour
journal
healthcare
context
process
impact
domains
services
using
innovation
building
health
based
policy
making
used
may
science
need
implementation
processes
across
research
barriers
levels
outcomes
theory
care
epis
new
system
approach
mechanisms
key
patient
practice
change
works
stakeholders
studies
settings
program
time
use
decision
frameworks
factors
work
social
understanding
multiple
innovations
medicine
adaptive
also
model
world
intervention
cfir
quality
people
community
guide
one
researchers
review
patients
evaluation
needs
explain
practices
organizations

Part I

Principles and concepts of implementation science

Setting the scene

Principles and concepts of implementation science

Frances Rapport, Robyn Clay-Williams,
and Jeffrey Braithwaite

In this very first section of the book, Part I, authors, individually or in collaboration, examine a wide range of issues that are fundamental to the reader's understanding of the principles and concepts of implementation science. This includes essays on how to get evidence into practice and the theories, models, and frameworks supporting evidence implementation. As Jeffrey Braithwaite reminds us in his opening essay, this is not as simple as it sounds. Moving evidence into practice, irrespective of its source, is not a "linear proposition", and as a result, implementation science is a considerably complex science – sometimes, infuriatingly so. Evidence often needs to be carefully deconstructed and intelligently reconstructed to ensure that a composite and comprehensive body of knowledge is put forward from which to build an implementation science study.

In this section authors also investigate the background to implementation science, not only to the benefit of newcomers to the subject but also to remind those more familiar with the topic as to where the "science" in implementation science derives and which key principles and practices drive the implementation. In Part I, authors examine the evidence that is vital for planning and preparing a coherent study, with essays from Ellen and Perlman and Woods and Rayo, taking a systems-view approach to understand potential improvement and sustained service delivery. Woods and Rayo, for example, consider how systems support resilient performance in enabling healthcare professionals to deal with both "successes and setbacks".

In examining the principles of implementation science in this first section, we learn from Kilbourne what implementation science really stands for; how it can most usefully function, flex, and adapt to different healthcare scenarios; and what purpose this serves. Clark takes us another step along the road to enquiry, describing humanism, in particular his expert understanding of medical humanism, to expand implementation science's strength of character. Clark describes the scope of implementation science as part of a medical humanism paradigm, which has the capacity to nurture the next generation of healthcare professionals and encourage them to uphold qualities of compassion and care.

Part I also pays homage to theory-building – seeing theory as the mainstay of methodological development while linking implementation science to the translation of research findings in real-world scenarios in clinical and non-clinical practice. In discussing theory, Kislov and Wilson and Nilsen adeptly present cases for implementation science models and frameworks which can guide the implementation of research findings, and which can also expand ideas and create knowledge, while helping others understand the effects of implementation outcomes. This section follows a clear pathway of discovery, through specific implementation science frameworks to implementable interventions. Damschroder describes the Consolidated Framework for Implementation Research (CFIR); Lorencatto updates us on

DOI: 10.4324/9781003109945-2

the Theoretical Domains Framework (TDF); Birken explores Organization Theory; Moullin and Aarons, the Exploration, Preparation, Implementation, Sustainment (EPIS) framework; and Yu, Diffusion of Innovation theory. All these authors offer clarifying depictions of ways of organizing and delivering healthcare and guiding implementation research, processes, and practices. Some frameworks, such as the TDF, for example, according to Lorencatto, concentrate on contextual influencers of behaviour, both "current and desired". Others, such as the CFIR, from Damschroder, guide the "assessment of context" and "constructs that have the potential to significantly affect implementation outcomes".

Smith and Durcinoska, taking a different angle, peer inside the health-related quality of life (HRQOL) black box and eloquently present the reader with the value of Patient Reported Outcome Measures, or PROMs, to evaluate HRQOL "in research, investigating the experience and treatment of various health conditions". They examine how implementation frameworks can guide PROM implementation as well as help overcome PROM implementation barriers and leverage enablers according to context and implementation stages. From this essay, we move on to Elwyn's strong reflection on the value of shared decision-making and Lamprell's considered view of "nudge" as a behaviour-change paradigm. Both Elwyn and Lamprell challenge us to think about who is making the decisions in the healthcare context and for what reason healthcare professionals hold on to old habits. In the case of Elwyn's essay, this refers to the lack of shared decision-making with patients and unresolved management of differing views of healthcare professionals and patients. In the case of Lamprell's essay, this refers to how compliance in workplace behaviour can be achieved and leads to commentary on the need to find adaptive processes to positively affect decision goals.

Finally, Part I turns to the challenge of moving from the theoretical to evidence building, design, and application. To link to Part II, *Methodology and Methods of Implementation Science*, Part I concludes with Hill and Knox's essay on pipeline and cyclical models of evidence building. In this piece the authors consider evidence building as a pipeline, moving from developing evidence to expanding knowledge, and somewhere at the end of the line, developing, testing, and creating an effective, long-lasting intervention.

Introduction to the book

This book is a compilation of 60 essays, each tackling a very different, unique, and singular "key concept" in implementation science, from the viewpoint of the author or authors. Collectively, the book aims to document the field's state of the art and convey the vocabulary of modern-day implementation science. The book has been carefully crafted so that every essay not only is a personalized piece about a topic close to the heart of the author but also represents a fascinating journey through the complex labyrinth that is implementation science.

Each essay, from brief 500-word testimonials to lengthier 1,000-word tomes, is expressive but is still able to distil wisdom for the widest of audiences – students, teachers, researchers, social scientists, implementation scientists, healthcare professionals, policymakers, and allied healthcare professionals.

The book has been edited to stand as a companion piece to the research literature as a compendium, expressing a multitude of theoretical, methodological, and practical insights. The way it has been written, including a mapping system to guide different audiences through the book, emphasizes essays of particular appeal to readers who are new to the topic and those more *au fait* with the subject.

It has been written for maximum interest by many of the "glitterati" of implementation science, brought together from the corners of the globe to discuss pure implementation science topics, such as translation, adoption, dissemination, diffusion, and take-up, through to many related and highly practical matters such as how to prepare for implementation, the politics and cultures of implementation settings, and the processes and practices involved in engagement. While authors have not shied away from deeply theoretical topics, some have reflected on tried and tested methods, while others have brought to attention new frameworks underpinning implementation science.

Writers have joined together from Australia and the United Kingdom, North America and Canada, South America, Europe, and Asia. Together this book delivers thoughtful and thought-provoking contributions that are versatile and inventive, academic and clinically excellent, and theoretically diverse. They include examples and case studies that illustrate a multitude of new ideas or take a fresh approach to an old concept. The book shines a light on Complex Adaptive Systems, service provision, and the receipt of care. There are essays ranging from behaviour change to adaptability and resilience and the importance of clear decision-making to patient-centred care.

We know that getting evidence into clinical practice may, on the surface, seem easy. Do the research, test it in the real world, implement it, spread the gains to every setting, and sit back and enjoy the shared benefits of evidence-based care. That is what the most optimistic amongst us believed at the beginning of the evidence-based movement. But alas, that was not to be. What appears to be a linear process is contested, challenging, tortuous, and political – governed more by the laws of complexity and chaos than those inherent in straight-line, formulaic models. That's where this book comes in – navigating between the world that insists on strict adherence to evidence-based protocols and the world that demands complete clinical freedom. Between medicine as science and medicine as art lie solutions, or at least tentative, and sometimes good answers to the thorny problem of how we can make care more evidence-informed.

So, with essays offering a perspective in clear commentary across medicine, implementation science, medical humanities, and the health services, the essays are richly realized, offering a dramatic departure from other "Introductions to Implementation Science" on the market today and methods-based dictionaries. Essays speak a very realistic language, examine a range of research methods applicable to implementation, and critique the field while offering vital insights into how research findings are derived from healthcare contexts that can help make sense of patient encounters. The essays reveal a very human side to caregiving but are also unafraid to broach its more complex, technological, adjunctive, or convoluted aspects, concentrating on not only what predominantly goes right in introducing a new intervention but also what can go wrong and how to face the challenges of that. Writers examine approaches that implementation scientists can and invariably do take to problem-solving in an attempt to improve care and save lives.

How to use this book

This edited book takes on the key concepts in implementation science and as such is an ideal guide to the discipline. Consider just some of the concepts explored:

> *Processes and practices, nudge as a solution, theoretical frameworks, evidence-synthesis, methodological diversity, walking methods, human factors and behaviour, agents of change, adaptability, and translation in the real world.*

Essays are cross-referenced to show the evidence base for ideas, their historical grounding, and future-orientation. As a result, we firmly believe that readers will find the work to be the

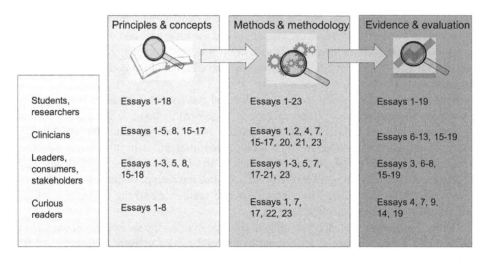

Figure 0.1 Mapping of essays

most useful of references. It can be read from cover to cover or dipped into as necessary. Whether for interest, professional development, or the completing of coursework in a degree program, we believe it will be an ideal resource. It has been purposefully crafted to suit the expert or layperson, the researcher, or those at the intersection of the art and science of clinical practice, those simply interested in implementation science, and those teaching and learning about translational research, its theories, notions, and methods. In Figure 0.1, we provide maps to guide students and researchers; clinicians; leaders, consumers, and other stakeholders; and those who are merely curious to learn more about the concepts of implementation with a healthcare focus along a more structured path through the book.

Conclusion

Implementation science is being explored here from its esoteric outer limits to its detailed human factors' aspects, in terms of root causes and effects, ideas and applications, and methodologies and methods.

The opportunities for a very original essay style have encouraged truly expressive, often quite profound narratives, neither rigid nor formulaic but free-flowing – and, often, gripping. Readers are in for a treat; a state of the art, multi-perspectival picture with intellectuals roaming free around the topic area, offering clear intuitions and sometimes groundbreaking understandings of healthcare situations, settings, and ecosystems. Join us for this deep dive into the richly realized accounts of the point at which evidence meets practice.

1 Complexity science

Jeffrey Braithwaite

To open this compendium of essays on implementation science (IS), it is important to say that IS is *centrally concerned with getting evidence into practice*. Its proponents are actively and often innovatively creating a discipline for how to accomplish this. One of the problems with this is the way this definition, at least on the surface, seems like a linear proposition. That is to say that the idea "getting evidence into practice" means for many implementation scientists a process involving assembling the evidence, carefully ensuring that it is as high-quality as possible, preferably from a randomized controlled trial (RCT), and then that it is put in place, adopted widely, scaled up, and practised uniformly (Figure 1.1).

Rapport and colleagues (Rapport et al. 2018) deconstructed the different ideas embedded in this linear model (Figure 1.2), highlighting the range of concepts inherent in a translation cycle, ranging from diffusion through to dissemination, to implementation, to adoption, and then take-up and scaling.

A model such as this helps us to understand that implementation is not linear, nor as it is displayed in this model, circular. Getting evidence into practice is in fact highly political, challenging, uncertain, culturally determined, value-laden, and multi-factorial. Challenges include that it is not clear how to access the evidence (e.g., there are over 28 million entries in Medline, the medical biographical database; so which evidence does a clinician choose?); not everything that is practised has evidence to support it; and of the care provided to adults and children, only around 60% consistently meets quality of care indicators enshrined in clinical guidelines (Runciman et al. 2012, Braithwaite et al. 2018a, 2018b). In short, the process of getting evidence into practice is complex, and the systems of care within which evidence is practised are Complex Adaptive Systems (CASs) (Lansing 2003). As a consequence, therefore, we need to shift thinking from an essentially linear paradigm to one that has a deep appreciation of complexity science if we are to understand the dimensions of the challenge of getting evidence into practice and create a science of implementation.

While there is no simplistic rendering of what complexity, complexity science, or CASs are, we can nevertheless discuss some of their core dimensions. A glossary of terms for the rest of this essay will be useful (Table 1.1).

While there are many definitions, a useful one is that complexity is "a dynamic and constantly emerging set of processes and objects that not only interact with each other, but come to be defined by those interactions" (Cohn et al. 2013, Greenhalgh and Papoutsi 2018), and complexity science is the rigorous study of complexity. So, in a healthcare context, agents and their artefacts (e.g., clinical professionals and the things they use by which to diagnose, treat, and care for patients such as stethoscopes, computers, MRI machines, beds in wards,

DOI: 10.4324/9781003109945-3

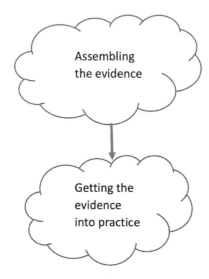

Figure 1.1 A linear conceptualization of evidence into practice
Source: Author

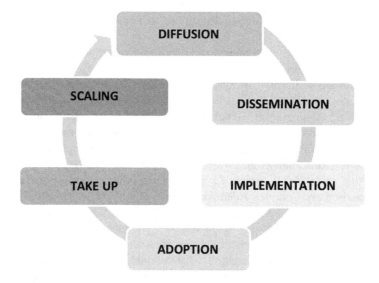

Figure 1.2 Translation cycle
Source: (Adapted from Rapport et al. 2018)

drugs, scalpels, and pens) interrelate. As they do, emergence occurs; various rules grow out of the interactions, which govern future behavioural activities; the boundaries within which participants enact their behaviours are fuzzy and indistinct; in essence, the actors adapt, co-evolve, interact, and are mutually interdependent. In such circumstances, work-life is political, and cultures and subcultures, and norms, beliefs, customs, and habits, all play a role in

Table 1.1 Glossary of terms

Glossary of terms	
Adaptation	The capacity to adjust to internal and external circumstances; usually thought of in terms of modifying behaviours over time.
Agents	The individual components of a complex system – typically, individuals, whose capacity for sensemaking means they can learn and adapt their behaviours across time, or artefacts.
Complex Adaptive System (CAS)	A dynamic, self-similar collective of interacting, adaptive agents and their artefacts.
Complexity	The behaviour embedded in highly composite systems or models of systems with large numbers of interacting components (e.g., agents, artefacts, and groups); their ongoing, repeated interactions create local rules and rich, collective behaviours.
Culture	The sum of the shared values, attitudes, and beliefs across part of or the whole of an organization (e.g., across the division of medicine or an entire hospital or health service).
Emergence	Behaviours that are built from smaller or simpler entities, the characteristics, or properties of which arise through the interactions of those smaller or simpler entities; the larger entities are one level up in scale and manifest as social structures, patterns, or properties.
Network	An interlocking web of relationships or connections at varying levels of scale in a system; the agents or artefacts are the nodes, and the relationships between them are lines or vectors, which together describe the structure of the interactions of the network's membership.
Self-organization	The way in which agents interact to coordinate their own circumstances, workplaces, processes, and procedures, such that they order their work and they autonomously, or semi-autonomously, organize their localized behaviour. This can occur passively or actively.
Social network	A set of people who have relationships, communications, ties, or interactions which connect them.
System dynamics	An analytical modelling methodology used for problem-solving, which combines qualitative and quantitative data and identifies the fundamental elements of a system, and how they influence one another over time.
Tipping point	A critical point in a system in which a kind of radical, potentially irreversible change may occur, resulting in a different state of system behaviour which can settle into a new equilibrium.

Source: Modified from Braithwaite et al. (2018a)

defining, enabling, and constraining behaviours and practices. And prediction – estimating or forecasting what is going to happen next – is very difficult. The CASs within which people are trying to get evidence into practice are dynamic, constituted by networks, subcultures, and shifting politics and power structures; people to a large extent self-organize within this milieu in order to get work done. Overarchingly, CASs are often labelled *non-linear dynamic systems* (Lansing 2003). In such ecosystems (to introduce a word using related terminology), there are always high degrees of uncertainty and unpredictability.

Occasionally, these interactive behaviours will build up a head of steam and reach a tipping point, and ultimately, a phase transition can occur whereby the system changes quickly from one state to another and then settles into the new state. Examples include the movement to laparoscopic surgery after decades of higher risk, invasive procedures (Fuchs 2002), the shift to day surgery when previously almost all patients were admitted for two or more days, and typically longer (Shnaider and Chung 2006), and the rapid transition from face-to-face consultations to telemedicine during COVID-19 (Smith et al. 2020). So, change occurs, and evidence gets into practice but often in irregular, unforeseeable ways – more like punctuated equilibrium than linear cause and effect.

One useful way to describe these interactions, interdependencies, and dynamism is through social network analyses (see essay 30; Long, Getting a handle on the social processes of implementation: social network research), which depict the structure of the relationships in the CASs to which we have an interest, particularly in terms of the ties and connections between them. Here are two examples (Figures 1.3 and 1.4). In Figure 1.3 we draw on work done in the Australian Genomics Health Alliance (AGHA) (Long et al. 2019). Before 2016, the network was flourishing and quite dense, but two years later, by 2018, there were substantial numbers of additional members, ties, and collaborations.

Such analyses can also be mapped longitudinally such as in the example of a Translational Cancer Research Network (TCRN) – a collaboration of researchers and practitioners in Eastern Sydney, Australia – where we showed increasingly extended and dense networks of influence as clinicians and researchers worked more collaboratively together from 2012 to 2017 (Figure 1.4). This illustrates the dynamism and collaborative capacity of the agents within the CAS at work, over time (Long, Hibbert, and Braithwaite 2015).

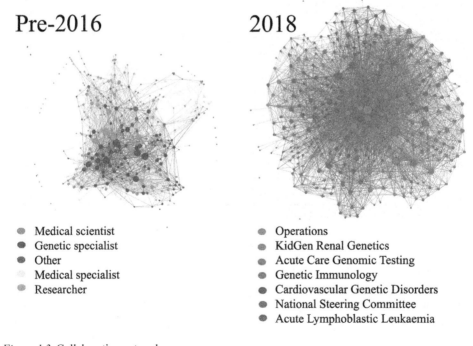

Pre-2016

- Medical scientist
- Genetic specialist
- Other
- Medical specialist
- Researcher

2018

- Operations
- KidGen Renal Genetics
- Acute Care Genomic Testing
- Genetic Immunology
- Cardiovascular Genetic Disorders
- National Steering Committee
- Acute Lymphoblastic Leukaemia

Figure 1.3 Collaboration network

Source: Originally published in Long et al. 2019

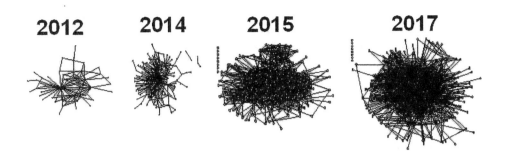

Figure 1.4 Networks of growing influence

Source: Originally published in Braithwaite, Glasziou, and Westbrook 2020

There are several take-home messages. Discussing the core challenges of translating research into practice in a nuanced way, as has been attempted here, means rejecting a linear depiction of the world in favour of a complexity science approach (Long et al. 2019). It means embracing ideas such as path dependence, adaptation over time, dynamic change, modelling behaviours via tools such as Social Network Analysis, and working through and with multiple stakeholders in complex ecosystems. It also means having a tolerance for uncertainty and unpredictability. Complex problems in complex settings are emergent and resist simplistic solutions. That's a lesson every implementation scientist needs to absorb.

References

Braithwaite, J., K. Churruca, J. C. Long, L. A. Ellis, and J. Herkes. 2018a. "When complexity science meets implementation science: A theoretical and empirical analysis of systems change." *BMC Medicine* 16 (1):63. doi: 10.1186/s12916-018-1057-z.

Braithwaite, J., P. Glasziou, and J. Westbrook. 2020. "The three numbers you need to know about healthcare: The 60–30–10 challenge." *BMC Medicine* 18:1–8.

Braithwaite, J., P. D. Hibbert, A. Jaffe, L. White, C. T. Cowell, M. F. Harris, W. B. Runciman, A. R. Hallahan, G. Wheaton, H. M. Williams, E. Murphy, C. J. Molloy, L. K. Wiles, S. Ramanathan, G. Arnolda, H. P. Ting, T. D. Hooper, N. Szabo, J. G. Wakefield, C. F. Hughes, A. Schmiede, C. Dalton, S. Dalton, J. Holt, L. Donaldson, E. Kelley, R. Lilford, P. Lachman, and S. Muething. 2018b. "Quality of health care for children in Australia, 2012–2013." *Journal of the American Medical Association* 319 (11):1113–1124. doi: 10.1001/jama.2018.0162.

Cohn, S., M. Clinch, C. Bunn, and P. Stronge. 2013. "Entangled complexity: Why complex interventions are just not complicated enough." *Journal of Health Services Research & Policy* 18 (1):40–43.

Fuchs, K. 2002. "Minimally invasive surgery." *Endoscopy* 34 (02):154–159.

Greenhalgh, T., and C. Papoutsi. 2018. "Studying complexity in health services research: Desperately seeking an overdue paradigm shift." *BMC Medicine* 16 (1):95. doi: 10.1186/s12916-018-1089-4.

Lansing, J. S. 2003. "Complex adaptive systems." *Annual Review of Anthropology* 32 (1):183–204.

Long, J. C., P. Hibbert, and J. Braithwaite. 2015. "Structuring successful collaboration: A longitudinal social network analysis of a translational research network." *Implementation Science* 11 (1):1–14.

Long, J. C., C. Pomare, S. Best, T. Boughtwood, K. North, L. A. Ellis, K. Churruca, and J. Braithwaite. 2019. "Building a learning community of Australian clinical genomics: A social network study of the Australian Genomic Health Alliance." *BMC Medicine* 17 (1):44.

Rapport, F., R. Clay-Williams, K. Churruca, P. Shih, A. Hogden, and J. Braithwaite. 2018. "The struggle of translating science into action: Foundational concepts of implementation science." *Journal of Evaluation in Clinical Practice* 24 (1):117–126.

Runciman, W. B., E. W. Coiera, R. O. Day, N. A. Hannaford, P. D. Hibbert, T. D. Hunt, J. I. Westbrook, and J. Braithwaite. 2012. "Towards the delivery of appropriate health care in Australia." *Medical Journal of Australia* 197 (2):78–81.

Shnaider, I., and F. Chung. 2006. "Outcomes in day surgery." *Current Opinion in Anesthesiology* 19 (6):622–629.

Smith, A. C., E. Thomas, C. L. Snoswell, H. Haydon, A. Mehrotra, J. Clemensen, and L. J. Caffery. 2020. "Telehealth for global emergencies: Implications for coronavirus disease 2019 (COVID-19)." *Journal of Telemedicine and Telecare*:1357633X20916567.

2 Taking a systems view

Moriah E. Ellen and Saritte Perlman

Health systems are multidimensional, multifaceted, dynamic, and complex, and implementation of interventions within them can occur at the micro (individual and teams), meso (institutional), and macro (whole system) levels. Interventions such as behaviour change and organizational change (at the micro and meso levels) and policymaking interventions (at the macro level) are common throughout the field of implementation science. Achieving successful implementation requires relevant and contextually adapted policy and buy-in from stakeholders, including engagement, involvement, and participation of patients, the public, and citizens (Cabassa and Baumann 2013, Ellen et al. 2017).

Systems research takes a holistic approach to health service interventions, using a broad perspective to study the different levels at which systems operate and the contexts within which they function. Theoretical frameworks and constructs for studying interventions such as the Consolidated Framework for Implementation Research (CFIR) (see essay 9; Damschroder, "The Consolidated Framework for Implementation Research (CFIR)") and the Context and Implementation of Complex Interventions (CICI) framework exist to facilitate the identification, understanding, interpretation, and application of research within various contextual dimensions (Damschroder et al. 2009, Nilsen and Bernhardsson 2019, Pfadenhauer et al. 2017).

The micro level of any health system is crucial for implementation science, since, at the end of the day, it is individuals or teams at this level who carry out the implementation of any particular intervention. Behaviour change must be a focus when designing and planning interventions. More thorough change processes increase the likelihood of successful and sustained implementation (Rycroft-Malone et al. 2004). Frameworks such as the Theoretical Domains Framework (TDF) (see essay 10/26; Lorencatto, TDF) can be used for data collection, examining relationships, evaluating processes, and synthesizing evidence to guide behaviour change measures at the micro level (Atkins et al. 2017).

However, many implementation science efforts are focused on the meso level of health systems research, and these approaches and activities need to account for the continual evolution of health systems themselves. The implementation of research findings into practice at the meso level can be facilitated by the implementation of appropriate infrastructures, both technological and organizational, such as structured databases to help users identify relevant research (Ellen et al. 2011).

Macro-level health systems research is crucial if we are to understand the bigger, strategic or policy perspective and improve the uptake of research evidence, meeting the challenge of implementation from the top of the infrastructure hierarchy. Studying systems from a macro level consists of context-specific, evidence-informed policymaking, aiming to take theoretical findings into practice by delivering interventions effectively in diverse settings and within

DOI: 10.4324/9781003109945-4

the wide range of existing health system contexts. The interconnectedness of health systems research and implementation science is highlighted at the macro level, using implementation strategies to promote evidence-informed policy and decision-making, while utilizing evidence-informed policies and decisions to improve intervention design and implementation.

Using a health systems research approach in implementation science allows for the participation, ownership, and engagement of multiple stakeholders and key partners across the different levels of the health system. This ensures better designed interventions and more successful implementation. By conducting health systems research, one can expect to gain a clearer understanding of the global context of the system, along with valuable knowledge and insight into the various system levels and key elements that function across disparate contexts. This can all contribute to more rigorous implementation.

References

Atkins, L., J. Francis, R. Islam, D. O'Connor, A. Patey, N. Ivers, R. Foy, E. M. Duncan, H. Colquhoun, and J. M. Grimshaw. 2017. "A guide to using the Theoretical Domains Framework of behaviour change to investigate implementation problems." *Implementation Science* 12 (1):1–18.

Cabassa, L. J., and A. A. Baumann. 2013. "A two-way street: Bridging implementation science and cultural adaptations of mental health treatments." *Implementation Science* 8 (1):1–14.

Damschroder, L. J., D. C. Aron, R. E. Keith, S. R. Kirsh, J. A. Alexander, and J. C. Lowery. 2009. "Fostering implementation of health services research findings into practice: A consolidated framework for advancing implementation science." *Implementation Science* 4 (1):1–15.

Ellen, M., R. Shach, M. C. Kok, and K. Fatta. 2017. "There is much to learn when you listen: Exploring citizen engagement in high-and low-income countries." *World Health & Population* 17 (3):31–42.

Ellen, M. E., J. N. Lavis, M. Ouimet, J. Grimshaw, and P.-O. Bédard. 2011. "Determining research knowledge infrastructure for healthcare systems: A qualitative study." *Implementation Science* 6 (1):1–5.

Nilsen, P., and S. Bernhardsson. 2019. "Context matters in implementation science: A scoping review of determinant frameworks that describe contextual determinants for implementation outcomes." *BMC Health Services Research* 19 (1):1–21.

Pfadenhauer, L. M., A. Gerhardus, K. Mozygemba, K. B. Lysdahl, A. Booth, B. Hofmann, P. Wahlster, S. Polus, J. Burns, and L. Brereton. 2017. "Making sense of complexity in context and implementation: The Context and Implementation of Complex Interventions (CICI) framework." *Implementation Science* 12 (1):1–17.

Rycroft-Malone, J., G. Harvey, K. Seers, A. Kitson, B. McCormack, and A. Titchen. 2004. "An exploration of the factors that influence the implementation of evidence into practice." *Journal of Clinical Nursing* 13 (8):913–924.

3 Resilience changes the lens for healthcare implementation systems

David D. Woods and Michael F. Rayo

Implementation systems are adaptive systems within the overall complex healthcare system. Implementation systems are subject to the laws that govern adaptive systems of all types and scales and can benefit from Complex Adaptive Systems' findings from other settings. These findings, when applied to implementation systems, will improve the ability of healthcare to learn and change to meet patient needs as knowledge and technologies change. The study of how adaptive systems function and malfunction has revealed the importance of sources for resilient performance to overcome the risks of brittle system collapse as stress builds. For example, adaptation to potential overload in an intensive care unit (ICU) or emergency department (ED) concerns individual, team, and unit adaptations, all operating in parallel relative to the changing tempo of operations (Wears et al. 2008, Woods and Branlat 2011).

The factors that support or undermine resilient system performance operate at multiple levels across biological and human systems. Different levels of physiological and healthcare systems where adaptive processes occur include the following:

- Healthy physiological systems such as bone recycling (Cook 2020) or how heart function shifts under increasing stress (Li et al. 2014).
- Clinicians anticipating and intervening to assist a sick heart or other malfunctioning physiological system (Cook, Render, and Woods 2000).
- Clinicians adapting to avoid or mitigate workload bottlenecks that can interfere with patient care (Patterson and Wears 2015, Perry and Wears 2012).
- EDs adapting to cope with high patient numbers and "beyond surge capacity" events (Chuang et al. 2019, Wears et al. 2008).
- Maladaptive processes when different parts of a hospital or hospital system fail to coordinate, such as when EDs and ICUs are heavily crowded (Stephens, Woods, and Patterson 2015).
- Adaptive and maladaptive interactions across roles at regional and national scales when infectious disease outbreaks, such as COVID-19, roll across a country.

Adaptive capacity

How adaptive systems function and malfunction is the subject matter of the field of resilience engineering. Although the term "resilience" is now used to refer to many different processes (Woods 2015), what matters most is understanding that resilience refers to the *potential* for adaptive action in the future when conditions change. The capabilities a system needs to respond to introduce inevitable surprises. Responding to surprises requires preparatory investments that provide the readiness to respond (Woods 2019).

DOI: 10.4324/9781003109945-5

Systems possess varieties of adaptive capacity, and resilience engineering seeks to understand how these are built, sustained, degraded, and lost. Adaptive capacity is the potential for adjusting patterns of activities to handle future changes in the kinds of events, opportunities, and disruptions experienced; therefore, adaptive capacities exist before changes and disruptions call upon those capacities. All systems are developed and operate in given finite resources and live in a changing environment. As a result, plans, procedures, automation, agents, and roles are inherently limited and unable to completely cover the complexity of activities, events, and demands. All systems operate under pressures and in degraded modes (Woods 2019). As a result, all systems are subject to the risk of "brittle collapse", and people adapt, stretch, and extend operations to meet the inevitable challenges, pressures, trade-offs, resource scarcity, uncertainties, and surprises (Cook, Render, and Woods 2000, Perry and Wears 2012, Cuvelier and Falzon 2011). This is resilience-as-extensibility, and this capability is necessary for resilient performance (Woods 2015).

Being *poised to adapt*, a system develops a readiness to revise how it currently works – its models, plans, processes, and behaviours (Woods 2019). Adaptation is not about always changing the plan, model, or previous approaches but about the *potential* to modify plans to continue to fit changing situations. Building a system that is poised to adapt requires investment to build a readiness to revise and a readiness to respond to events and contexts that challenge the boundaries of normal work as specified in rules, policies, standard practices, and contingency plans. Space mission control is the definitive exemplar for this capability, especially how space shuttle mission control developed its skill at handling anomalies, even as they expected that the next anomaly to be handled would not match any of the ones they had planned and practised for (Watts-Perotti and Woods 2009). However, one of the most productive natural laboratories for learning the basic patterns and laws of adaptation are customers of the healthcare implementation system: emergency and critical care medicine (e.g., Chuang et al. 2019, Patterson and Wears 2015, Stephens, Woods, and Patterson 2015, Wears et al. 2008, Woods and Branlat 2011).

Three basic patterns in how adaptive systems fail

The studies in critical care medicine, among other settings, reveal three basic, durable patterns of how adaptive systems break down (Woods and Branlat 2011):

1   Decompensation – when the system exhausts its capacity to adapt as disturbances or challenges grow and cascade over time.
2   Working at cross purposes – when roles exhibit behaviours that are locally adaptive for their role and its rules but globally maladaptive from broader or multiple perspectives.
3   Getting stuck in outdated or "stale" behaviours – when the system over-relies on past models and fails to revise when conditions change.

Studies of sources of resilient performance have revealed how to design and operate systems to mitigate the risk of these failure modes.

Decompensation: exhausting capacity to adapt as disturbances or challenges cascade

In this pattern, breakdown occurs when challenges grow and cascade faster than responses can be decided upon and deployed to effect. A variety of cases from supervisory control of dynamic processes provide the archetype for the basic pattern. One example of this decompensation occurs in human cardiovascular physiology (e.g., the Starling curve in cardiology (Klabunde 2021a, 2021b)). When physicians manage sick hearts, they can miss signals that the cardiovascular system is running out of control capability and fail to intervene early enough to avoid a physiological crisis (Feltovich, Spiro, and Coulson 1988). In these situations, the critical information is not the abnormal process symptoms *per se* but the increasing efforts required to resist the process of deterioration. This failure mode refers to the inability to keep pace with changing situations.

Countermeasure

Anticipation is the key capability to produce resilient performance by mitigating the risk of this failure mode. The ability to *anticipate* allows systems to keep pace with increasing demands (Hollnagel 2009).

For implementation systems, anticipation can be achieved by monitoring for unanticipated effects in the aftermath of implementing changes and checking periodically thereafter. Changes, however planned, can produce forms of stress and pressure that lead to unexpected effects and adaptations. Stress symptoms include increased effort and increased use of workarounds to maintain performance (see essay 4; Rayo, "Implementation Systems That Support Resilient Performance").

Working at cross purposes: behaviour that is locally adaptive but globally maladaptive

This refers to the inability to coordinate and synchronize different groups at different echelons as goals conflict and crunches build. As a result of mis-synchronization, the groups work at cross purposes. Each group works hard to achieve the local goals defined for their scope of responsibility, but these activities make it more difficult for other groups to meet the responsibilities of their roles or undermine the global or long-term goals that all groups recognize. This failure mode includes common concerns about silos and fragmentation across roles in organizations.

Countermeasure

Synchronization across roles is the key capability to produce resilient performance by mitigating the risk of this failure mode. Ability to coordinate and *synchronize* across roles and across levels in an organization counteracts fragmentation and working at cross purposes (Woods 2019). Synchronization refers to when coordination across roles is needed and refers to the signals which indicate the need for different roles or levels to coordinate given changing situations.

For implementation systems, synchronization can be achieved by the implementation team staying in close contact with those affected by the implementation, probing for changing goals or conditions that are leading to unexpected adaptations that reveal the gap between the effects on work as envisioned and the adaptations that result (see essay 4; Rayo, Implementation Systems That Support Resilient Performance).

Getting stuck in outdated behaviours: the world changes, but the system remains stuck in previously successful adaptive strategies (over-relying on past successes)

This pattern relates to breakdowns in how systems learn. What was previously adaptive can become rigid at the level of individuals, groups, or organizations. These behaviours can persist even as information builds that the environment, relationships, risks, and opportunities are changing. This failure mode leads systems to get stuck in "stale" approaches even though events reveal that usual behaviours or processes are not working to produce desired effects or goals.

Countermeasure

Continuous and proactive learning is the key capability to produce resilient performance by mitigating the risk of this failure mode. Investments in mechanisms to learn from smaller earlier signals, rather than waiting for failures to occur, stimulate adoption of new practices as conditions continue to change (Hollnagel 2009).

For implementation systems, continuous learning depends on searching out early signals of emerging issues in order to reframe and revise previous priorities and directions (Klein et al. 2005).

References

Chuang, S., K.-S. Chang, D. D. Woods, H.-C. Chen, M. E. Reynolds, and D.-K. Chien. 2019. "Beyond surge: Coping with mass burn casualty in the closest hospital to the Formosa Fun Coast Dust Explosion." *Burns* 45 (4):964–973.

Cook, R. I. 2020. "A few observations on the marvelous resilience of bone and resilience engineering." *Adaptive Capacity Lab*, New York, USA, September 1.

Cook, R. I., M. Render, and D. D. Woods. 2000. "Gaps in the continuity of care and progress on patient safety." *BMJ* 320 (7237):791–794.

Cuvelier, L., and P. Falzon. 2011. "Coping with uncertainty: Resilient decisions in anaesthesia." In *Resilience Engineering in Practice*, edited by E. Hollnagel, J. Paries, D. D. Woods and J. Wreathall, 127–143. Aldershot, UK: Ashgate.

Feltovich, P. J., P. J. Spiro, and R. L. Coulson. 1988. "The nature of conceptual understanding in biomedicine: The deep structure of complex ideas and the development of misconceptions." In *Cognitive Science in Medicine: Biomedical Modeling,* edited by D. A. Evans and V. L. Patel, 113–172. The MIT Press.

Hollnagel, E. 2009. "The four cornerstones of resilience engineering." In *Resilience Engineering Perspectives, Volume 2: Preparation and Restoration*, 117–134. Surrey, UK: Ashgate.

Klabunde, R. E. 2021a. "Frank-Starling mechanism." In *Cardiovascular Physiology Concepts*. Philadelphia, PA: Wolters Kluwer.

Klabunde, R. E. 2021b. "Pathophysiology of heart failure." In *Cardiovascular Physiology Concepts*. Philadelphia, PA: Wolters Kluwer.

Klein, G., R. Pliske, B. Crandall, and D. Woods. 2005. "Problem detection." *Cognition, Technology & Work* 7 (1):14–28.

Li, N., J. Cruz, C. S. Chien, S. Sojoudi, B. Recht, D. Stone, M. Csete, D. Bahmiller, and J. C. Doyle. 2014. "Robust efficiency and actuator saturation explain healthy heart rate control and variability." *Proceedings of the National Academy of Sciences* 111 (33):E3476–E3485.

Patterson, M. D., and R. L. Wears. 2015. "Resilience and precarious success." *Reliability Engineering & System Safety* 141:45–53.

Perry, S. J., and R. L. Wears. 2012. "Underground adaptations: Case studies from health care." *Cognition, Technology & Work* 14 (3):253–260.

Stephens, R. J., D. D. Woods, and E. S. Patterson. 2015. "Patient boarding in the emergency department as a symptom of complexity-induced risks." In *Resilience in Everyday Clinical Work*, edited by R. L. Wears, E. Hollnagel and Jeffrey Braithwaite, 129–144. Farnham, UK: Ashgate.

Watts-Perotti, J., and D. D. Woods. 2009. "Cooperative advocacy: An approach for integrating diverse perspectives in anomaly response." *Computer Supported Cooperative Work (CSCW)* 18 (2–3): 175–198.

Wears, R. L., S. J. Perry, S. Anders, and D. D. Woods. 2008. "Resilience in the emergency department." In *Resilience Engineering Perspectives 1: Remaining Sensitive to the Possibility of Failure*, edited by E. Hollnagel, C. Nemeth, and S. W. A. Dekker. Aldershot, UK: Ashgate.

Woods, D. D. 2015. "Four concepts for resilience and the implications for the future of resilience engineering." *Reliability Engineering & System Safety* 141:5–9.

Woods, D. D. 2019. "Essentials of resilience, revisited." In *Handbook on Resilience of Socio-Technical Systems*, edited by M. Ruth and S. G. Reisemann, 52–56. Cheltenham: Edward Elgar Publishing.

Woods, D. D., and M. Branlat. 2011. "How adaptive systems fail." In *Resilience Engineering in Practice*, edited by E. Hollnagel, J. Paries, D. Woods and J. Wreathall, 127–143. Aldershot, UK: Ashgate.

4 Implementation systems that support resilient performance

Michael F. Rayo

Studies that distinguish between brittle and resilient systems emphasize that the latter are poised to adapt by building a readiness to revise, reframe, and respond when conditions, challenges, and opportunities change. The difference between brittle and resilient systems is captured in three forms of adaptive system breakdowns and the corresponding countermeasures (see essay 3; Woods and Rayo, Resilience Changes the Lens for Healthcare Implementation Systems). This essay provides a case in healthcare that illustrates how to engineer better implementation systems despite the trade-offs and pressures that will inevitably occur. The case in question reviews a set of implementation successes and setbacks, revealing how iterative loops of initial research, design, implementation, and assessment led to improvements in the patient care system being able to detect and respond to signs of patient decompensation (Horwood, Moffatt-Bruce, and Rayo 2019, Rayo et al. 2016, Rayo et al. 2019).

The goal of the studies was to improve the organization's ability to monitor and respond to patients at risk of physiological collapse. This risk is an example of one of the general forms of adaptive system breakdown, decompensation, and its countermeasure, to support anticipation (Woods and Branlat 2011). The risk of decompensation originates at the level of a patient's physiology, which occurs when the patient's body can no longer fully regulate critical physiological functions (e.g., cardiac, respiratory) which then begin to fail. The risk of decompensation also arises at the patient care level, where the care team needs the ability to anticipate and respond to early signs of decompensation, especially because physiological systems can deteriorate quickly. All patients in an acute care or intensive care unit are at some risk of experiencing a decompensation event. As a result, the care system should work to mitigate this risk.

At a third level, the patient care system is assisted by an implementation system. This includes deciding to purchase or develop new technologies, intervening to manage clinician workload and patient-to-staff ratios, and many more. Implementation systems influence all these factors as hospitals carry out efforts to improve efficiency, learn from adverse events, invest in team building, purchase and modify alerting systems, and create new policies and other initiatives intended to produce changes that improve patient care.

Interactions between the patient care and implementation systems illustrate the effects of the other two general risks of adaptive system breakdown and their corresponding countermeasures: fragmentation versus synchronization across roles and levels and becoming stuck in "stale models" versus a readiness to learn and revise as conditions change (Woods and Branlat 2011).

The goal of the implementation system research was to increase the anticipatory power of monitoring systems in order to reduce late responses to signs of physiological decompensation. The line of implementation system research began with studies to determine 1) the

DOI: 10.4324/9781003109945-6

current strategies and capabilities for early detection of patient decompensation (Horwood et al. 2018a) and 2) how current tools supported and sometimes hobbled clinician monitoring tactics (Horwood et al. 2018b). The research showed that effective anticipation was based on clinicians' ability to recognize change over time and departures from the patient-specific, context-aligned baseline. The factors shown to hobble anticipation and slow recognition depended on staffing, patient numbers, documentation demands, coordination across unit staff, and design of monitoring technology including alarms and displays. Importantly, the research showed that alarms and displays meant to improve anticipation often actually hobbled it. The studies also revealed ways that clinicians adapted their work and interactions to demonstrate resilient performance most of the time despite system characteristics that impaired anticipation, particularly with respect to poor alerts and displays.

Based on the empirical results, the researchers used the relevant science on alarm, alerts and displays in human-machine systems (Woods 1995) to develop new alerts, and information displays and policies (Rayo et al. 2016). The team then tested the new designs to check if these enhanced anticipation of physiological decompensation and received positive results (Rayo et al. 2019).

However, implementing the changes more widely met with reluctance due to conflicting views across the implementation system on how best to solve the problems that were discovered. Fragmentation across different parts of the hospital and the implementation system impeded change. Fragmentation led one group to push for simplification of alerts and sounds and a reluctance to change from the current alarm sounds. Another group pushed for uniformity and compliance with a new set of monitoring policies for the entire organization (Fitzgerald 2019). Both ignored the science on how to improve anticipation and resilience in cognitive work systems. Instead, these groups relied on their previous model of how they thought nurses use alarms to monitor rather than the empirical results from the studies on how nurses actually monitor patients, given weaknesses in the alerts. These types of misunderstandings reveal how the gap between Work-as-Imagined and Work-as-Done can be common in implementation systems (see essay 58; Sklar and Aarons, "Scaling-Out" Evidence-based Practices).

Fragmentation across implementation groups contributed to the struggle to act on the research and design results from the first phase. Each unit stayed within the scope of their own role within the implementation system. Miscoordination between groups responsible for policy dissemination, alarm management, and alarm implementation led to confusion about the purpose of the initiative: was the goal to reduce alarms (it wasn't) or to improve them (it was!)? The lack of ability to develop a coordinated response across the different roles and perspectives highlights the risk of the second form of adaptive system breakdown: working at cross purposes. This breakdown has been observed in poor coordination across units in hospitals (e.g., Stephens, Woods, and Patterson 2015), and the countermeasure can be seen in effective and rapid re-configuration across units in "beyond surge capacity" medical emergencies (Chuang et al. 2019).

After the alert changes new policy implementation, it became unambiguously clear that the simple alarms were counterproductive to anticipation, and benefits from the policy change were limited overall and uneven across units. This first round of change incurred significant financial cost and reputational cost to the implementation system. The poor results reduced the ability of the frontline clinical systems to accommodate further change.

The disappointing results led to increased coordination and support to implement the science-influenced versions of the original alarm and display design (Rayo et al. 2016, Rayo et al. 2019). The impact was tracked in a three-year study which showed tangible and sustained improvements in anticipation and monitoring, particularly in the cardiac units (Horwood, Moffatt-Bruce, and Rayo 2019).

The third general form of adaptive system breakdown, noted by Woods and Branlat (2011), is also highlighted by this case. Different groups appeared to be stuck in past models, even as evidence became available that these needed to be revised. First, several groups in the implementation system had mental models of nurses' work that were shown to be mismatched to how nurses actually monitor for physiological decompensation. This was also true of models of physicians' work not matching how they actually anticipated physiological decompensation. In addition, research results in general, confirmed by the results in this particular case, on how technology supports or hinders anticipation, did not match several groups' models of the impact of alarm system design on cognitive factors. However, all these mental models that were challenged or refuted outright by empirical findings and relevant literature were resistant to revision (Rayo and Moffatt-Bruce 2015). The irony is that the implementation system is in principle tasked with aiding organizational learning. This persistence of "stale models" and the fragmentation across roles 1) reduced the organization's ability to recognize the gap and the *opportunity* to improve, 2) slowed the organization's response once recognized, and 3) increased the cost of change.

This case demonstrates how people provide the ad hoc source of resilient performance to bridge gaps in a system despite being hobbled by aspects of system design (Cook, Render, and Woods 2000). The implementation systems can miss the sources of resilient performance, the gaps, and the constricting factors. As a result, their model of work differs substantially from how actual practice has adapted to gaps, risks, load, and conflicts (Braithwaite, Wears, and Hollnagel 2016). Adverse events still occur, which surprise and puzzle stakeholders. They interpret the adverse events as failures to work to rule, to roll, and to plan, which produces increased reliance on standards and increased pressure to comply with standards (Perry and Fairbanks 2017). These steps undermine sources of resilient performance, leaving the system more brittle than realized or desired (Woods and Branlat 2011).

This case also illustrates how implementation systems are subject to the laws of adaptive systems in complex worlds. Explicitly considering these laws can help implementation systems reconfigure to facilitate learning and adaptation. This is particularly important as systems in healthcare and other industries become increasingly complex with greater interdependencies across multiple levels (Braithwaite et al. 2018). Resilient implementation systems provide a reflective integrated perspective to help overloaded units recognize how to coordinate and anticipate, to build a readiness to revise and a readiness to respond that benefits patients. Early recognition of potential problems and active effort to mitigate fragmentation and reveal stale models among the team are critically important to the sustained success of the implementation system.

References

Braithwaite, J., K. Churruca, J. C. Long, L. A. Ellis, and J. Herkes. 2018. "When complexity science meets implementation science: A theoretical and empirical analysis of systems change." *BMC Medicine* 16 (1). doi: 10.1186/s12916-018-1057-z.

Braithwaite, J., R. L. Wears, and E. Hollnagel. 2016. *Reconciling Work-as-Imagined and Work-as-Done*. Vol. 3, *Resilient Health Care*. Boca Raton, FL: CRC Press.

Chuang, S., K.-S. Chang, D. D. Woods, H.-C. Chen, M. E. Reynolds, and D.-K. Chien. 2019. "Beyond surge: Coping with mass burn casualty in the closest hospital to the Formosa Fun Coast Dust Explosion." *Burns* 45 (4):964–973.

Cook, R. I., M. Render, and D. D. Woods. 2000. "Gaps in the continuity of care and progress on patient safety." *BMJ* 320 (7237):791–794.

Fitzgerald, M. C. 2019. *The IMPActS Framework: The Necessary Requirements for Making Science-Based Organizational Impact*. Columbus, OH: The Ohio State University.

Horwood, C. R., S. D. Moffatt-Bruce, M. Fitzgerald, and M. F. Rayo. 2018a. "A qualitative analysis of clinical decompensation in the surgical patient: Perceptions of nurses and physicians." *Surgery* 164 (6):1311–1315.

Horwood, C. R., S. D. Moffatt-Bruce, and M. F. Rayo. 2019. "Continuous cardiac monitoring policy implementation: Three-year sustained decrease of hospital resource utilization." In *Structural Approaches to Address Issues in Patient Safety*. Bradford: Emerald Publishing Limited.

Horwood, C. R., M. F. Rayo, M. Fitzgerald, E. A. Balkin, and S. D. Moffatt-Bruce. 2018b. "Gaps between alarm capabilities and decision-making needs: An observational study of detecting patient decompensation." Proceedings of the International Symposium on Human Factors and Ergonomics in Health Care.

Perry, S. J., and R. J. Fairbanks. 2017. "Tempest in a teapot: Standardisation and workarounds in everyday clinical work." In *Resilient Health Care, Volume 2*, 193–206. Boca Raton, FL: CRC Press.

Rayo, M. F., J. Mansfield, D. Eiferman, T. Mignery, S. White, and S. D. Moffatt-Bruce. 2016. "Implementing an institution-wide quality improvement policy to ensure appropriate use of continuous cardiac monitoring: A mixed-methods retrospective data analysis and direct observation study." *BMJ Quality & Safety* 25 (10):796–802.

Rayo, M. F., and S. D. Moffatt-Bruce. 2015. "Alarm system management: Evidence-based guidance encouraging direct measurement of informativeness to improve alarm response." *BMJ Quality & Safety* 24 (4):282–286.

Rayo, M. F., E. S. Patterson, M. Abdel-Rasoul, and S. D. Moffatt-Bruce. 2019. "Using timbre to improve performance of larger auditory alarm sets." *Ergonomics*:1–33. doi: 10.1080/00140139.2019.1676473.

Stephens, R. J., D. D. Woods, and E. S. Patterson. 2015. "Patient boarding in the emergency department as a symptom of complexity-induced risks." In *Resilience in Everyday Clinical Work*, edited by R. L. Wears, E. Hollnagel and J. Braithwaite, 129–144. Farnham, UK: Ashgate.

Woods, D. D. 1995. "The alarm problem and directed attention in dynamic fault management." *Ergonomics* 38 (11):2371–2393.

Woods, D. D., and M. Branlat. 2011. "How adaptive systems fail." In *Resilience Engineering in Practice*, edited by E. Hollnagel, J. Paries, D. Woods, and J. Wreathall, 127–143. Aldershot, UK: Ashgate.

5 Principles of implementation science

Amy M. Kilbourne

Implementation science is the process of solving complex healthcare problems by motivating providers to use effective treatments for their patients, especially when faced with resource limitations. Interdisciplinary in nature, implementation science draws its foundations from public health, psychology, the health professions, social sciences, and business. These multiple perspectives are vital to enable implementation scientists to face the daunting challenge of changing provider behaviour especially when faced with organizational constraints and competing demands. The ability to understand, motivate, and inspire providers and healthcare teams to take on something new is a core component of implementation science. Not surprisingly, many of the lessons from community-engaged research (Jones and Wells 2007), business management, including Transformational (Servant) Leadership (Avolio 2011), and even from Dale Carnegie (Carnegie 1936) parallel those garnered from the field of implementation science.

Implementation strategies are highly specified, theory-based tools or methods for promoting provider behaviour change to facilitate adoption of effective treatments (Bauer et al. 2015). It is well known that it can take years for a fraction of effective healthcare treatments to reach patients who need them the most. Despite documentation of recent implementation success stories (Kilbourne, Glasgow, and Chambers 2020), there is little definitive research on which implementation strategies work for different treatments or settings. Results from these studies have also not been widely replicated or applied outside of the scientific research-funded world, which supports a major portion of implementation science development. Key reasons for this implementation-to-real-world gap is the lack of incentives for implementation researchers to engage with routine care practices in an ongoing manner in order to ensure treatment sustainment over time (e.g., through ongoing provider training, technical support, and surveillance) (Kilbourne, Jones, and Atkins 2020). Academic medical centres, the principal employers of implementation researchers in the United States (US), measure success through promotion and tenure when researchers publish more papers and acquire more competitive federal grant funding. The field of implementation science can get pulled into the academic "ivory tower" mindset, with its own guild and language that can leave out those with a less academic approach, leaning towards real-world experiences or with diverse perspectives. Without a dramatic shift in the way real-world implementation research is recognized and rewarded, the field risks further drift away from its original purpose of solving real-world problems, ultimately becoming irrelevant to the needs of providers and patients in community-based settings.

To ensure implementation science is relevant to the needs of patients, providers, other stakeholders, and community-based health systems, academic medical centres and federal funders (such as in the US context) need to promote incentives to ensure that implementation

DOI: 10.4324/9781003109945-7

studies of effective treatments involve these multilevel stakeholders on an ongoing basis, from the inception of the research ideal to dissemination of results. Moreover, the effective treatment needs to be adapted so it can be feasible enough to be implemented by existing providers, without having to hire new staff.

In addition, implementation researchers need incentives to work on solving healthcare problems identified by external health systems or community partners, who may have some of the best ideas for addressing complex health problems. In solving these problems, researchers should be encouraged to maximize impact, especially by encouraging the implementation of effective treatments created by other research teams and not just regarding their own research.

So how can implementation science get back to its roots and address healthcare problems in the real world? The VA Quality Enhancement Research Initiative (QUERI) program provides an Implementation Roadmap for involving stakeholders and planning rigorous implementation research that is relevant to real-world health problems. The mission of QUERI is to improve veteran health by accelerating the adoption of effective treatments in routine practice. The QUERI Implementation Roadmap (Figure 5.1) communicates implementation processes to stakeholders using a Learning Health System framework,

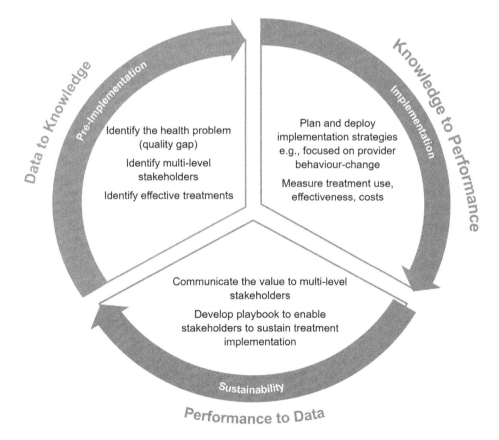

Figure 5.1 QUERI Implementation Roadmap

Source: Adapted from Goodrich et al. 2020

which emphasizes continuous quality improvement and knowledge generation through the continuous ascertainment of data which inform implementation and evaluation (Kilbourne et al. 2019). Through active implementation, evaluation, and ongoing training and support, QUERI promotes more providers deploying effective treatments using rigorous implementation methods. QUERI's core principles strive to make implementation science more relevant to the real world. First, there is a strong emphasis on the application of implementation strategies to promote the uptake of effective treatments and benchmarking on meaningful outcomes to patients, providers, and health system leaders. Second, QUERI focuses on rigorous and rapid evaluation of national healthcare priorities, where many of its centres have investigators on "retainer" to deploy Rapid Response Teams to address time-sensitive implementation needs identified by stakeholders. Third, QUERI is committed to maximizing diversity among its investigators, VA leadership partners, and sites. QUERI centres are strongly encouraged to prioritize quality improvement at sites that have experienced disparities in healthcare and include multilevel stakeholders including frontline providers, mid-level managers, consumers, and healthcare leaders throughout the implementation process. Fourth, QUERI, notably through its funding mechanisms and centres' mentoring cores, are encouraged to identify and promote leaders from underrepresented backgrounds (e.g., the majority of QUERI projects are led by women, and about a quarter are led by people of colour). Finally, QUERI commits to sustainment over time by ensuring that stakeholders have the tools and methods to support ongoing implementation and trains practitioners and researchers on implementation strategies through its Implementation Strategy Learning Hubs.

Ultimately, QUERI rewards its investigators through a combination of stable funding to devote the time to build relationships across multiple stakeholders and the use of competitive federal funding mechanisms that are recognized by US academic medical centres as centre grants. QUERI's devotion to ongoing learning, improvement, and partnership with healthcare leaders enables investigators to have the opportunity to spend essential time cultivating strong and lasting relationships with clinical operations partners. To this end, QUERI can serve as a model for operationalizing principles of implementation science in the real world, especially by encouraging researchers to address problems identified by healthcare providers and the communities they serve and by rewarding them along with their community health partners for successful spread and sustainment of effective treatments and quality and outcomes improvement for the people they serve.

References

Avolio, B. 2011. *Full Range Leadership Development*. 2nd ed. Thousand Oaks, CA: Sage Publications.

Bauer, M., L. Damschroder, H. Hagedorn, J. Smith, and A. Kilbourne. 2015. "An introduction to implementation science for the non-specialist." *BMC Psychology* 3 (1):32. doi: 10.1186/s40359-015-0089-9.

Carnegie, D. 1936. *How to Win Friends and Influence People*. New York: Simon & Schuster.

Goodrich, D. E., I. Miake-Lye, M. Z. Braganza, N. Wawrin, and A. M. Kilbourne. 2020. *QUERI Roadmap for Implementation and Quality Improvement*. Washington, DC: United States Department of Veterans Affairs Veterans Health Administration Office of Research and Development Health Services Research and Development.

Jones, L., and K. Wells. 2007. "Strategies for academic and clinician engagement in community-participatory partnered research." *Journal of the American Medical Association* 297 (4):407–410. doi: 10.1001/jama.297.4.407.

Kilbourne, A., R. Glasgow, and D. Chambers. 2020. "What Can Implementation Science Do for You? Key Success Stories from the Field." *Journal of General Internal Medicine*. doi: 10.1007/s11606-020-06174-6.

Kilbourne, A., D. Goodrich, I. Miake-Lye, M. Braganza, and N. Bowersox. 2019. "Quality enhancement research initiative implementation roadmap: Toward sustainability of evidence-based practices in a learning health system." *Medical care* 10 (Suppl 3):S286–S293. doi: 10.1097/MLR.0000000000001144.

Kilbourne, A., P. Jones, and D. Atkins. 2020. "Accelerating implementation of research in Learning Health Systems: Lessons learned from VA health services research and NCATS clinical science translation award programs." *Journal of Clinical and Translational Science* 4 (3):195–200. doi: 10.1017/cts.2020.25.

6 Medical humanism

The role of character in implementation science

Mark Clark

The Medical Humanities is an interdisciplinary field that uses the humanities' methods of inquiry to analyse, critique, and improve the practice of medicine. Numerous practitioners in the field have particular interests related to narrative and rhetorical issues in medicine as well as the ethical action following from processes of interpretation, representation, and persuasion (Brody 2009, Carson 1997, Charon and Montello 2002, Nelson 1997). Such practitioners would be inclined to regard the project of implementation science as a rhetorical endeavour: the aim is, by means of representation and translation, to persuade non-scientists of the value of scientific conceptualization and of subsequent action – making choices in life – grounded in this understanding. If I, as a physician, enter conscientiously into a conversation that results in informed consent, I may need to re-present complex scientific concepts in a fashion that my patients will understand such that they are able to choose, with freedom, the path of treatment they wish. If I wish to administer a vaccine to a relatively undereducated Nicaraguan woman, I may need to explain the nature and function of the vaccine by means of a metaphor – a White Cadejo and a Black Cadejo, for instance: a Good Spirit and a Bad Spirit[1] – such that the woman and I communicate on a common ground of understanding (Chase et al. 2020). If, through the means of the metaphor, the woman grasps the good of the vaccine, she will probably be more willing to accept the treatment. Implementation science is interested in the efficacy of such a rhetorical act: the effective construction of a metaphor that brings about an understanding of the vaccine and a willingness to accept vaccination.

In reflecting further upon this Nicaraguan woman and my interaction with her as a rhetorical endeavour aimed at persuasion, my thoughts turn to Aristotle and his considerations of effective rhetoric not simply as an exercise of pure logic but also as an act that integrates *ethos* (the Aristotelian appeal to the presenter's authority), *pathos* (appealing to the receiver's emotions), and *logos* (appeal to the logic which supports the presenter's argument). Effective persuasion is to be achieved through a wholeness of person, an exhibition of integrated being. What occurs when I construct the metaphor of the White Cadejo and the Black Cadejo? Motivated by some sort of compassion or care about a fellow human being in need, I find my moral imagination engaged, wonder what the experience of another is like, and demonstrate the generosity of spirit to construct a common ground of understanding. My credibility with the woman arises not simply from exercises of reason but also through a demonstrated generosity of spirit (*ethos*) and fellow-feeling (*pathos*). A trustworthy person of integrity cares for this woman: the act of metaphor construction communicates this in addition to the nature and function of the vaccine. She is persuaded to accompany me in treatment because I engage the wholeness of my person with the wholeness of her being.

Clinical medicine, practised as such, *is* implementation science. And implementation science, realized in this way, is an art of rhetoric that relies on the demonstration of good

DOI: 10.4324/9781003109945-8

character: *ethos*. A medical education engaged in the formation of good doctors ought to be a process, then, that actively cultivates a generous spirit who exercises, by habit, the moral imagination, who truly listens to the voice of another, however broken and alien it may be, and who relishes the vulnerability to fall into compassion with those who suffer. Clinical vignettes and cases – the stories through which so much of medical education is accomplished – do not foster such an *ethos*, though. They depict patients as little more than biological puzzles who lack voices and agency and depict doctors who work efficiently within a linear time that has no tolerance for the messy, experiential time of illness. Students learn to assume identities as scientists, not clinicians (Montgomery 2006), and learn to develop a *character* that is narcissistic – demanding *adherence* to its understanding of illness experience – and not the generous spirit of ethical doctoring.

The rhetorical project of implementation science, as it is to be conducted in clinical medicine, needs to take a careful look at the cultivation of good character. A good, compassionate, caring person has the credibility to be believed as a prophet of the benefits of science. Such a person testifies, through *character*, that scientific understanding may be a dimension of a person who is the embodiment of goodness and moral beauty.

Note

1 I am grateful to my student, Melanie Musselman, for providing me with this image, a discussion of which we were able to publish in the referenced article.

References

Brody, H. 2009. *The Future of Bioethics*. New York: Oxford University Press.

Carson, R. 1997. "Medical ethics as reflective practice." In *Philosophy of Medicine and Bioethics: A Twenty Year Retrospective and Critical Appraisal*, edited by R. A. Carson and C. R. Burns. Dordrecht, Netherlands: Kluwer.

Charon, R., and M. Montello. 2002. *Stories Matter: The Role of Narrative in Medical Ethics*. New York: Routledge.

Chase, A., M. Clark, A. Rogalska, and M. Musselman. 2020. "Cultivating physician-patient communication about vaccination through vaccine metaphor." *Medical Science Educator* 30:1015–1017. doi: 10.1007/s40670-020-00981-6.

Montgomery, K. 2006. *How Doctors Think: Clinical Judgment and the Practice of Medicine*. New York: Oxford University Press.

Nelson, H. 1997. *Stories and their limits: Narrative Approaches to Bioethics*. New York: Routledge.

7 Theorizing

Roman Kislov and Paul Wilson

Theory provides a lens through which we can explore, explain, and predict implementation. It can be defined as "an ordered set of assertions about a generic behaviour or structure assumed to hold throughout a significantly broad range of specific instances" (Weick 1989). By developing concepts and explicating their interrelationships, theory seeks to explain how and why a phenomenon occurs (Corley and Gioia 2011).

Despite its ordered and abstract nature, which can occasionally alienate researchers and practitioners, theory should not be treated as an isolated, static, reified source ready to be plucked off the shelf and used to guide implementation. Instead, we call for a change of perspective from "theories" as finished products created by the leading lights of our discipline to "theorizing" as the process of developing, refining, and expanding theoretical knowledge in which all implementation researchers can and should engage (Kislov et al. 2019).

As shown in Figure 7.1, theorizing involves moving back and forth between empirical data and theories at different levels of abstraction:

- Program, or "small", theories that explain how a specific policy, intervention, or project is supposed to function and achieve its objectives (e.g., establishment of university-industry partnerships may be underpinned by an assumption that collaboration leads to the development of knowledge that is more implementable (Rycroft-Malone et al. 2013)).
- Mid-range theories whose application is restricted to a certain subset of social phenomena relevant to a particular range of contexts (e.g., Normalization Process Theory (May et al. 2009)).
- Grand theories, aiming to construct all-encompassing meta-narratives that span space and time (e.g., theoretical oeuvres of Marx and Bourdieu).

Constant dialogue between the empirical and the theoretical (particularly at the level of mid-range theory) is a cornerstone of so-called theoretically informative, as opposed to merely theoretically informed, research (Kislov 2019). Although guided by existing theory, this approach aims to yield new theoretical insights applicable to a broader range of settings. A *particular* empirical case or set of cases is used as an opportunity for refining previous conceptualizations of the *general* processes contained in the earlier theoretical accounts. Theorizing is, therefore, an iterative and recursive process: theory is no longer seen as "fixed and immutable" but as "a fluid collection of principles and hypotheses" (Lewis and Ritchie 2003).

How can we engage with theorizing when designing or evaluating implementation interventions? First of all, even in the absence of an explicitly adopted theoretical approach, all

DOI: 10.4324/9781003109945-9

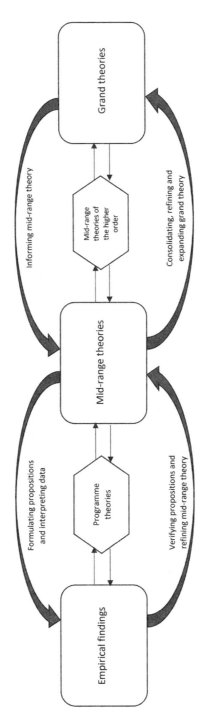

Figure 7.1 Theorizing in implementation science

Source: Adapted from Kislov et al. 2019

empirical observations are inherently theory laden as they draw on implicit "theories in use", that is, ideas about what makes certain settings, interventions, and approaches operate in a certain way. Eliciting, articulating, and comparing "theories in use" espoused by reflective stakeholders, recipients, and researchers of implementation and linking them with relevant mid-range theories can help to frame and analyse an empirical case under investigation ("What is going on here?") as an example of a broader social phenomenon ("What is this a case of?") (Tsoukas 2009).

Second, a theoretically informative approach involves discussing what the resulting empirical findings mean for theory. To achieve this, an empirical case under investigation should be positioned against, and compared with, previous studies that have contributed to the formulation and development of the relevant theory. Analysis and interpretation of findings should not be limited to identifying similarities between the empirical case and extant theory but should aim to identify the differences and/or omissions, express them in theoretical terms, and use these newly identified variations to refine previous theoretical knowledge. These insights do not have to be large-scale and transformative to be revelatory and original, though they do need to represent more than tinkering, navel-gazing or adding terminological clutter. When undertaking data analysis, it is important to avoid producing "shopping lists" of themes that are purely descriptive or simply catalogue multiple contextual factors or processes of change. Themes and propositions should evolve from the data that link different determinants, concepts, or factors together, thus reflecting relationships between them and uncovering generative mechanisms of social phenomena.

Finally, theorizing often involves choosing – and adjudicating – between alternative theoretical approaches, some of which can be more relevant to an implementation problem at hand than others. Practical adequacy of a theory can be assessed by its ability to explain the phenomena observed and to assist problem-solving (Brodie and Peters 2020). Empirical data can help researchers to elucidate in which respects one theory is preferable to others. Engaging with this aspect of theorizing can prevent a commonly observed mismatch between implementation problems and solutions proposed to address them (Wensing and Grol 2019).

It is through the verification, refinement, and consolidation of theoretical knowledge that social science disciplines develop. Engaging with the processes of theorizing can help researchers gain new insights and contribute to advancing the knowledge base of implementation science.

References

Brodie, R. J., and L. D. Peters. 2020. "New directions for service research: Refreshing the process of theorizing to increase contribution." *Journal of Services Marketing* 34 (3):415–428.

Corley, K. G., and D. A. Gioia. 2011. "Building theory about theory building: What constitutes a theoretical contribution?" *Academy of Management Review* 36 (1):12–32.

Kislov, R. 2019. "Engaging with theory: From theoretically informed to theoretically informative improvement research." *BMJ Quality & Safety* 28 (3):177–179.

Kislov, R., C. Pope, G. P. Martin, and P. M. Wilson. 2019. "Harnessing the power of theorising in implementation science." *Implementation Science* 14 (1):103.

Lewis, J., and J. Ritchie. 2003. "Generalising from qualitative research." In *Qualitative Research Practice: A Guide for Social Science Students and Researchers*, edited by J. Ritchie and J. Lewis. London: Sage Publications.

May, C., F. Mair, T. Finch, A. MacFarlane, C. Dowrick, S. Treweek, T. Rapley, L. Ballini, B. N. Ong, A. Rogers, E. Murray, G. Elwyn, F. Légaré, J. Gunn, and V. M. Montori. 2009. "Development of a theory of implementation and integration: Normalisation Process Theory." *Implementation Science* 4 (29). doi: 10.1186/1748-5908-4-29.

Rycroft-Malone, J., J. Wilkinson, C. R. Burton, G. Harvey, B. McCormack, I. Graham, and S. Staniszewska. 2013. "Collaborative action around implementation in Collaborations for Leadership in Applied Health Research and Care: Towards a programme theory." *Journal of Health Services Research & Policy* 18(Suppl 3):13–26.

Tsoukas, H. 2009. "Craving for generality and small-N studies: A Wittgensteinian approach towards the epistemology of the particular in organization and management studies." In *SAGE Handbook of Organizational Research Methods*, edited by David Buchanan and A. Bryman, 285–301. London: Sage Publications.

Weick, K. E. 1989. "Theory construction as disciplined imagination." *Academy of Management Review* 14 (4):516–531.

Wensing, M., and R. Grol. 2019. "Knowledge translation in health: How implementation science could contribute more." *BMC Medicine* 17:88.

8 Theories, models, and frameworks in implementation science

A Taxonomy

Per Nilsen

Implementation science has increasingly emphasized the importance of establishing the theoretical bases of implementation processes and strategies to facilitate implementation. In fact, there are now so many theoretical approaches that some researchers have complained about the difficulties of choosing the most appropriate (Cane, O'Connor, and Michie 2012, Martinez, Lewis, and Weiner 2014, Rycroft-Malone and Bucknall 2010b). This essay provides a brief overview of categories of theories, models, and frameworks (TMFs) used in this research field.

A theory in implementation science usually implies some predictive capacity and attempts to explain the causal mechanisms of implementation. Models in implementation science are commonly used to describe and/or guide the process of translating research into practice. Frameworks in implementation science often have a descriptive purpose by pointing to factors believed or found to influence implementation outcomes. Neither models nor frameworks specify the mechanisms of change; they are typically more like checklists of factors relevant to various aspects of implementation.

TMFs have three overarching aims in implementation science: 1) describing and/or guiding the process of translating research into practice, 2) understanding and/or explaining what influences implementation outcomes, and 3) evaluating implementation. TMFs that aim at understanding and/or explaining influences on implementation outcomes (i.e., aim 2) can be broken down into 2a) determinant frameworks, 2b) classic theories, and 2c) implementation theories. Thus, on this account, there are five TMF categories used in implementation science.

Process models (category 1) outline phases or stages of the research-to-practice process, from discovery and production of research-based knowledge to implementation and use of research (e.g., in the form of an evidence-based intervention or program). So-called action models are process models that facilitate implementation by offering practical guidance in the planning and execution of implementation endeavours. Action models elucidate important aspects that need to be considered and usually prescribe a number of activities that should be undertaken in the process of translating research into practice. Action models have been described as "active" by Graham et al. (2009) because they are used to cause change. However, the terminology is not fully consistent, because some process models are referred to as frameworks – for example, the Knowledge-to-Action Framework (Rycroft-Malone and Bucknall 2010a).

Determinant frameworks (category 2a) describe general types (also referred to as classes or domains) of determinants that are hypothesized or have been found to influence implementation outcomes. Each type of determinant typically comprises a number of individual barriers and/or facilitators, which are seen as independent variables that impact implementation

DOI: 10.4324/9781003109945-10

outcomes, that is, the dependent variable. Some frameworks also hypothesize relationships between these determinants (e.g., Gurses et al. 2010), whereas others recognize such relationships without clarifying them (e.g., Cochrane et al. 2007). Two of the most applied determinant frameworks are Consolidated Framework for Implementation Research (CFIR) (Damschroder et al. 2009) (see essay 9; Damschroder, "The Consolidated Framework for Implementation Research (CFIR)") and Promoting Action on Research Implementation in Health Services (PARIHS) (Rycroft-Malone 2010). Determinant frameworks do not address how change takes place or any causal mechanisms, underscoring that they should not be considered theories. Many frameworks are multilevel, identifying determinants at different levels, from the individual user or adopter (e.g., healthcare practitioner) to the organization and beyond.

Theories borrowed from other fields such as psychology, sociology, and organizational theory may be referred to as classic theories (category 2b) since they are established, already-existing theories. They might be considered passive in relation to action models because they describe change mechanisms and explain how change occurs without ambitions to bring about change.

Implementation theories (category 2c) have been developed or adapted by researchers for potential use in implementation science to achieve enhanced understanding and explanation of certain aspects of implementation. Some of these have been developed by modifying certain features of existing classic theories or concepts – for example, concerning organizational climate (Weiner 2009). The adaptation allows researchers to prioritize aspects considered to be most critical to analyse issues related to the how and why of implementation, thus improving the relevance and appropriateness of the particular circumstances at hand.

Evaluation frameworks (category 3) provide a structure for evaluating implementation endeavours. Two common frameworks that originated in public health are RE-AIM (Reach, Effectiveness, Adoption, Implementation, Maintenance) (Glasgow, Vogt, and Boles 1999) and PRECEDE-PROCEED (Predisposing, Reinforcing, and Enabling Constructs in Educational Diagnosis and Evaluation-Policy, Regulatory, and Organizational Constructs in Educational and Environmental Development) (Green and Kreuter 2005). Both frameworks specify implementation aspects that should be evaluated as part of intervention studies. Proctor et al. (2010) have developed a framework of implementation outcomes that can be applied to evaluate implementation endeavours. They propose eight conceptually distinct outcomes for potential evaluation: acceptability, adoption (also referred to as uptake), appropriateness, costs, feasibility, fidelity, penetration (integration of a practice within a specific setting), and sustainability (also referred to as maintenance or institutionalization).

Although evaluation frameworks may be considered in a category of their own, TMFs from the other four categories (1, 2a, 2b, 2c) can also be applied for evaluation purposes because they specify concepts and constructs that may be operationalized and measured. Furthermore, many TMFs have spawned instruments that serve evaluation purposes – for example, tools linked to CFIR (Damschroder and Lowery 2013) and Theoretical Domains Framework (Dyson et al. 2013). Other examples include the BARRIERS Scale to identify barriers to research use (Kajermo et al. 2010) and instruments to operationalize theories such as Implementation Climate (Jacobs, Weiner, and Bunger 2014) and Organizational Readiness (Gagnon et al. 2011).

There is overlap between some of the categories (Figure 8.1). Thus, determinant frameworks, classic theories, and implementation theories can also help to guide implementation practice (i.e., functioning as process models), because they identify potential barriers and

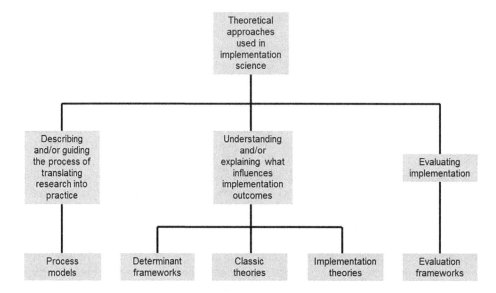

Figure 8.1 Three aims of the use of theoretical approaches in implementation science and the five categories of theories, models, and frameworks

Source: Originally published in Nilsen 2015

enablers that might be important to address when undertaking an implementation endeavour. They can also be used for evaluation because they describe aspects that might be important to evaluate.

References

Cane, J., D. O'Connor, and S. Michie. 2012. "Validation of the theoretical domains framework for use in behaviour change and implementation research." *Implementation Science* 7 (1):1–17.

Cochrane, L. J., C. A. Olson, S. Murray, M. Dupuis, T. Tooman, and S. Hayes. 2007. "Gaps between knowing and doing: Understanding and assessing the barriers to optimal health care." *Journal of Continuing Education in the Health Professions* 27 (2):94–102.

Damschroder, L. J., D. C. Aron, R. E. Keith, S. R. Kirsh, J. A. Alexander, and J. C. Lowery. 2009. "Fostering implementation of health services research findings into practice: A consolidated framework for advancing implementation science." *Implementation Science* 4 (1):1–15.

Damschroder, L. J., and J. C. Lowery. 2013. "Evaluation of a large-scale weight management program using the consolidated framework for implementation research (CFIR)." *Implementation Science* 8 (1):1–17.

Dyson, J., R. Lawton, C. Jackson, and F. Cheater. 2013. "Development of a theory-based instrument to identify barriers and levers to best hand hygiene practice among healthcare practitioners." *Implementation Science* 8 (1):1–9.

Gagnon, M.-P., J. Labarthe, F. Légaré, M. Ouimet, C. A. Estabrooks, G. Roch, and J. Grimshaw. 2011. "Measuring organizational readiness for knowledge translation in chronic care." *Implementation Science* 6 (1):1–10.

Glasgow, R. E., T. M. Vogt, and S. M. Boles. 1999. "Evaluating the public health impact of health promotion interventions: The RE-AIM framework." *American journal of public health* 89 (9):1322–1327.

Graham, I. D., J. Tetroe, and KT Theories Group. 2009. "Planned action theories." In *Knowledge Translation in Health Care: Moving from Evidence to Practice,* edited by Sharon Straus, Jacqueline Tetroe and Ian D Graham. Hoboken, NJ: John Wiley & Sons.

Green, L. W., and M. W. Kreuter. 2005. *Health Program Planning: An Educational and Ecological Approach.* 4th ed. Boston: McGraw-Hill.

Gurses, A. P., J. A. Marsteller, A. A. Ozok, Y. Xiao, S. Owens, and P. J. Pronovost. 2010. "Using an interdisciplinary approach to identify factors that affect clinicians' compliance with evidence-based guidelines." *Critical Care Medicine* 38:S282–S291.

Jacobs, S. R., B. J. Weiner, and A. C. Bunger. 2014. "Context matters: Measuring implementation climate among individuals and groups." *Implementation Science* 9 (1):1–14.

Kajermo, K. N., A.-M. Boström, D. S. Thompson, A. M. Hutchinson, C. A. Estabrooks, and L. Wallin. 2010. "The BARRIERS scale – the barriers to research utilization scale: A systematic review." *Implementation Science* 5 (1):1–22.

Martinez, R. G., C. C. Lewis, and B. J. Weiner. 2014. "Instrumentation issues in implementation science." *Implementation Science* 9 (1):1–9.

Nilsen, P. 2015. "Making sense of implementation theories, models and frameworks." *Implementation Science* 10 (1):53. doi: 10.1186/s13012-015-0242-0.

Proctor, E., H. Silmere, R. Raghavan, P. Hovmand, G. Aarons, A. Bunger, R. Griffey, and M. Hensley. 2010. "Outcomes for implementation research: Conceptual distinctions, measurement challenges, and research agenda." *Administration and Policy in Mental Health and Mental Health Services Research* 38 (2):65–76.

Rycroft-Malone, J. 2010. "Promoting action on research implementation in health services (PARIHS)." *Models and Frameworks for Implementing Evidence-based Practice: Linking Evidence to Action* 109:135.

Rycroft-Malone, J., and T. Bucknall. 2010a. *Analysis and Synthesis of Models and Frameworks.* Edited by J. Rycroft-Malone and T Bucknall, *Models and Frameworks for Implementing Evidence-based Practice: Linking Evidence to Action.* Chichester: Wile-Blackwell.

Rycroft-Malone, J., and T. Bucknall. 2010b. "Theory, frameworks, and models." *Models and Frameworks for Implementing Evidence-based Practice: Linking Evidence to Action:*23.

Weiner, B. J. 2009. "A theory of organizational readiness for change." *Implementation Science* 4 (1):1–9.

9 The Consolidated Framework for Implementation Research (CFIR)

Laura Damschroder

The overarching aim of health and medical research is to find innovative, breakthrough discoveries for the benefit of human beings. The number of randomized controlled trials (RCTs) that test innovations is proliferating exponentially (Bastian, Glasziou, and Chalmers 2010). Though RCTs produce knowledge of *what* works within highly controlled settings, they fail to guide *where* the innovation will work and *why* and *how* to implement in real-world clinical settings for sustained routine use (Green and Glasgow 2006). This gap has contributed to the vast lack of use of beneficial innovations within healthcare settings.

To help address this gap, hybrid trial designs have been proposed, which include dual aims focusing on *both* innovation effectiveness *and* implementation context, processes, and outcomes (Curran et al. 2012). This shift in trial design highlights the importance of context. When contexts of studies are fully reported, the scope and limits of transferability to other settings can be determined. Knowledge of context is necessary to adapt innovations, tailor strategies, and monitor and respond based on progress of implementation.

The Consolidated Framework for Implementation Research (CFIR) (Damschroder et al. 2009) is a determinant framework (Damschroder 2020, Nilsen 2020) that helps guide assessment of context. It provides terms and definitions for constructs that have the potential to significantly affect implementation outcomes. In recognition of the foundational role of context and the imperative to understand its interplay with implementation efforts, it is one of the most widely applied frameworks within implementation science. The CFIR is "meta-theoretical". It is designed to address widespread construct fallacies, where inconsistent naming and defining contributed to confusion and a proliferation of studies with insightful findings that were difficult to compare and advance theory to inform implementations. Thus, the CFIR provides much-needed clarity in naming and classification (Wacker 1998) by organizing, labelling, and describing the wide and complex array of constructs that contribute to the dynamic process of implementation.

Table 9.1 lists CFIR's five domains, with constructs listed within each. Detailed descriptions have been published (Damschroder et al. 2009) and are available on our technical website (www.cfirguide.org); the website also provides detailed guidance, templates, and tools to aid users in applying the CFIR, based on published methods (e.g., Damschroder et al. 2017).

Conceptualization of CFIR's domains was influenced by Pettigrew and Whipp (1992) who emphasized the essential interactive dimensions of content of the innovation, context (inner and outer settings), and the process of implementation more than 30 years ago. This basic structure is echoed by the Promoting Action on Research Implementation in Health Services (PARIHS) framework, which describes three domains including evidence, context, and facilitation (Kitson et al. 2008). The seminal work by Greenhalgh and colleagues provided

DOI: 10.4324/9781003109945-11

Table 9.1 Domains of CFIR

CFIR Domain	Description	Constructs
Innovation Characteristics	Aspects, including quality and content, of the "thing" that is being implemented	Intervention Source, Evidence Strength and Quality, Relative Advantage, Adaptability, Trialability, Complexity, and Design Quality and Packaging
Outer Setting	The economic, political, and social context within which an organization resides	Patient Needs and Resources, Cosmopolitanism, Peer Pressure, and External Policy and Incentives
Inner Setting	Structural, political, cultural, and organizational features within which the implementation process will proceed	Structural Characteristics, Networks and Communications, Culture, Implementation Climate (subconstructs include Tension for Change, Compatibility, Relative Priority, Organizational Incentives and Rewards, Goals and Feedback, Learning Climate), and Readiness for Implementation (subconstructs include Leadership Engagement, Available Resources, Access to Knowledge and Information)
Characteristics of Individuals	Concepts that potentially explain individual actors' ability to make the behavioural changes necessary to support implementation efforts	Knowledge and Beliefs about the Intervention, Self-efficacy, Individual Stage of Change, Individual Identification with Organization, and Other Personal Attributes
Process	Intentional activities that are executed to accomplish implementation goals	Planning, Engaging (subconstructs include Opinion Leaders, Formally appointed Internal Implementation Leaders, Champions, External Change Agents), Executing, and Reflecting and Evaluating

Source: Created by author

rich content on a wide array of constructs, drawn from nearly 500 sources across 13 scientific fields (Greenhalgh, Macfarlane, and Bate 2004).

CFIR's highly operationalized constructs simplify use and promote comparisons of findings across studies that use the CFIR. Multiple systematic reviews have tallied use of each construct across a diversity of settings (e.g., Kirk et al. (2015)) and synthesized shared barriers to implementation. This information is essential to tailor implementation strategies to address these barriers (Waltz et al. 2019) and guide adaptations for optimal fit within local settings. A published tool (available online at www.cfirguide.org) helps users select implementation strategies based on knowledge of CFIR barriers (Waltz et al. 2019).

Though the CFIR provides an ordered set of constructs, these must be applied, recognizing the layers of complexity that challenge implementation efforts: complexities related to multiple interacting components of innovations; complexities related to multiple levels involved, including teams within service units, within medical settings, within systems, within state, and national regulatory structures; complexities related to multi-component implementation strategies; complexities related to feedback loops and dynamic interplay between mediators and moderators; and complexities related to populations who may benefit from implementation efforts. The CFIR helps to navigate these complexities, but boundaries are fuzzy between inner and outer setting – sometimes researchers must consider evaluating multiple contexts. Future research must continue to develop theories and methods to embrace these complexities to continue to better inform implementation efforts.

The CFIR will continue to evolve as implementation science advances. We need to push beyond the boundary of active implementation and into *sustained* use of the innovation. Too often, implementation efforts are "spotlighted" with attention, priority, and resources which then die away, leaving efforts unfinished and a sub-optimized innovation that fails to achieve expected benefits.

The CFIR will include guidance for assessing sustainability of innovations, beyond the focus on initial implementation. Four evaluations of lifestyle behaviour change program implementations, all using the CFIR within the US Veterans Affairs system; reveal the need for strategies to build capacity in frontline teams to plan; engage key leaders and peers; and reflect, evaluate, and adjust based on progress (e.g., Damschroder et al. 2017). This is a pervasive need, mirrored in systematic reviews across a diversity of other healthcare settings (Means et al. 2020). Not only are these factors central for implementing innovations but they are also central to *sustained* use of the innovation. One example of a packaged strategy that was designed to address these CFIR-based findings is the Learn. Engage. Act. Process. (LEAP) Program. LEAP draws on quality improvement principles to build team-based skills through hands-on learning with a coach (Damschroder et al. 2021). A key goal of LEAP is to engage teams in continued optimization of innovations for long-term sustainment. The value of this type of program is further reinforced alignment with long-term transformation goals of many healthcare delivery systems for becoming learning organizations, high reliability organizations, and/or build cultures of total quality improvement, all of which identify similar barriers and the need for similar strategies.

Further research, beyond needs described above, includes addressing equity issues. Contextual structures are at the heart of addressing inequities and protecting against disparities in outcomes across populations. Consideration of equity issues needs to be "baked into" implementation frameworks including the CFIR.

A decade after CFIR's publication, its value has been demonstrated by wide adoption by users across multiple, diverse settings to help guide implementation efforts. Its coherence in terminology and language is a likely contributor. As evidenced by many published reviews, the CFIR has promoted comparison of results across studies, contributing to a rapidly growing knowledge base, and it has stimulated new theoretical developments through adaptations, measurement, and strategies to improve implementation outcomes.

References

Bastian, H., P. Glasziou, and I. Chalmers. 2010. "Seventy-five trials and eleven systematic reviews a day: How will we ever keep up?" *PLoS Medicine* 7 (9):e1000326.

Curran, G. M., M. Bauer, B. Mittman, J. M. Pyne, and C. Stetler. 2012. "Effectiveness-implementation hybrid designs: Combining elements of clinical effectiveness and implementation research to enhance public health impact." *Medical Care* 50 (3):217.

Damschroder, L. J. 2020. "Clarity out of chaos: Use of theory in implementation research." *Psychiatry Research* 283:112461.

Damschroder, L. J., D. C. Aron, R. E. Keith, S. R. Kirsh, J. A. Alexander, and J. C. Lowery. 2009. "Fostering implementation of health services research findings into practice: A consolidated framework for advancing implementation science." *Implementation Science* 4 (1):1–15.

Damschroder, L. J., C. M. Reardon, N. Sperber, C. H. Robinson, J. J. Fickel, and E. Z. Oddone. 2017. "Implementation evaluation of the telephone lifestyle coaching (TLC) program: Organizational factors associated with successful implementation." *Translational Behavioral Medicine* 7 (2):233–241.

Damschroder, L. J., N. R. Yankey, C. H. Robinson, M. B. Freitag, J. A. Burns, S. D. Raffa, and J. C. Lowery. 2021. "The LEAP program: Quality improvement training to address team readiness gaps identified by implementation science findings." *Journal of General Internal Medicine* 36 (2):288–295.

Green, L. W., and R. E. Glasgow. 2006. "Evaluating the relevance, generalization, and applicability of research: Issues in external validation and translation methodology." *Evaluation and the Health Professions* 29 (1):126–153.

Greenhalgh, T., R. Macfarlane, and P. Bate. 2004. "Conceptual model for considering the determinants of diffusion, dissemination, and implementation of innovations in health service delivery and organization." *The Milbank Quarterly* 82:581–582.

Kirk, M. A., C. Kelley, N. Yankey, S. A. Birken, B. Abadie, and L. Damschroder. 2015. "A systematic review of the use of the consolidated framework for implementation research." *Implementation Science* 11 (1):1–13.

Kitson, A. L., J. Rycroft-Malone, G. Harvey, B. McCormack, K. Seers, and A. Titchen. 2008. "Evaluating the successful implementation of evidence into practice using the PARiHS framework: Theoretical and practical challenges." *Implementation Science* 3 (1):1–12.

Means, A. R., C. G. Kemp, M.-C. Gwayi-Chore, S. Gimbel, C. Soi, K. Sherr, B. H. Wagenaar, J. N. Wasserheit, and B. J. Weiner. 2020. "Evaluating and optimizing the consolidated framework for implementation research (CFIR) for use in low-and middle-income countries: A systematic review." *Implementation Science* 15 (1):1–19.

Nilsen, P. 2020. "Making sense of implementation theories, models, and frameworks." In *Implementation Science 3.0*, 53–79. Cham: Springer.

Pettigrew, A., and R. Whipp. 1992. "Managing change and corporate performance." In *European Industrial Restructuring in the 1990s*, 227–265. New York: Springer.

Wacker, J. G. 1998. "A definition of theory: Research guidelines for different theory-building research methods in operations management." *Journal of Operations Management* 16 (4):361–385.

Waltz, T. J., B. J. Powell, M. E. Fernández, B. Abadie, and L. J. Damschroder. 2019. "Choosing implementation strategies to address contextual barriers: Diversity in recommendations and future directions." *Implementation Science* 14 (1):1–15.

10 The Theoretical Domains Framework

Fabiana Lorencatto

Implementation of anything different or new always requires someone to do something differently. This can involve adopting entirely new practices (e.g., uptake of new diagnostic tests), doing more of existing practices (e.g., increasing referral rates), doing less of existing practices (e.g., reducing inappropriate use of antibiotics), or discontinuing a practice altogether (e.g., de-implementation of low value care) (Patey et al. 2018). Such actions are forms of human behaviour. Implementation therefore requires behaviour change, often in individual and collective behaviours as well as at organization, service, and system levels (Francis, O'Connor, and Curran 2012, Ferlie and Shortell 2001).

Designing interventions to change behaviour and improve implementation processes first requires understanding the influences on current and desired behaviours in the context in which they occur (Michie, Atkins, and West 2014). This can be facilitated through the application of evidence-based theories and frameworks from behavioural science, which provide explicit statements regarding processes hypothesized to regulate behaviour, and can thus be used to explain and predict human behaviours (Atkins et al. 2017). The use of a theory enables drawing from, and contributing to, the wider literature and evidence base on what influences behaviour and practice change. While the benefits of theory are widely recognized (Michie and Prestwich 2010), the reality of applying theory in practice is often far from straightforward. There is a plethora of behaviour change theories. A systematic review of behaviour change theories across disciplines identified 83 theories (Davis et al. 2015). There is limited guidance for selecting among the numerous potentially relevant, yet sometimes overlapping, theories. It is perhaps unsurprising that theory has consequently been deemed "mystifying" to non-specialists (Davidoff et al. 2015). This is a challenge relevant to the multidisciplinary implementation research community and is reflected in the findings from systematic reviews of implementation interventions which have identified limited application of theory to guide intervention design (Davies, Walker, and Grimshaw 2010).

The Theoretical Domains Framework (TDF) was developed in collaboration by behavioural and implementation researchers in recognition of these issues and in an effort to render theory more accessible (Michie et al. 2005). The TDF aims to provide an integrated theoretical framework and was developed by extracting and synthesizing 128 constructs from 33 multidisciplinary behaviour change theories. Similar constructs were grouped into theoretical domains, which represent the potential mediators of behaviour change. For instance, the constructs "social support", "group norms", "social pressure", and "social comparison" were synthesized into the domain *Social Influences*, representing the interpersonal processes that can cause individuals to change their thoughts, feelings, or behaviours (Cane, O'Connor, and Michie 2012). The first version of the TDF was published in 2005 and included 12 domains (Michie et al. 2005). An updated version was published in 2012 following an expert validation exercise which resulted in a revised structure of 14 domains (Table 10.1) (Cane,

DOI: 10.4324/9781003109945-12

Table 10.1 The Theoretical Domains Framework (V2) (Cane, O'Connor, and Michie 2012) with definitions, component constructs, and example survey items to investigate each domain[1] [*Example interview items are published in Michie et al. 2005.*]

Domain (definition)	Constructs	Example Survey Items
Knowledge (An awareness of the existence of something)	Knowledge (including knowledge of condition/scientific rationale) Procedural knowledge Knowledge of task environment	I am familiar with the content and objectives of [innovation/guideline]
Skills (An ability or proficiency acquired through practice)	Skills Skills development Competence Ability Interpersonal skills Practice Skill assessment	I have been trained how to [A] in [C, T] with [Ta]*
Beliefs about capabilities (Acceptance of the truth, reality, or validity about an ability, talent, or facility that a person can put to constructive use)	Self-confidence Perceived competence Self-efficacy Perceived behavioural control Beliefs Self-esteem Empowerment Professional confidence	I am confident that if I wanted, I could [A] in [C, T] with [Ta]
Beliefs about consequences (Acceptance of the truth, reality, or validity about outcomes of a behaviour in a given situation)	Beliefs Outcome expectancies Characteristics of outcome expectancies Anticipated regret Consequents	If I [A] in [C, T] with [Ta], it will benefit public health
Optimism (The confidence that things will happen for the best or that desired goals will be attained)	Optimism Pessimism Unrealistic optimism Identity	With regard to [A] in [C, time] with [Ta], I'm always optimistic about the future
Intentions (A conscious decision to perform a behaviour or a resolve to act in a certain way)	Stability of intentions Stages of change model Transtheoretical model and stages of change	I will definitely [A] in [C] with [Ta] in the next [T]
Goals (Mental representations of outcomes or end states that an individual wants to achieve)	Goals (distal/proximal) Goal priority Goal/target setting Goals (autonomous/controlled) Action planning Implementation intention	I have a clear plan for how often I will [A] in [C, T] with [Ta]**
Reinforcement (Increasing the probability of a response by arranging a dependent relationship, or contingency, between the response and a given stimulus)	Rewards (proximal/distal, valued/not valued, probable/improbable) Incentives Punishment Consequents Reinforcement Contingencies Sanctions	Whenever I [A] in [C, T] with [Ta], I get recognition from professionals who are important to me**

(Continued)

Table 10.1 (Continued)

Domain (definition)	Constructs	Example Survey Items
Memory, Attention, Decision-Making (The ability to retain information, focus selectively on aspects of the environment, and choose between two or more alternatives)	Memory Attention Attention control Decision-making Cognitive overload/tiredness	When concentrating on [A] in [C, T] with [Ta], I can focus my attention so that I become unaware of what's going on around me
Emotions (A complex reaction pattern, involving experiential, behavioural, and physiological elements, by which the individual attempts to deal with a personally significant matter or event)	Fear Anxiety Affect Stress Depression Positive/negative affect Burnout	Have you recently, during the past two weeks, been feeling unhappy and depressed?
Social Professional Role/Identity (A coherent set of behaviours and displayed personal qualities of an individual in a social or work setting)	Professional identity Professional role Social identity Identity Professional boundaries Professional confidence Group identity Leadership Organizational commitment	It is my responsibility as a [profession] to [A] in [C, T] with [Ta]
Environmental Context and Resources (Any circumstance of a person's situation or environment that discourages or encourages the development of skills and abilities, independence, social competence, and adaptive behaviour)	Environmental stressors Resources/material resources Organizational culture/climate Salient events/critical incidents Person × environment interaction Barriers and facilitators	Within the sociopolitical context, there is sufficient financial support (e.g., from local authorities, insurance companies, the government) for [innovation/guideline]
Social Influences (Those interpersonal processes that can cause individuals to change their thoughts, feelings, or behaviours)	Social pressure Social norms Group conformity Social comparisons Group norms Social support Power Intergroup conflict Alienation Group identity Modelling	Most people whose opinion I value would approve me of [A] in [C, T] with [Ta]

Domain *(definition)*	Constructs	Example Survey Items
Behavioural Regulation (Anything aimed at managing or changing objectively observed or measured actions)	Self-monitoring Breaking habit Action planning	I keep track of my overall progress towards [A] in [C, T] with [Ta]**

Source: Adapted from Atkins et al. (2017)

1   Rated on 5-point Likert-type scales from 1 Strongly Disagree → 5 Strongly agree. Example survey items from Huijg et al. (2014)
*   *Note.* [A], action (behaviour); [C], context (where); [T], time (when); [Ta], target (to/with whom)
** Discriminant content validity not demonstrated for items measuring these domains.

O'Connor, and Michie 2012). The domains represent factors influencing behaviour at the individual (e.g., knowledge, intention, emotions, beliefs about consequences), sociocultural (e.g., social influences, professional role, identity), and environmental (e.g., environmental context, resources) levels. It is important to note that the TDF, by definition, is not a theory as it does not specify testable relationships between the domains; rather, within the array of theoretical approaches in implementation science, the TDF is classed as a determinant framework (Nilsen 2015).

The TDF has primarily been used to conduct a "behavioural diagnosis", to identify barriers and enablers to changing behaviours and improving implementation. A detailed guide for collecting and analysing data using the TDF has been published (Atkins et al. 2017). The TDF is commonly used in semi-structured qualitative interview studies, whereby the interview topic guide questions are structured around the 14 domains to explore the role each domain plays in facilitating or hindering implementation in the context of interest. Example TDF-based interview questions for each domain have been published (Michie et al. 2005), and many papers reporting the findings of TDF-based interviews also publish interview topic guides as supplementary files (e.g., Patey et al. 2012). The TDF is subsequently applied during analysis as a coding framework following a combined deductive framework and inductive thematic analysis approach (Atkins et al. 2017). A validated questionnaire to measure TDF-based determinants of healthcare professionals' implementation behaviours has also been developed (Huijg et al. 2014). This can be applied to investigate barriers and enablers in larger samples and to statistically examine associations between domains and implementation outcomes. Table 10.1 includes sample survey questions for each domain (Huijg et al. 2014). The TDF has also been applied in systematic reviews, as a framework for synthesizing published evidence on barriers and enablers to behaviours such as increasing attendance for diabetic retinopathy screening (Graham-Rowe et al. 2018) and implementation of pregnancy weight management guidelines (Heslehurst et al. 2014).

References

Atkins, L., J. Francis, R. Islam, D. O'Connor, A. Patey, N. Ivers, R. Foy, E. M. Duncan, H. Colquhoun, and J. M. Grimshaw. 2017. "A guide to using the Theoretical Domains Framework of behaviour change to investigate implementation problems." *Implementation Science* 12 (1):77.

Cane, J., D. O'Connor, and S. Michie. 2012. "Validation of the theoretical domains framework for use in behaviour change and implementation research." *Implementation Science* 7 (1):37.

Davidoff, F., M. Dixon-Woods, L. Leviton, and S. Michie. 2015. "Demystifying theory and its use in improvement." *BMJ Quality & Safety* 24 (3):228–238.

Davies, P., A. E. Walker, and J. M. Grimshaw. 2010. "A systematic review of the use of theory in the design of guideline dissemination and implementation strategies and interpretation of the results of rigorous evaluations." *Implementation Science* 5 (1):14.

Davis, R., R. Campbell, Z. Hildon, L. Hobbs, and S. Michie. 2015. "Theories of behaviour and behaviour change across the social and behavioural sciences: A scoping review." *Health Psychology Review* 9 (3):323–344.

Ferlie, E. B., and S. M. Shortell. 2001. "Improving the quality of health care in the United Kingdom and the United States: A framework for change." *The Milbank Quarterly* 79 (2):281–315.

Francis, J. J., D. O'Connor, and J. Curran. 2012. "Theories of behaviour change synthesised into a set of theoretical groupings: Introducing a thematic series on the theoretical domains framework." *Implementation Science* 7 (1):35.

Graham-Rowe, E., F. Lorencatto, J. Lawrenson, J. Burr, J. Grimshaw, N. Ivers, J. Presseau, L. Vale, T. Peto, and C. Bunce. 2018. "Barriers to and enablers of diabetic retinopathy screening attendance: A systematic review of published and grey literature." *Diabetic Medicine* 35 (10):1308–1319.

Heslehurst, N., J. Newham, G. Maniatopoulos, C. Fleetwood, S. Robalino, and J. Rankin. 2014. "Implementation of pregnancy weight management and obesity guidelines: A meta-synthesis of healthcare professionals' barriers and facilitators using the Theoretical Domains Framework." *Obesity Reviews* 15 (6):462–486.

Huijg, J. M., W. A. Gebhardt, M. R. Crone, E. Dusseldorp, and J. Presseau. 2014. "Discriminant content validity of a theoretical domains framework questionnaire for use in implementation research." *Implementation Science* 9 (1):11.

Michie, S., L. Atkins, and R. West. 2014. "The behaviour change wheel." In *A Guide to Designing Interventions*. 1st ed., 1003–1010. Great Britain: Silverback Publishing.

Michie, S., M. Johnston, C. Abraham, R. Lawton, D. Parker, and A. Walker. 2005. "Making psychological theory useful for implementing evidence based practice: A consensus approach." *BMJ Quality & Safety* 14 (1):26–33.

Michie, S., and A. Prestwich. 2010. "Are interventions theory-based? Development of a theory coding scheme." *Health Psychology* 29 (1):1.

Nilsen, P. 2015. "Making sense of implementation theories, models and frameworks." *Implementation Science* 10 (1):53. doi: 10.1186/s13012-015-0242-0.

Patey, A. M., C. S. Hurt, J. M. Grimshaw, and J. J. Francis. 2018. "Changing behaviour 'more or less' – do theories of behaviour inform strategies for implementation and de-implementation? A critical interpretive synthesis." *Implementation Science* 13 (1):134.

Patey, A. M., R. Islam, J. J. Francis, G. L. Bryson, and J. M. Grimshaw. 2012. "Anesthesiologists' and surgeons' perceptions about routine pre-operative testing in low-risk patients: Application of the Theoretical Domains Framework (TDF) to identify factors that influence physicians' decisions to order pre-operative tests." *Implementation Science* 7 (1):52.

11 Organization theory for implementation science

Sarah A. Birken and Emily R. Haines

Nuanced explanations of how organizations' external environments influence the implementation of evidence-based interventions (EBIs) are generally lacking in implementation research (Damschroder et al. 2009, Powell et al. 2016, Raghavan, Bright, and Shadoin 2008, Raghavan et al. 2007). Implementation researchers may benefit from organization theories, which offer a host of existing, highly relevant, and heretofore largely untapped explanations of the dynamic interactions between organizations and their environments (Birken et al. 2017). Organization theories, which have roots in management and sociology (Daft 2015), can describe, explain, and predict the complex relationships between organizations and features of their external context. For example, they can shed light on the role of legislation, institutions, funding fluctuations, contracting and procurement processes, and workforce dynamics in implementation. Organization theories have been used to explain phenomena in a variety of fields, including human services, education, and health services research (Bonner, Koch, and Langmeyer 2004, Hunter 2006, Payne and Leiter 2013). Organizational sociologists and others urging researchers studying implementation in healthcare organizations to take advantage of organization theory and the application of organization theory in implementation research remain scant. There are a few notable exceptions (Novotná, Dobbins, and Henderson 2012, Shearer, Dion, and Lavis 2014, Shortell 2016, Borghi et al. 2013, Clauser et al. 2009). For example, studies have used organization theory to help explain the role of an organization's external environment in the translation of research into practice (Novotná, Dobbins, and Henderson 2012) and the differential sustainment of certain intervention components versus others (Clauser et al. 2009). Studies have used transaction cost economics to explain the creation of organizational networks (Shearer, Dion, and Lavis 2014), the evaluation of accountable care organization (Shortell 2016), and why some organizations' pay-for-performance systems inflate performance scores to increase payment (Borghi et al. 2013).

We propose that implementation researchers apply organization theories to advance rigorous and theoretically grounded studies of the interplay between external context and implementation (Birken et al. 2017). To exemplify, we applied several organization theories to discuss the implementation of SafeCare (Lutzker and Chaffin 2012), a child maltreatment prevention program that has been implemented in 23 US states, largely by state- and county-level child welfare agencies (Box 11.1). Rather than adopting models for the use of SafeCare "in-house", many child welfare agencies contract with private community-based organizations to implement SafeCare (Collins-Camargo, McBeath, and Ensign 2011). Further, some of these contracted, community-based organizations have formed interagency collaborative teams to administer SafeCare (Chaffin et al. 2016). The complex organizational relationships inherent to this public–private child welfare system offer a useful example of how organizational theories can further our understanding of the influence of the external environment on SafeCare implementation.

DOI: 10.4324/9781003109945-13

Box 11.1   SafeCare® description (Lutzker and Chaffin 2012)

Developed in 1979, SafeCare® is an evidence-based behavioural parent training model that targets the proximal parenting behaviours that lead to the neglect and abuse of children 0 to 5 years old with at-risk parents (i.e., typically those involved in child welfare or intensive prevention settings). Trained SafeCare providers deliver in-home parent training across three core content areas: 1) child health, 2) home safety, and 3) parent–child interactions. This is typically done through 18 weekly one-hour sessions. Providers are usually professionals with bachelors or masters degrees who are employed by an agency that contracts with a state or county government to deliver child welfare services. SafeCare has been implemented in a range of service settings (e.g., child welfare, education) in 30 US states, 6 of which executed statewide or regional rollouts. Seven other countries (Belarus, Spain, Israel, England, Australia, Kenya, and Canada) have also implemented SafeCare. Within US child welfare settings, SafeCare may be implemented by public child welfare agencies, contracted private community-based organizations, or some combination of both (Collins-Camargo, McBeath, and Ensign 2011, McBeath et al. 2014).

Source: Adapted from Birken et al. (2017)

In Table 11.1, we use organizational theories to help explain 1) why public child welfare agencies increasingly contract with community-based organizations to administer EBIs, 2) why SafeCare is often the EBI of choice, and 3) the role of interagency collaborative teams in addressing local community-based organizations' needs and resource constraints, thereby facilitating SafeCare implementation.

Table 11.1 Organization theory descriptions and applications to SafeCare® (Lutzker and Chaffin 2012)

Theory	Main Propositions	Applications to SafeCare
Transaction cost economics	• Transaction costs influence an organization's decision on whether to contract with another organization to implement an evidence-based intervention (EBI). • Decreases in transaction frequency will increase the likelihood that organizations contract with other organizations to implement an EBI. • Familiarity between organizations reduces the costs and uncertainty associated with contracting.	Adoption: • Cost likely influenced child welfare agencies' decision to contract with community-based organizations to administer EBIs rather than administering EBIs internally. • The cost of EBI administration depends on the frequency of collaboration between community-based organizations and child welfare agencies and the familiarity of child welfare agencies with community-based organizations.

Theory	*Main Propositions*	*Applications to SafeCare*
Institutional theory	• Organizations implement EBIs that are regarded as legitimate by institutions within their environment. • Organizations adopt some EBIs because of strong pressure to adhere to rules, mandates, and regulations. • Organizations mimic the structures and behaviours of other successful organizations in their environment (e.g., the adoption of certain EBIs). • Organizations adopt EBIs that align with professional norms.	Adoption: • Child welfare agencies' decision to adopt SafeCare may have been influenced by pressure from policymakers to implement EBIs, perceptions of SafeCare as the norm, and advocacy from child welfare professional communities for SafeCare adoption. Sustainment: • Efforts to maintain SafeCare contracts may have put pressure on community-based organizations to sustain SafeCare by establishing rules, regulations, and mandates set forth in contracts. • The contracts generated support for SafeCare, resulting in normative pressure on community-based organizations to sustain SafeCare.
Contingency theories	• Organizations' design decisions are contingent upon the organization's internal and external contexts. • The compatibility of an EBI with an organization's internal context influences EBI implementation. • EBI implementation is influenced by the extent to which organizations' can adapt to their external context.	Implementation: • The use of interagency collaborative teams allowed child welfare systems to respond to features of external contexts (e.g., local client needs). • Larger, governmental organizations had less flexibility in implementing SafeCare, demonstrating the role of internal context in implementation.
Resource dependency theory	• Organizations' design decisions are influenced by the extent to which they depend on other organizations, their ability to maintain autonomy, and their relationships with other organizations. • Organizations form relationships with other organizations to obtain and maintain autonomy and resources.	Implementation: • Community-based organizations depended on the funding organizations and the expertise of SafeCare developers, reducing their autonomy and power. • Community-based organizations often negotiated the balance of autonomy and dependence on other organizations by creating interagency collaborative teams, which decreased the resources required for individual community-based organizations to implement SafeCare. Sustainment: • Policymakers could have set aside funds for contracts that would have supported SafeCare's sustainment. • Train-the-trainer models decreased community-based organizations' reliance on SafeCare developers, allowing their staff to sustain the practice autonomously.

Source: Adapted from Birken et al. (2017)

References

Birken, S. A., A. C. Bunger, B. J. Powell, K. Turner, A. S. Clary, S. L. Klaman, Y. Yu, D. J. Whitaker, S. R. Self, and W. L. Rostad. 2017. "Organizational theory for dissemination and implementation research." *Implementation Science* 12 (1):1–15.

Bonner, M., T. Koch, and D. Langmeyer. 2004. "Organizational theory applied to school reform: A critical analysis." *School Psychology International* 25 (4):455–471.

Borghi, J., I. Mayumana, I. Mashasi, P. Binyaruka, E. Patouillard, I. Njau, O. Maestad, S. Abdulla, and M. Mamdani. 2013. "Protocol for the evaluation of a pay for performance programme in Pwani region in Tanzania: A controlled before and after study." *Implementation Science* 8 (1):1–12.

Chaffin, M., D. Hecht, G. Aarons, D. Fettes, M. Hurlburt, and K. Ledesma. 2016. "EBT fidelity trajectories across training cohorts using the interagency collaborative team strategy." *Administration and Policy in Mental Health and Mental Health Services Research* 43 (2):144–156.

Clauser, S. B., M. R. Johnson, D. M. O'Brien, J. M. Beveridge, M. L. Fennell, and A. D. Kaluzny. 2009. "Improving clinical research and cancer care delivery in community settings: Evaluating the NCI community cancer centers program." *Implementation Science* 4 (1):1–11.

Collins-Camargo, C., B. McBeath, and K. Ensign. 2011. "Privatization and performance-based contracting in child welfare: Recent trends and implications for social service administrators." *Administration in Social Work* 35 (5):494–516.

Daft, R. L. 2015. *Organization Theory & Design*. Boston, MA: Cengage learning.

Damschroder, L. J., D. C. Aron, R. E. Keith, S. R. Kirsh, J. A. Alexander, and J. C. Lowery. 2009. "Fostering implementation of health services research findings into practice: A consolidated framework for advancing implementation science." *Implementation Science* 4 (1):1–15.

Hunter, D. E. 2006. "Using a theory of change approach to build organizational strength, capacity and sustainability with not-for-profit organizations in the human services sector." *Evaluation and Program Planning* 29 (2):193–200.

Lutzker, J. R., and M. Chaffin. 2012. "Safecare®: An evidence-based constantly dynamic model to prevent child maltreatment." *World Perspectives on Child Abuse*:93–96.

McBeath, B., C. Collins-Camargo, E. Chuang, R. Wells, A. C. Bunger, and M. P. Jolles. 2014. "New directions for research on the organizational and institutional context of child welfare agencies: Introduction to the symposium on 'The Organizational and Managerial Context of Private Child Welfare Agencies'." *Children and Youth Services Review* 38:83–92.

Novotná, G., M. Dobbins, and J. Henderson. 2012. "Institutionalization of evidence-informed practices in healthcare settings." *Implementation Science* 7 (1):1–8.

Payne, J., and J. Leiter. 2013. "Structuring agency: Examining healthcare management in the USA and Australia using organizational theory." *Journal of Health Organization and Management* 27 (1):106–126.

Powell, B. J., R. S. Beidas, R. M. Rubin, R. E. Stewart, C. B. Wolk, S. L. Matlin, S. Weaver, M. O. Hurford, A. C. Evans, and T. R. Hadley. 2016. "Applying the policy ecology framework to Philadelphia's behavioral health transformation efforts." *Administration and Policy in Mental Health and Mental Health Services Research* 43 (6):909–926.

Raghavan, R., C. L. Bright, and A. L. Shadoin. 2008. "Toward a policy ecology of implementation of evidence-based practices in public mental health settings." *Implementation Science* 3 (1):1–9.

Raghavan, R., M. Inkelas, T. Franke, and N. Halfon. 2007. "Administrative barriers to the adoption of high-quality mental health services for children in foster care: A national study." *Administration and Policy in Mental Health and Mental Health Services Research* 34 (3):191–201.

Shearer, J. C., M. Dion, and J. N. Lavis. 2014. "Exchanging and using research evidence in health policy networks: A statistical network analysis." *Implementation Science* 9 (1):1–12.

Shortell, S. M. 2016. "Applying organization theory to understanding the adoption and implementation of accountable care organizations: Commentary." *Medical Care Research and Review* 73 (6):694–702.

12 Exploration, Preparation, Implementation, Sustainment (EPIS) framework

Joanna C. Moullin and Gregory A. Aarons

The Exploration, Preparation, Implementation, Sustainment (EPIS) framework is a multiphasic, multilevel implementation framework developed to guide implementation research and practice (Figure 12.1) (Aarons, Hurlburt, and Horwitz 2011, Moullin et al. 2019). EPIS may be used to understand the implementation process (phases), identify determinants (implementation factors) and mechanisms (mediators and moderators) or implementation outcomes, and to guide evaluation.

Implementation phases

EPIS stages the implementation process in four phases: Exploration, Preparation, Implementation, and Sustainment. As shown in Figure 12.1, the implementation process is illustrated as a circle around the outside of the figure, with double arrows indicating the recursive or bidirectional and iterative nature of implementation. Furthermore, the phases are not isolated and may have overlapping processes.

The exploration phase is the beginning of an implementation process, in which stakeholders consider the health and contextual needs, the problem or gap they are trying to solve and decide which innovations may be best suited to the purpose or is appropriate to adopt. Exploration also considers the context in which innovations are to be implemented and the need to adapt outer system or inner organizational context to support implementation and sustainment. The exploration process should include stakeholders who will be directly involved in the innovation's implementation and delivery or use (e.g., providers, consumers, administrators, intermediaries) and those with oversight or influence on the providing organizations (e.g., supervisors/managers, executives, policymakers, funding bodies).

Following a decision to adopt an innovation, the preparation phase begins. With ongoing stakeholder collaboration, implementation strategies are planned, and through this process, ownership and buy-in to the implementation process are fostered. Preparation may involve developing a program logic that describes the inputs, activities, outputs, and outcomes. In addition, an initial assessment of implementation determinants and mechanisms may be conducted to develop hypothesized change mechanisms and to assist in the selection and tailoring of implementation strategies.

The Implementation phase occurs when providers are being trained and are beginning to use the innovation. EPIS has an explicit focus on promoting the "fit" between the innovation and the context in which implementation occurs, and as such, throughout the implementation phase, adaptation of the innovation and implementation strategies ensue (von Thiele Schwarz, Aarons, and Hasson 2019).

DOI: 10.4324/9781003109945-14

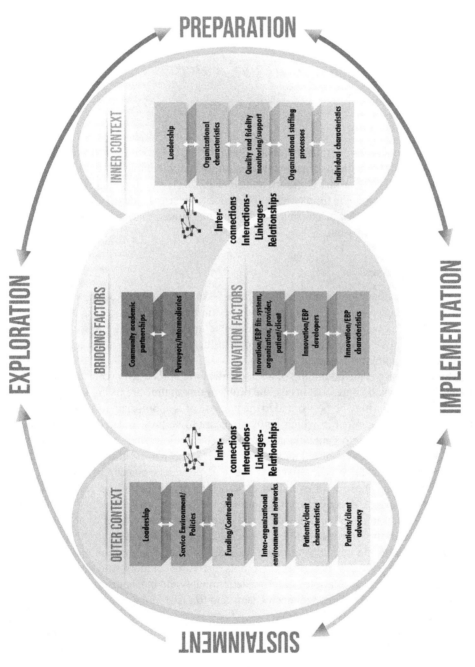

Figure 12.1 Exploration, Preparation, Implementation, Sustainment (EPIS) framework including phases, outer/inner context, bridging factors, and innovation factors

Source: Originally published in Moullin et al. 2019, Aarons, Hurlburt, and Horwitz 2011

In the Sustainment phase, the innovation is being delivered, routinized, or institutionalized; however, ongoing monitoring, evaluation, adaptation, and improvement of both the setting and the innovation should receive continued attention. The process should encourage ongoing use that continues through changing circumstances, through maintenance of capacity support and benefits, and through necessary adaptation (Chambers, Glasgow, and Stange 2013).

Implementation determinants and mechanisms

The EPIS framework constructs consist of key implementation factors associated with the outer system context, the inner organizational context, bridging factors (i.e., bidirectional influences between outer and inner contexts), and the innovation being implemented. Implementation factors may act as either barriers or facilitators that affect implementation and are likely to be determinants or mechanisms of the implementation process. Their weight and nature may vary across the implementation phase. As such, implementation factors should ideally be assessed at multiple time points for longitudinal evaluations but also to select implementation strategies and develop implementation plans and then to adapt these plans throughout the implementation process. Implementation factors are important in order to specify likely determinants (factors that impact implementation outcomes) and to explain mechanisms that can mediate or moderate effects of determinants on implementation outcomes.

Outer context factors are those external to implementing organizations. These include the broader service (e.g., health system, education system), political, funding and community influences, as well as the characteristics of the target of the innovation (e.g., patients, clients, consumers).

Inner context factors are those that are qualities and features of the organization(s) implementing the innovation, including the characteristics of the employees. Within an organization multiple layers manifest, from board directors and executives to managers, supervisors, team leaders, direct service providers, and administrators.

Bridging factors connect the outer and inner contexts. They may be relational ties (e.g., partnerships or an individual), formal arrangements (e.g., a funding contract or incentive), or processes (e.g., accreditation or data sharing). Identifying and specifying bridging factors is a distinctive priority of EPIS that allows greater understanding of the mechanisms of how an implementation effort was successful or unsuccessful.

Innovation factors relate to the characteristics of the innovation, its fit with the inner context, and the ways in which innovation developers consider fit with outer and inner contexts. We recommend that developers take the approach of "designing for dissemination" and implementation as recommended by Brownson and colleagues (2013).

Linkages

In addition to bridging factors, EPIS conveys the importance of inter-connections, interactions, linkages, and relationships within contextual levels. It is often the case that networks and relationships across the outer context (e.g., between different governmental departments or organizations) or within the inner context (e.g., across levels within an organization) are enablers of implementation. Furthermore, a principal objective of the EPIS framework is to facilitate examination and promotion of the "fit" between an innovation and the settings in which implementation occurs.

Implementation strategies

EPIS does not include implementation strategies, but rather it is a framework that is used to guide the selection of implementation strategies, development of implementation plans, and creation of program logics.

Tailored implementation strategies should employ identified facilitators and address identified barriers at each phase to advance implementation. Furthermore, as the EPIS framework spans multiple levels of implementation (system, community, organization, individual), EPIS encourages a selection of implementation strategies for a given level and across levels.

Implementation evaluation

EPIS enables qualitative (e.g., interviews, focus groups, and document analysis), quantitative (e.g., surveys), and mixed method assessment of the implementation process and implementation factors. Implementation factors may act as either mediators or moderators and may be tested longitudinally for both formative and summative evaluations. Comprehensive implementation evaluation allows for testing hypotheses, studying implementation strategies and their mechanisms, and subsequently cultivating generalizable implementation evidence. The EPIS website (www.episframework.com) provides tools for both qualitative assessment and quantitative assessment.

Movement through EPIS phases may be evaluated as a process outcome. For example, when an organization is aware of, or shows interest in, using an evidence-based practice (EBP), they enter the Exploration phase. Subsequently, if they make the decision to adopt the EBP, then they would move into the Preparation phase. First use of the EBP would signify transition into the Implementation phase. Lastly, continued use over a designated period of time may be defined as being in the Sustainment phase. For each phase a number of other measures may be included such as the rate of movement through the stages or the duration in the stages (Becan et al. 2018). In addition, more detailed and comprehensive measures may be used to evaluate the implementation factors associated with particular phases.

Application of EPIS framework

As illustrated in this essay, and explored in detail in a systematic review of the use of the EPIS framework (Moullin et al. 2020), EPIS has broad and wide-reaching applicability and utility. Central features and benefits of applying EPIS include the following:

- The phases of EPIS may be used to engage stakeholders (policy, provider, community, purveyors, intervention developers, etc.) in understanding the implementation process.
- Bridging factors emphasize the importance of collaboration from the beginning of the implementation process.
- Assessment of an implementation context using EPIS aids the identification and specification of implementation factors that can then be incorporated into an implementation plan. As such, EPIS may be used to develop research and practice-based projects.
- EPIS acknowledges and encourages the dynamic nature of implementation and the need for adaptation to fit an innovation to a context.
- EPIS allows for measurement of implementation process. In addition, definitions for qualitative work and measures for quantitative work are provided on the EPIS website.
- EPIS is a living theory that is constantly studied, tested, revised, and improved.

References

Aarons, G. A., M. Hurlburt, and S. M. Horwitz. 2011. "Advancing a conceptual model of evidence-based practice implementation in public service sectors." *Administration and Policy in Mental Health and Mental Health Services Research* 38 (1):4–23.

Becan, J. E., J. P. Bartkowski, D. K. Knight, T. R. Wiley, R. DiClemente, L. Ducharme, W. N. Welsh, D. Bowser, K. McCollister, and M. Hiller. 2018. "A model for rigorously applying the Exploration, Preparation, Implementation, Sustainment (EPIS) framework in the design and measurement of a large scale collaborative multi-site study." *Health and Justice* 6 (1):9.

Brownson, R. C., J. A. Jacobs, R. G. Tabak, C. M. Hoehner, and K. A. Stamatakis. 2013. "Designing for dissemination among public health researchers: Findings from a national survey in the United States." *American Journal of Public Health* 103 (9):1693–1699.

Chambers, D. A., R. E. Glasgow, and K. C. Stange. 2013. "The dynamic sustainability framework: Addressing the paradox of sustainment amid ongoing change." *Implementation Science* 8 (1):1–11.

Moullin, J. C., K. S. Dickson, N. A. Stadnick, B. Albers, P. Nilsen, S. Broder-Fingert, B. Mukasa, and G. A. Aarons. 2020. "Ten recommendations for using implementation frameworks in research and practice." *Implementation Science Communications* 1:1–12.

Moullin, J. C., K. S. Dickson, N. A. Stadnick, B. Rabin, and G. A. Aarons. 2019. "Systematic review of the Exploration, Preparation, Implementation, Sustainment (EPIS) framework." *Implementation Science* 14 (1):1–16.

von Thiele Schwarz, U., G. A. Aarons, and H. Hasson. 2019. "The Value Equation: Three complementary propositions for reconciling fidelity and adaptation in evidence-based practice implementation." *BMC Health Services Research* 19 (1):1–10.

13 Implementation science as process ecology

Normalization Process Theory

Carl May

Normalization Process Theory (NPT) helps us to understand how new ways of organizing and delivering healthcare become routinely embedded – or not – in everyday practice (May 2006, 2013, May and Finch 2009, May, Johnson, and Finch 2016). It has important applied relevance in understanding and evaluating the implementation of innovations and interventions across a range of settings. Implementation processes are characterized by the translation of the strategic intentions of one group of actors into the everyday practices of others. In healthcare, these processes usually come about as "deliberately initiated attempts to introduce new, or modify existing, ways of delivering and organising care in practice. Implementation processes of this kind are normally institutionally sanctioned; formally defined; consciously planned; and intended to lead to some improvement in outcome" (May et al. 2007).

They are brought about through collective action and collaborative work. Such processes are very common, and they comprise three phenomena of interest. These are *implementation:* the social organization of work to bring an innovation into use; *embedding:* the extent to which an innovation becomes routinely incorporated in everyday work; and *integration:* the processes by which an embedded innovation is sustained by its users (May et al. 2009). The theory helps us to understand these phenomena by identifying, characterizing, and explaining the core components of implementation processes. It focuses on what people actually *do* – rather than on what their beliefs or intentions are – as they engage in the implementation, embedding, and integration of innovations in the organization and delivery of care. Here it draws attention to

> the work that actors do as they engage with some ensemble of activities (that may include new or changed ways of thinking, acting, and organising) and . . . becomes routinely embedded in the matrices of already existing, socially patterned, knowledge and practice.
>
> (May and Finch 2009, 540)

To do this, NPT deals with work that takes place in relation to objects, actors, and contexts. *Objects* are the ensembles of practices and things – for example, the components of a complex intervention – that are enacted by participants in implementation processes. NPT specifies four generative mechanisms that characterize the capabilities that stem from these objects (May, Finch, and Rapley 2020, 149):

1 *Interactional workability*: capabilities that *enable* participants in an implementation process to operationalize intervention components in practice.

DOI: 10.4324/9781003109945-15

2   *Skill-set workability*: capabilities that *equip* participants in an intervention process to perform the work associated with intervention components and which are distributed in a division of labour.

3   *Relational integration*: capabilities that *promote* knowledge about intervention components within networks of participants in an implementation process and which mediate trust and confidence.

4   *Contextual integration*: capabilities that *support* intervention components through resource allocation and mobilization and that link them to their contexts of action.

In NPT, we understand objects in terms of the qualities that determine their workability and integration in practice. These are qualities of objects in use. Their users are *actors*, and these are the people implicated in an implementation process. Their agency is expressed when they make things happen. NPT specifies emergent *contributions* to collective action and collaborative work through a further set of generative mechanisms through which people not only enact innovations but also make their activities meaningful and build commitments to them (May, Finch, and Rapley 2020, 149–150):

1   *Coherence-building* that makes interventions and their components *meaningful*: participants contribute to enacting intervention components by working to make sense of its possibilities within their field of agency. They work to understand how intervention components are different from other practices, and they work to make them a coherent proposition for action.

2   *Cognitive Participation* that forms *commitment* around an intervention and its components: participants contribute to enacting intervention components through work that establishes its legitimacy and that enrols themselves and others into an implementation process. This work frames how participants become members of a specific community of practice.

3   *Collective Action* through which *effort* is invested in an intervention and its components: participants mobilize skills and resources and collaboratively make a complex intervention workable. This work frames how participants realize and perform intervention components in practice.

4   *Reflexive Monitoring* through which the effects of an intervention and its components are *appraised*: participants contribute to enacting intervention components through work that assembles and appraises information about their effects and utilize that knowledge to reconfigure social relations and action.

These mechanisms form the *implementation core*, and their analysis provides the foundation of its analytic purchase on practice. But these must be placed in context. *Contexts* are the dynamic and emergent process ecologies in which actors and objects interact (May 2013). They confer *capacity* on actors through the social structural resources that circulate within them (these include informational and material resources and social norms and roles). They also confer *potential* on actors through social cognitive resources that actors possess (these include knowledge and beliefs and individual intentions and shared commitments). These resources are mobilized by actors when they invest in the ensembles of practices that are the objects of implementation processes.

NPT characterizes contexts as dynamic, so the implementation of innovations involves participants in *normative restructuring* – changes in the conventions, rules, and resources that are the framework for everyday action. Implementation processes also lead to *relational restructuring* – changes in the structure and meaning of relationships between people that are implicated in them. This reveals a further fundamental feature of implementation. The translation of strategic intentions to everyday practices involves multiple negotiation pathways as objects, actors, and contexts interact. This means that the outcomes of implementation processes are highly situational. As instruments to measure variables defined by NPT mechanisms are developed (Rapley et al. 2018, Finch et al. 2018) and they themselves become normalized in practice, quantitative researchers will increasingly use NPT to make predictions about the direction and outcome of implementation processes.

Acknowledgement

The author gratefully acknowledges support from NIHR ARC North Thames. The views expressed in this publication are those of the author and not necessarily those of the National Health Service (NHS), NIHR, or the Department of Health and Social Care, England.

References

Finch, T. L., M. Girling, C. R. May, F. S. Mair, E. Murray, S. Treweek, E. McColl, I. N. Steen, C. Cook, C. R. Vernazza, N. Mackintosh, S. Sharma, G. Barbery, J. Steele, and T. Rapley. 2018. "Improving the normalization of complex interventions: Part 2 – Validation of the NoMAD instrument for assessing implementation work based on normalization process theory (NPT)." *BMC Medical Research Methodology* 18 (1). doi: 10.1186/s12874-018-0591-x.

May, C. 2006. "A rational model for assessing and evaluating complex interventions in health care." *BMC Health Services Research* 6 (86):1–11. doi: 10.1186/1472-6963-6-86.

May, C. 2013. "Towards a general theory of implementation." *Implementation Science* 8 (1):18.

May, C., and T. Finch. 2009. "Implementing, embedding, and integrating practices: An outline of normalization process theory." *Sociology* 43 (3):535–554.

May, C., T. Finch, F. Mair, L. Ballini, C. Dowrick, M. Eccles, L. Gask, A. MacFarlane, E. Murray, and T. Rapley. 2007. "Understanding the implementation of complex interventions in health care: The normalization process model." *BMC Health Services Research* 7 (1):148.

May, C., T. Finch, and T. Rapley. 2020. "Normalization process theory." In *Handbook on Implementation Science*, edited by Per Nilsen and Sarah Birken, 144–167. Cheltenham: Edward Elgar Publishing Limited.

May, C., F. S. Mair, T. Finch, A. MacFarlane, C. Dowrick, S. Treweek, T. Rapley, L. Ballini, B. N. Ong, A. Rogers, E. Murray, G. Elwyn, F. Legare, J. Gunn, and V. M. Montori. 2009. "Development of a theory of implementation and integration: Normalization Process Theory." *Implementation Science* 4 (29). doi: 10.1186/1748-5908-4-29.

May, C. R., M. Johnson, and T. Finch. 2016. "Implementation, context and complexity." *Implementation Science* 11 (1):141. doi: 10.1186/s13012-016-0506-3.

Rapley, T., M. Girling, F. S. Mair, E. Murray, S. Treweek, E. McColl, I. N. Steen, C. R. May, and T. L. Finch. 2018. "Improving the normalization of complex interventions: Part 1 – Development of the NoMAD instrument for assessing implementation work based on normalization process theory (NPT)." *BMC Medical Research Methodology* 18 (1). doi: 10.1186/s12874-018-0590-y.

14 Diffusion of Innovation theory

Ping Yu

Diffusion of Innovations is among the most influential of theories; it explains how, why, and at what rate new ideas, processes, and technology spread through a population or community. Everett Rogers, a professor of communication studies, puts forward this theory in his landmark book *Diffusion of Innovations* in 1962. The book, in its fifth edition in 2003, is the standard text and referenced in multiple fields such as implementation science, Diffusion of Innovation, and marketing (Rogers 1995). The famous innovation S-curve (Figure 14.1) shows that an innovative technology, process, or service starts slowly at the early stage. It goes through an acceleration phase (a steeper line) to mature. This is followed by a flattening, stabilization phase, over time, to keep the momentum going. The S-curve has helped generations to conceive the rate at which innovations are spread.

According to the theory Rogers propounds, diffusion is the process by which information about the innovation is communicated from one person to another over time across a community (Rogers 1995). There are four main determining factors for the success of any innovation: good communication channels, the attributes of the innovation, the characteristics of the adopters, and the social system. The communication channels refer to the medium through which people obtain the information about the innovation and perceive its usefulness. This can be mass media, social media, or interpersonal communication. The attributes of an innovation include five user-perceived qualities: relative advantage, compatibility, complexity, trialability, and observability. Relative advantage is the degree of benefits or improvements that the innovation will bring upon the existing idea, process, or technology. Compatibility captures the extent to which an innovation is consistent with the existing social technical environment. The more successfully that an innovation can align with, or fit in to the existing values, needs, and experiences of the community, the greater its chance for diffusion and adoption. Complexity measures how difficult it is for the community to understand, adopt, or use an innovation. The less complex an innovation, the larger its chance to be accepted by the end users, and vice versa. Trialability is the effort required to test the innovation. Generally speaking, complex innovations are less easily adopted than less complex innovations. Finally, observability is the visibility of the innovation for the potential users. Only when the community see the benefits will an innovation be accepted, adopted, and used. The structure of a community affects individuals' attitudes toward innovation, and as a result, an innovation must fit with the perceived needs, values, and beliefs of key stakeholders in the community for it to be accepted.

Rogers categorizes people in a community into five groups based on their attitude, sequence and time to adopt an innovation: innovators, early adopters, earlier majority, later majority, and laggards (Rogers 1995). Innovators occupy 2.5 per cent of the community. They are the risk takers and entrepreneurs who have the appetite to invent or introduce an

DOI: 10.4324/9781003109945-16

innovation into the community. They are courageous to introduce new concepts, ideas, and technology and are willing to break with the status quo, taking risks, and being prepared to fail or be rejected by the community. The next 13.5 per cent of the community are the early adopters. They tend to be open-minded and are willing to give innovation a chance. They are also better connected with the rest of the community supporting the spread of the innovation. The early majority is the next 34 per cent of the group; they are the mainstream adopters. The next 34 per cent, the later majority, are the cautious observers. They learn from peers and will come on board after ensuring that the innovation is fully functional. The final 16 per cent of the individuals, laggards, are the strongest resisters to any change. They stick with tradition or habit, are very slow to adopt, or may never adopt the innovation (Rogers 1995).

The S-curve explains how the innovation embeds (Rogers 1995). For any given innovation at the start, a handful of innovators will try hard to make it work (Figure 14.1). The innovation grows slowly in popularity. When early adopters get involved, exponential growth starts, even though the innovation can still disrupt the community. When the early majority are on board, the innovation becomes part of the norm, and then the later majority will follow. The laggards will always fall behind. The innovation S-curve allows us to understand, who, through which sequence, and at which speed, adoption occurs.

Diffusion of Innovation theory has provided guidance for generations of policymakers, managers, and researchers worldwide to conceive, design, and roll out interventions in fields such as implementation science, marketing, and technology transfer. For example, Yenglier, Frederick, and Ziem (2020) applied it as the theoretical framework to explain the challenges for the implementation of evidence-based nursing practice in rural Ghana and put forward recommendations for policymakers to improve evidence uptake. Bayram et al. (2020) applied it to design, implement, and explain their social marketing program of "mask-wearing", "physical distancing", and "staying at home" during the COVID-19 pandemic in Turkey, informative research that was also guided by the Health Belief Model. Kelly et al. (2020) reported the application of popular opinion leader interventions to facilitate population-level

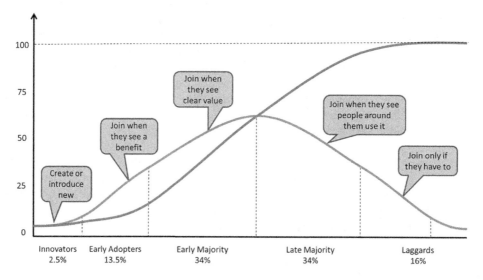

Figure 14.1 The S-curve of innovation

Source: Created by author

HIV behaviour change in the United States. Quinn (2020) further suggested the transfer of Kelly's implementation method to public education about COVID-19. Zhang et al. (2015) applied Diffusion of Innovation theory to explain the factors impacting patient acceptance and use of an online patient appointment system in a primary care clinic in a regional town in Australia. Marshall et al. (2020) applied the theory to identify the challenges for widespread implementation of antiviral therapies for hepatitis C virus infection in general practice in Australia.

As of mid-2021, according to Google Scholar, Roger's original book "Diffusion of Innovations" published in 1962 (Rogers 1962) has attracted more than 126,000 citations, endorsing this landmark masterpiece. The continuing growth in citation numbers reflects the tremendous utility and social value of the Diffusion of Innovation theory. It has offered human society a useful framework to conceive, design, implement, and evaluate the introduction of innovations in all walks of life.

References

Bayram, T., A. Camcıoğlu, G. Keskiner, and İ. Başıbüyük. 2020. "Social marketing of 'mask-wearing', 'physical distancing' and 'staying at home' during the COVID-19 pandemic: A study from Turkey." *Turkish Journal of Public Health* 18:112–119.

Kelly, J. A., Y. A. Amirkhanian, J. L. Walsh, K. D. Brown, K. G. Quinn, A. E. Petroll, B. M. Pearson, A. N. Rosado, and T. Ertl. 2020. "Social network intervention to increase pre-exposure prophylaxis (PrEP) awareness, interest, and use among African American men who have sex with men." *AIDS Care* 32 (Suppl 2):40–46. doi: 10.1080/09540121.2020.1739207.

Marshall, A. D., M. Hopwood, J. Grebely, and C. Treloar. 2020. "Applying a diffusion of innovations framework to the scale-up of direct-acting antiviral therapies for hepatitis C virus infection: Identified challenges for widespread implementation." *International Journal of Drug Policy* 86:102964. doi: /10.1016/j.drugpo.2020.102964.

Quinn, K. G. 2020. "Applying the popular opinion leader intervention for HIV to COVID-19." *AIDS and Behavior* 24 (12):3291–3294. doi: 10.1007/s10461-020-02954-7.

Rogers, E. 1962. *Diffusion of Innovations*. 1st ed. New York: The Free Press of Glencore.

Rogers, E. 1995. *Diffusion of Innovations*. 4th ed. New York: Free Press.

Yenglier, Y., D. Frederick, and B. Samuel Ziem. 2020. "Evidence-based practice and rural health service delivery: Knowledge and barriers to adoption among clinical nurses in Ghana." *Rural Society* 29 (2):134–149. doi: 10.1080/10371656.2020.1795350.

Zhang, X., P. Yu, J. Yan, and I. Ton A M Spil. 2015. "Using diffusion of innovation theory to understand the factors impacting patient acceptance and use of consumer e-health innovations: A case study in a primary care clinic." *BMC Health Services Research* 15 (1):71. doi: 10.1186/s12913-015-0726-2.

15 Health-related quality of life

Ben Smith and Ivana Durcinoska

Health-related quality of life (HRQOL) can be defined as the "the subjective assessment of the impact of disease and treatment across the physical, psychological, social and somatic domains of functioning and well-being" (Revicki et al. 2000). Patient Reported Outcome Measures (PROMs) have long been used to evaluate HRQOL in research investigating the experience and treatment of various health conditions. Since the advent of electronic data collection systems, using PROMs to collect HRQOL data to inform and enhance routine clinical care has become increasingly common, particularly in oncology (Howell et al. 2015).

Electronic PROM systems typically use online surveys to collect HRQOL and other Patient Reported Outcome (PRO) data from patients, either at home or during clinic visits. These data are then provided to the clinical team so that patients' HRQOL and other issues of concern can be discussed, enabling patient-centred care (Velikova et al. 2004). Patients are sometimes also provided with relevant recommendations to enable self-management of symptoms affecting HRQOL (Girgis et al. 2017). Studies have found that routine electronic collection and clinical use of PROMs can improve patient HRQOL, treatment adherence, and survival and reduce emergency department presentations (Absolom et al. 2021, Girgis et al. 2020, Graupner et al. 2021). Despite these benefits, implementation of PROMs in routine care has been patchy. Implementation science is playing a growing role in addressing this evidence-practice gap, providing a framework to systematically evaluate PROMs' implementation barriers and enablers and apply strategies to overcome barriers and leverage enablers.

Various implementation frameworks have been used to guide PROMs' implementation. One of the most commonly used frameworks (Stover et al. 2020) is the Consolidated Framework for Implementation Research (CFIR) (Damschroder et al. 2009) (see Essay 9; Damschroder, "The Consolidated Framework for Implementation Research (CFIR)"), which comprises 39 constructs drawn from multiple frameworks grouped into five multilevel domains: the intervention itself (e.g., PROMs), outer setting (e.g., national policies), inner setting (e.g., clinic readiness for change), characteristics of individual implementers (e.g., healthcare and administrative staff), and the implementation process (Figure 15.1). A CFIR guide helps fit implementation strategies to barriers (see https://cfirguide.org/choosing-strategies/).

Research on the implementation of PROMs in routine care is still maturing, but several common barriers have been identified across varied contexts (Foster et al. 2018, Howell et al. 2015, Stover et al. 2020). The additional time and resources needed for PROMs' implementation is a key concern for both clinicians and administrators. Many clinicians feel uncertainty around PROMs' interpretation and worry about usage of PROMs increasing their workload

DOI: 10.4324/9781003109945-17

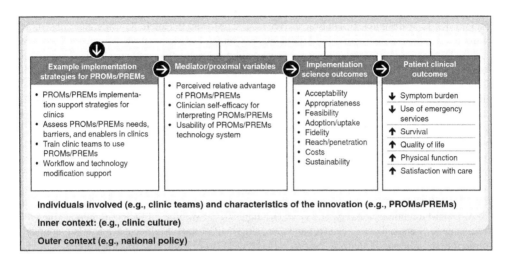

Individuals involved (e.g., clinic teams) and characteristics of the innovation (e.g., PROMs/PREMs)

Inner context: (e.g., clinic culture)

Outer context (e.g., national policy)

Figure 15.1 Key factors involved in PROMs/Patient Reported Experience Measures implementation according to the CFIR

Source: Originally published in Stover et al. 2020

and consultation length. These issues may be compounded by lack of PROMs' integration with electronic health record systems.

Reported PROMs' implementation enablers seem less consistent and more context dependent, highlighting the need for co-design of context-specific PROMs' implementation strategies with clinics involved in implementation. Some more common enablers include automatic scoring of PROMs and flagging of clinically significant scores for access by clinicians at point of care and incorporating the service user (both patient and clinician) perspective into the development of PROMs' systems (Foster et al. 2018, Howell et al. 2015, Stover et al. 2020).

Evidence is emerging regarding the utility of strategies to overcome PROMs' implementation barriers and leverage enablers, which vary considerably according to the context and implementation stage. During pre-implementation, for example, engaging the clinical team and establishing their needs seem critical (Foster et al. 2018, Stover et al. 2020). Throughout implementation, training clinical teams on using and interpreting PROMs and providing technical support appear to be key (Foster et al. 2018, Stover et al. 2020). Engaging with clinical teams at these earlier stages may prevent later problems (Foster et al. 2018). To sustain implementation, a feedback and refinement process seems important (Foster et al. 2018, Stover et al. 2020). To maximize HRQOL benefits to patients through broadscale PROMs' implementation, further research is needed to identify 1) optimal levels of technology and workflow support for implementation of PROMs and 2) strategies suited to initial versus sustained implementation of PROMs. Using an implementation science framework to guide this research will aid tailoring and refinement of PROMs' systems and implementation strategies to suit different contexts and maximize the likelihood that they are embedded as part of routine care. Routine usage of PROMs to assess HRQOL will enable more patient-centred care and help ensure the HRQOL benefits of PROMs' collection, and clinical use moves beyond research studies to the real world.

References

Absolom, K., L. Warrington, E. Hudson, J. Hewison, C. Morris, P. Holch, R. Carter, A. Gibson, M. Holmes, B. Clayton, Z. Rogers, L. McParland, M. Conner, L. Glidewell, B. Woroncow, B. Dawkins, S. Dickinson, C. Hulme, J. Brown, and G. Velikova. 2021. "Phase III randomized controlled trial of eRAPID: eHealth intervention during chemotherapy." *Journal of Clinical Oncology* 38 (15_ suppl):7002. doi: 10.1200/JCO.20.02015.

Damschroder, L. J., D. C. Aron, R. E. Keith, S. R. Kirsh, J. A. Alexander, and J. C. Lowery. 2009. "Fostering implementation of health services research findings into practice: A consolidated framework for advancing implementation science." *Implementation Science* 4 (1):50. doi: 10.1186/1748-5908-4-50.

Foster, A., L. Croot, J. Brazier, J. Harris, and A. O'Cathain. 2018. "The facilitators and barriers to implementing patient reported outcome measures in organisations delivering health related services: A systematic review of reviews." *Journal of Patient-Reported Outcomes* 2 (1):46. doi: 10.1186/s41687-018-0072-3.

Girgis, A., I. Durcinoska, A. Arnold, J. Descallar, N. Kaadan, E.-S. Koh, A. Miller, W. Ng, M. Carolan, S. A. Della-Fiorentina, S. Avery, and G. P. Delaney. 2020. "Web-based Patient-Reported Outcome Measures for Personalized Treatment and Care (PROMPT-Care): Multicenter pragmatic nonrandomized trial." *Journal of Medical Internet Research* 22 (10):e19685. doi: 10.2196/19685.

Girgis, A., I. Durcinoska, J. V. Levesque, M. Gerges, T. Sandell, A. Arnold, and G. P. Delaney. 2017. "eHealth system for collecting and utilizing Patient Reported Outcome Measures for Personalized Treatment and Care (PROMPT-Care) among cancer patients: Mixed methods approach to evaluate feasibility and acceptability." *Journal of Medical Internet Research* 19 (10):e330. doi: 10.2196/jmir.8360.

Graupner, C., M. L. Kimman, S. Mul, A. H. M. Slok, D. Claessens, J. Kleijnen, C. D. Dirksen, and S. O. Breukink. 2021. "Patient outcomes, patient experiences and process indicators associated with the routine use of patient-reported outcome measures (PROMs) in cancer care: A systematic review." *Supportive Care in Cancer* 29 (2):573–593. doi: 10.1007/s00520-020-05695-4.

Howell, D., S. Molloy, K. Wilkinson, E. Green, K. Orchard, K. Wang, and J. Liberty. 2015. "Patient-reported outcomes in routine cancer clinical practice: A scoping review of use, impact on health outcomes, and implementation factors." *Annals of Oncology* 26 (9):1846–1858. doi: 10.1093/annonc/mdv181.

Revicki, D. A., D. Osoba, D. Fairclough, I. Barofsky, R. Berzon, N. K. Leidy, and M. Rothman. 2000. "Recommendations on health-related quality of life research to support labeling and promotional claims in the United States." *Quality of Life Research* 9 (8):887–900. doi: 10.1023/a:1008896223999.

Stover, A. M., L. Haverman, H. A. van Oers, J. Greenhalgh, C. M. Potter, S. Ahmed, J. Greenhalgh, E. Gibbons, L. Haverman, K. Manalili, C. Potter, N. Roberts, M. Santana, A. M. Stover, H. van Oers, and I. P. P. i. C. P. I. S. W. G. On behalf of the. 2020. "Using an implementation science approach to implement and evaluate patient-reported outcome measures (PROM) initiatives in routine care settings." *Quality of Life Research*. doi: 10.1007/s11136-020-02564-9.

Velikova, G., L. Booth, A. B. Smith, P. M. Brown, P. Lynch, J. M. Brown, and P. J. Selby. 2004. "Measuring quality of life in routine oncology practice improves communication and patient well-being: A randomized controlled trial." *Journal of Clinical Oncology* 22 (4):714–724. doi: 10.1200/jco.2004.06.078.

16 Shared decision-making

Consider context

Glyn Elwyn

Shared decision-making

"Shared decision-making" has become a widely used term in healthcare communication, while there's some debate about when exactly the term arrived and was first used. The term definitely appears in Jay Katz's seminal book "The Silent World of Doctor and Patient" (Katz 1984). Most cite the prominent use in a presidential commission on ethics (Commission 1982). And so, the term arises from ideas of informed consent and the ethical concept of autonomy and agency. Although the term did not come into common use until the early 1990s, the concept of involving patients in decision-making was proposed at more or less the same time as the ideas of patient-centred care (Balint 1969) and the biopsychosocial model arrived (Engel 1977). The concept was foreshadowed by Emanuel and colleagues when they described four models of patient–physician communication (Emanuel and Emanuel 1992). Their "deliberative" approach stops short of regarding the informed views and preferences of the patient as key factors to be considered in arriving at decisions, and the patient does not have decision-making agency. Charles partly addressed the issue of agency by saying that "both parties take steps to build a consensus about the preferred treatment", noting that agreement had to be reached. There was no room in the model for patients to have a different view to that of the clinician (Charles, Gafni, and Whelan 1997). Many definitions followed, and Makoul provided an integrated view which summarizes the main components (Makoul and Clayman 2006). In sum, shared decision-making is viewed as a process of communication between those who are collaboratively engaged in making a decision in a healthcare setting. That much everyone agrees on.

Countercultural

The problem, however, is that it has been extremely difficult to instantiate shared decision-making. Numerous measures exist, though they are plagued with problems. Those that are based on perceptions of people who might or might not have experienced a decision shared have the most challenges of validity and reliability. Can a decision ever be truly shared? What if a person decides, despite what is said by the professional, to disagree with their "decision"? There is a perception problem here: who's making the decision, and when? Is a decision a set of thoughts? Or does a decision need to be enacted for it to become a decision? When does a thought become an intention, and when does an intention become an action? Such are the challenges of measuring this from the perspective of a person receiving attention from a healthcare professional, who is normally feeling like a stranger in an unfamiliar world of medicine, slightly anxious at best, bewildered often, and, at times full of dread

DOI: 10.4324/9781003109945-18

about an uncertain future. The norm for this world is for experts to occupy decision-making roles and convey them with confidence. People expect this, and introducing a different decision dynamic is countercultural.

If making shared decisions in healthcare settings is countercultural for most people, so it is for health professionals. Trained to be experts, knowledgeable, and conveying certainty, most health professionals find it intractably difficult to make people aware of options, even where reasonable alternatives should be considered. Measures based on observation, using audio or video tapes, bear witness to the inability of clinicians to introduce the idea of supporting a process of deliberation, to convey the existence of options, to compare them using trustworthy information, and to then elicit individuals' preferences. Attempts to make this concept simple, such as the *three-talk model* (Figure 16.1) (Elwyn et al. 2017), do not seem to make the task any easier for clinicians.

Consider context

Perhaps a solution to this intractable countercultural problem is to set a goal that is likely to be much easier to understand and culturally far more acceptable to both health professionals

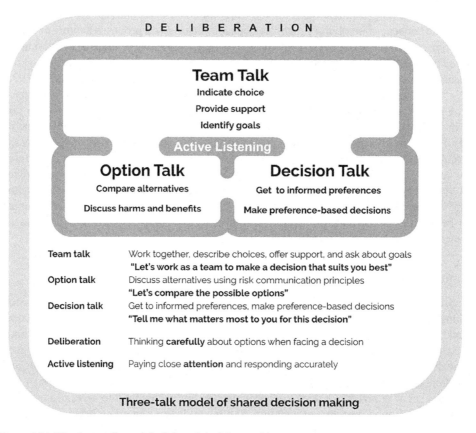

Figure 16.1 The three-talk model of shared decision-making

Source: Reprinted from *Patient Education and Counseling*, Glyn Elwyn, "Shared decision making: what is the work?", 2021, with permission from Elsevier

and others. Gerwing and Gulbrandsen write about "contextualizing decisions" (Gerwing and Gulbrandsen 2019). I might go further and use the term "consider context". Put an emphasis on always understanding what Mishler aptly called the *person's lifeworld* (Mishler 1984). What brings them joy? What do they fear (Matthys et al. 2009)? What are they able to consider in terms of action or cost or extra work? If decisions are made in as best an understanding of context as is possible, it is highly likely that the psychosocial dimensions of a person's existence, and not just the clinical problem or basic age and gender, will have been given attention. To consider context, deeply, are the prerequisites of a good decision, whoever makes it.

References

Balint, E. 1969. "The possibilities of patient-centered medicine." *The Journal of the Royal College of General Practitioners* 17 (82):269.

Charles, C., A. Gafni, and T. Whelan. 1997. "Shared decision-making in the medical encounter: What does it mean?(or it takes at least two to tango)." *Social Science & Medicine* 44 (5):681–692.

Commission, U. S. P. s. 1982. *United States President's Commission for the Study of Ethical Problems in Medicine Biomedical, Behavioral, Research. Making Health Care Decisions: The Ethical and Legal Implications of Informed Consent in the Patient-practitioner Relationship.* Washington, DC: US Code Annot.

Elwyn, G. 2021. "Shared decision making: What is the work?" *Patient Education and Counseling* 104 (7):1591–1595. doi: 10.1016/j.pec.2020.11.032.

Elwyn, G., M. A. Durand, J. Song, J. Aarts, P. J. Barr, Z. Berger, N. Cochran, D. Frosch, D. Galasiński, and P. Gulbrandsen. 2017. "A three-talk model for shared decision making: Multistage consultation process." *BMJ* 359:j4891.

Emanuel, E. J., and L. L. Emanuel. 1992. "Four models of the physician-patient relationship." *Journal of the American Medical Association* 267 (16):2221–2226.

Engel, G. L. 1977. "The need for a new medical model: A challenge for biomedicine." *Science* 196 (4286):129–136.

Gerwing, J., and P. Gulbrandsen. 2019. "Contextualizing decisions: Stepping out of the SDM track." *Patient Education and Counseling* 102 (5):815.

Katz, J. 1984. *The Silent World of Doctor and Patient.* New York: Free Press.

Makoul, G., and M. L. Clayman. 2006. "An integrative model of shared decision making in medical encounters." *Patient Education and Counseling* 60 (3):301–312.

Matthys, J., G. Elwyn, M. Van Nuland, G. Van Maele, A. De Sutter, M. De Meyere, and M. Deveugele. 2009. "Patients' ideas, concerns, and expectations (ICE) in general practice: Impact on prescribing." *British Journal of General Practice* 59 (558):29–36.

Mishler, E. G. 1984. *The Discourse of Medicine: Dialectics of Medical Interviews.* Norwood, NJ: Ablex.

17 Core aspects of nudge as a behaviour change paradigm in implementation science

Klay Lamprell

Until the advent of germ theory and antibiotics, post-partum infections, also known as "puer-peral fever", regularly swept through hospital maternity wards, killing up to 70 per cent of new mothers (Hallett 2005). The deaths were attributed to miasmas, or unhealthy vapours. In the mid-1800s, Ignaz Semmelweis, a young obstetrician working in Vienna, Austria, observed that the highest mortality rates were in clinics staffed by physicians and medical students who also performed autopsies. He proposed that disease particles from cadavers were being transmitted to patients, and he implemented a program of hand scrubbing with chlorinated lime solution. Maternal mortality rates dropped to around 2 per cent (Best and Neuhauser 2004, Ataman, Vatanoğlu-Lutz, and Yıldırım 2013).

His fellow physicians, however, soon began to evade the protocol (Best and Neuhauser 2004, Ataman, Vatanoğlu-Lutz, and Yıldırım 2013). They disputed the validity of his evidence given the current paradigm that disease was airborne (Ataman, Vatanoğlu-Lutz, and Yıldırım 2013), they found the process to be time-consuming, and they were insulted at the implication that they were unclean (Best and Neuhauser 2004). Though the death rate rose again, Semmelweis could not persuade physicians to participate in hand scrubbing (Ataman, Vatanoğlu-Lutz, and Yıldırım 2013).

Perhaps surprisingly, even today we struggle to achieve compliance with hand sanitization programs in hospitals (Ataman, Vatanoğlu-Lutz, and Yıldırım 2013). It is part of the larger problem of poor adherence to clinical practice guidelines across all areas of medical practice and across all health systems (Braithwaite et al. 2018).

Innovation emerging from the "choice architecture" movement may hold promise for shifting physicians' behaviours, at least in some aspects of medical practice. Choice architecture is a term used in the best-selling 2008 book "Nudge: Improving Decisions about Health, Wealth and Happiness" (Thaler and Sunstein 2008). It describes the design and implementation of choice situations that use behavioural insights to predictably nudge decision-makers towards a preferred option, without removing the right to choose otherwise (Johnson et al. 2012, Hansen 2016). The action achieved by this choice architecture is a "nudge".

A nudge aims to achieve an immediate change in behaviour (Dolan et al. 2012). It stimulates reflexive, instinctive decision-making. Though the outcome can be long-term attitudinal and preference change (Huh, Vosgerau, and Morewedge 2014, Olshan, Rareshide, and Patel 2019), the simplicity and immediacy of a nudge differentiates it from interventions seeking deliberative shifts in mindsets over time, such as education. Nudging may be an apt approach to influencing physicians because it preserves the decision-maker's autonomy, which is a crucial element in the practice of safe, patient-centred medicine (Jones et al. 2017).

The choice architecture movement promoted the proposition of nudging as "libertarian paternalism" (Thaler and Sunstein 2008), a paradigm that preserves freedom of choice but

DOI: 10.4324/9781003109945-19

authorizes institutions to steer people in a direction that promotes the welfare of self and others (Thaler and Sunstein 2008, Hansen 2016). Promoting evidence-based care using simple nudges to reflexively shift behaviour is a pragmatic deployment of this philosophical construct. As yet, however, implementation scientists working in healthcare are not well versed in the causal pathways by which a nudge influences behaviour and the assumptions about cognitive processing that inform a nudge (Hertwig and Grüne-Yanoff 2017).

The assumption underpinning a nudge is that decision-making is an *adaptive* process. Decision-makers must adapt their decision goals to the limitations on their time, their access to knowledge, and their computational power to process knowledge. It is rarely feasible to evaluate all factors and all possible alternatives. Reflexively, in most circumstances, seeks a decision that will 'satisfice' – a portmanteau of the meanings of 'satisfy' and 'suffice' (Simon 1955).

In order to satisfice, decision-making has to be a *heuristic* process. Decision-makers rely on intuitive shortcuts to make a good-enough decision (Hertwig and Grüne-Yanoff 2017, Croskerry 2013). Those shortcuts take the form of biases that are preconfigured cognitively to rapidly validate deviations from rationality in judgement. Decisions that satisfy cognitive biases can be made quickly, such as decisions anchored to the status quo (Saposnik et al. 2016, Croskerry 2013), or decisions that will avert a loss in the short term, which is instinctively more important than achieving a gain in the long term (Croskerry 2013). Decision-making environments such as clinical information systems (Patel, Navathe, and Liao 2020) can support rapid choices by satisfying cognitive biases for streamlined, prominently presented, and easily selected options (Saposnik et al. 2016).

The reliance on heuristics makes decision-making an inherently *subjective* process. Decision-makers are influenced by social and professional interaction and cultures and by physical and informational environments that satisfy their cognitive biases. Additionally, decisions become subject to idiosyncratic routines and habits (Bierbaum et al. 2020), personal passions and interests, and the innate motivation to serve one's own utility (Saposnik et al. 2016). Cognitive dissonance draws decision-makers away from challenging ideas and the prospect of change towards choices that are comfortable and that do not conflict with their cognitive biases.

Dr Semmelweis would have appreciated the innovation of nudging physicians to adhere to evidence-based guidelines and the understanding of decision-making as an adaptive, heuristic, and biased process. Having spent years trying to convince the medical establishment that post-partum infection was transmitted through person-to-person contact, he died in a psychiatric asylum, aged 47, two decades short of the dawn of germ theory. He did eventually receive recognition. He is now known as the "saviour of mothers" (Best and Neuhauser 2004) and the originator of infection control (Ataman, Vatanoğlu-Lutz, and Yıldırım 2013).

References

Ataman, A. D., E. E. Vatanoğlu-Lutz, and G. Yıldırım. 2013. "Medicine in stamps-Ignaz Semmelweis and puerperal fever." *Journal of the Turkish German Gynecological Association* 14 (1):35–39. doi: 10.5152/jtgga.2013.08.

Best, M., and D. Neuhauser. 2004. "Ignaz Semmelweis and the birth of infection control." *Quality and Safety in Health Care* 13 (3):233. doi: 10.1136/qshc.2004.010918.

Bierbaum, M., J. Braithwaite, G. Arnolda, G. P. Delaney, W. Liauw, R. Kefford, Y. Tran, B. Nic Giolla Easpaig, and F. Rapport. 2020. "Clinicians' attitudes to oncology clinical practice guidelines and the barriers and facilitators to adherence: A mixed methods study protocol." *BMJ Open* 10 (3):e035448. doi: 10.1136/bmjopen-2019-035448.

Braithwaite, J., K. Churruca, J. C. Long, L. A. Ellis, and J. Herkes. 2018. "When complexity science meets implementation science: A theoretical and empirical analysis of systems change." *BMC Medicine* 16 (1):63. doi: 10.1186/s12916-018-1057-z.

Croskerry, P. 2013. "From mindless to mindful practice – cognitive bias and clinical decision making." *The New England Journal of Medicine* 368 (26):2445–2448.

Dolan, P., M. Hallsworth, D. Halpern, D. King, R. Metcalfe, and I. Vlaev. 2012. "Influencing behaviour: The mindspace way." *Journal of Economic Psychology* 33 (1):264–277. doi: 10.1016/j.joep.2011.10.009.

Hallett, C. 2005. "The attempt to understand puerperal fever in the eighteenth and early nineteenth centuries: The influence of inflammation theory." *Medical History* 49 (1):1–28. doi: 10.1017/s0025772730000119.

Hansen, P. G. 2016. "The definition of nudge and libertarian paternalism: Does the hand fit the glove?" *European Journal of Risk Regulation* 7 (1):155–174. doi: 10.1017/S1867299X00005468.

Hertwig, R., and T. Grüne-Yanoff. 2017. "Nudging and boosting: Steering or empowering good decisions." *Perspectives on Psychological Science* 12 (6):973–986. doi: 10.1177/1745691617702496.

Huh, Y. E., J. Vosgerau, and C. K. Morewedge. 2014. "Social defaults: Observed choices become choice defaults." *Journal of Consumer Research* 41 (3):746–760. doi: 10.1086/677315.

Johnson, E. J., S. B. Shu, B. G. C. Dellaert, C. Fox, D. G. Goldstein, G. Häubl, R. P. Larrick, J. W. Payne, E. Peters, D. Schkade, B. Wansink, and E. U. Weber. 2012. "Beyond nudges: Tools of a choice architecture." *Marketing Letters* 23 (2):487–504. doi: 10.1007/s11002-012-9186-1.

Jones, M., J. Butler, C. J. Graber, P. Glassman, M. H. Samore, L. A. Pollack, C. Weir, and M. B. Goetz. 2017. "Think twice: A cognitive perspective of an antibiotic timeout intervention to improve antibiotic use." *Journal of Biomedical Informatics* 71:S22–S31. doi: 10.1016/j.jbi.2016.06.005.

Olshan, D., C. A. L. Rareshide, and M. S. Patel. 2019. "Longer-term durability of using default options in the electronic health record to increase generic prescribing rates." *Journal of General Internal Medicine* 34 (3):349–350. doi: 10.1007/s11606-018-4719-9.

Patel, M. S., A. S. Navathe, and J. M. Liao. 2020. "Using nudges to improve value by increasing imaging-based cancer screening." *Journal of the American College of Radiology* 17 (1 Pt A):38–41. doi: 10.1016/j.jacr.2019.08.025.

Saposnik, G., D. Redelmeier, C. C. Ruff, and P. N. Tobler. 2016. "Cognitive biases associated with medical decisions: A systematic review." *BMC Medical Informatics and Decision Making* 16 (1):138. doi: 10.1186/s12911-016-0377-1.

Simon, H. A. 1955. "A behavioral model of rational choice." *The Quarterly Journal of Economics* 69 (1):99–118. doi: 10.2307/1884852.

Thaler, R. H., and C. R. Sunstein. 2008. *Nudge: Improving Decisions about Health, Wealth, and Happiness*. New Haven and London: Yale University Press.

18 Pipeline and cyclical models of evidence building

The roles of implementation research

Carolyn J. Hill and Virginia Knox

How do we build evidence about effective policies and programs? The process is commonly depicted as a pipeline: from developing a new intervention to testing it on a small scale, to conducting impact studies in new locations, to expanding effective interventions. But an updated depiction of evidence building could better reflect realities of decision-making and practice in the field. Under a cyclical evidence-building, implementation, and adaptation paradigm, researchers and funders create more information that is attuned to the real-world needs of users of evidence (the implementers of the programs they are studying) (Knox, Hill, and Berlin 2018).

Implementation research has always been a key part of impact studies and evidence building. It takes on a central role in an updated cyclical model of evidence building as program operators systematically consider how, for whom, and where they operate programs; decide what adaptations they should make; and build new evidence about the effectiveness of those adaptations.

The pipeline paradigm of evidence building

The prevailing paradigm for building evidence about programs or policies is a linear one, as depicted in Figure 18.1: a new intervention is developed and undergoes early tests of its effectiveness. These tests attempt to ascertain the intervention's *impact*, that is, the value added of the intervention over and above what would have occurred in the absence of the intervention (see Box 18.1). If early tests find favourable impacts, replication studies ascertain if the initial impacts occur in new locations. If findings from the replication studies are favourable, funders support scale-up or further expansion, expecting to see similar effects as long as future versions implement the core elements of the intervention (Institute of Education Science 2016).

Box 18.1 Impact studies and evidence-based interventions

We refer to *impact studies* as those that use well-implemented experimental or non-experimental designs. Experimental designs (also called randomized controlled trials) compare the outcomes of a group of people assigned at random to receive an intervention with the outcomes of a control group whose members may often receive other available services but do not receive the intervention being studied. Because they were assigned at random, the two groups' measurable and unmeasurable characteristics should be similar, on average, at the outset of the study. The design allows researchers to be confident that any differences in the outcomes of the two groups that emerge over time are caused by the program group's participation in the intervention. For this reason, we use the term "evidence-based" to refer to interventions that have favourable findings from rigorous impact studies.

Source: Created by authors

DOI: 10.4324/9781003109945-20

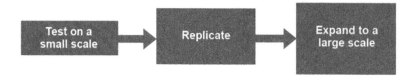

Figure 18.1 Evidence building as a pipeline

Source: Reprinted from Knox, Hill, and Berlin 2018, with permission from SAGE publishing

Often, researchers focus on building evidence about individual program models or interventions, not on building evidence about effective strategies or components.[1] The underlying assumption is that a policy or program that works in one location will continue to work when it is replicated elsewhere. The process often ends in disappointment, in part because that assumption is naïve. It ignores or underestimates the challenges of replicating a program at a larger scale, where interventions are embedded in organizations or systems (McCarthy 2014). Moreover, even if it is implemented well, an intervention that shows impacts in one context may not bring greater benefits to participants in another context compared with the policies and programs that are already available.

Implementation research often accompanies impact studies to provide insight into the steps and mechanisms involved in an intervention. Though they vary in emphasis and comprehensiveness, implementation analyses use both qualitative and quantitative information to analyse the following:

- Policy, political, economic, and social contexts in which interventions take place.
- Organizations and systems in which interventions are embedded.
- Differences between the services received by intervention and control group members, in the case of a randomized controlled trial (also known as service contrast) (Hamilton and Scrivener 2018).
- Characteristics of staff members and participants, as well as their perceptions about and experiences in the program.
- Factors that may influence effectiveness in different contexts (Manno 2018).

Relatively sparse systematic information is available about whether and how evidence-based practices maintain, decrease, or increase their effects as they are widely implemented. Initiatives under the umbrella of "implementation science" at least initially focused on how evidence-based policy interventions were disseminated, implemented, and adapted over time (Fixsen et al. 2005). And, frameworks such as Getting to Outcomes are designed to guide local organizations as they adopt, adapt, and implement evidence-based interventions (RAND Health 2017).

An updated cyclical paradigm

Updating the pipeline paradigm of evidence building prompts closer connections between research and practice over time and across settings. It stretches intervention-centric understandings to envision robust systems that can evolve and improve over time (Coburn 2003).

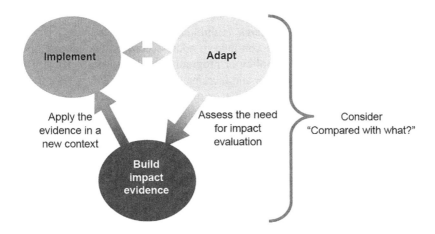

Figure 18.2 Evidence building as a cycle

Source: Reprinted from Knox, Hill, and Berlin 2018, with permission from SAGE publishing

As Figure 18.2 depicts, it requires reimagining rigorous evidence building as part of a cycle of program innovation that furthers the research process by:

- Building impact evidence about new approaches to social programs.
- Implementing evidence-based programs and supporting their expansion in ways that recognize the complexity inherent in replication.
- Encouraging adaptations and improvements.
- Assessing the need for further impact evidence.

Through iteration, this process promotes innovation in a changing environment and continues to build credible evidence about whether and how programs bring down costs or have greater effects than the status quo. It has two key features that distinguish it from the pipeline framework: first, it emphasizes the value of considering service contrast at every stage, not just in the evidence-building stage of impact studies. Second, the implementation of an evidence-based program is not the end point, as it is in the pipeline framework. Instead, the cyclical framework assumes that the intervention will be adapted over time and across settings so that impacts can be sustained or increased under changing circumstances. Innovation, learning, and building new evidence are part of the cycle.

Adaptations are necessary components for continued learning. But there are also risks because there is no "effectiveness guarantee" for new approaches or existing approaches for new populations. Strong rationales, transparent data collection, and study should accompany any adaptations so that they can be used for learning (Balu 2017, Chambers and Norton 2016, Durlak and DuPre 2008). One way to ensure that such strong rationales are present is by periodically reassessing services, clients, and contexts – that is, what, who, and where – while asking, "Compared with what?"

At some point, an intervention may reflect substantial modifications that arise from new service technologies, new constraints, and new challenges. Organizations and funders could agree on conditions that define when an evidence-based model has advanced far enough from its originally tested service contrast, client population, or context that a new rigorous impact evaluation should be conducted.

The nature of implementation research is unlikely to change drastically in a cyclical evidence-building framework. It will continue to address core contextual and operational questions about new approaches to policy or programs. But because a cyclical framework explicitly includes phases of adaptation and incremental improvement, at least five specific aspects of implementation research become even more consequential.

1   Understanding and documenting service contrast, in both impact studies and when implementing in new settings.
2   Documenting and communicating clearly about the environment in which a study is conducted: the context, systems, communities, organizations, program components, and populations involved.
3   Articulating the program's theory of change, and how it is used (or not) to guide implementation and adaptations.
4   Detecting and tracking program adaptations by program decision-makers and frontline staff members.
5   Integrating implementation and impact research, with audiences of potential adopters and adapters in mind.

Conclusion

Viewing program development as a cycle of evidence building, implementation, and adaptation provides a foundation for learning agendas that are attuned to the real-world needs of the people who will implement and adopt the programs. Implementation researchers have a key role to play as program operators systematically consider how, for whom, and where they operate programs; decide what adaptations they should make; and build new evidence about the effectiveness of those adaptations.

Note

1   However, efforts are increasing around identifying "key components" across interventions. See, for example, https://opremethodsmeeting.org/meetings/2020/.

References

Balu, R. 2017. "Anticipating variation in implementation: The multistate evaluation of response to intervention practices." www.mdrc.org/sites/default/files/IRI-2017-04_May_AnticipatingVariation_0.pdf.

Chambers, D. A., and W. E. Norton. 2016. "The adaptome: Advancing the science of intervention adaptation." *American Journal of Preventive Medicine* 51 (4 Suppl 2):S124–S131. doi: 10.1016/j.amepre.2016.05.011.

Coburn, C. E. 2003. "Rethinking scale: Moving beyond numbers to deep and lasting change." *Educational Researcher* 32 (6):3–12. doi: 10.3102/0013189X032006003.

Durlak, J. A., and E. P. DuPre. 2008. "Implementation matters: A review of research on the influence of implementation on program outcomes and the factors affecting implementation." *American Journal of Community Psychology* 41 (3–4):327–350. doi: 10.1007/s10464-008-9165-0.

Fixsen, D. L., S. F. Naoom, R. M. Friedman, and F. Wallace. 2005. *Implementation Research: A Synthesis of the Literature*. Tamps, FL: University of South Florida, Louis de la Parte Florida Mental Health Institute, National Implementation Research Network.

Hamilton, G., and S. Scrivener. 2018. "The central role of implementation research in understanding treatment contrast." www.mdrc.org/sites/default/files/TreatmentContrast_revised.pdf.

Institute of Education Science. 2016. *Non-Regulatory Guidance: Using Evidence to Strengthen Education Investments*. Edited by U.S. Department of Education. Washington, DC: Department of Education.

Knox, V., C. J. Hill, and G. Berlin. 2018. "Can evidence-based policy ameliorate the nation's social problems?" *The ANNALS of the American Academy of Political and Social Science* 678 (1):166–179. doi: 10.1177/0002716218769844.

Manno, M. S. 2018. "How early implementation research can inform program scale-up efforts." www.mdrc.org/publication/how-early-implementation-research-can-inform-program-scale-efforts.

McCarthy, P. T. 2014. "The road to scale runs through public systems." *Stanford Social Innovation Review* 12 (2):12A.

RAND Health. 2017. "Getting to outcomes: Improving community-based prevention." www.rand.org/health-care/projects/getting-to-outcomes.html.

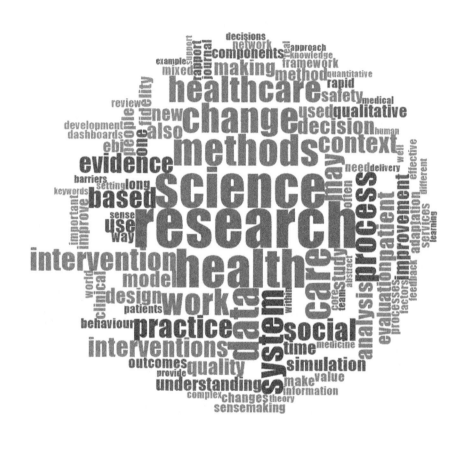

Part II

Methodology and methods of implementation science

Now that we have an understanding of some of the core principles and concepts of implementation science (IS), including knowledge about some of the models and frameworks that underpin IS, we can turn our thinking to application and design. We may have an intervention in mind to solve a pressing workplace problem, but how do we design the implementation process for the complex environments that we see in healthcare systems today? How do we apply IS thinking to implement our intervention in ways that guarantee the best chance of uptake? Furthermore, how do we develop an implementation strategy that will enable us to scale and spread our successful interventions to other areas in our healthcare system? To help answer these questions, and more, read on.

This section opens with a discussion of methodology in all its diversity. Sevdalis and Hull frame the discussion with an essay about the importance of recognizing IS as an *applied* science. Braithwaite then introduces Deming's foundation concept of the Plan, Do, Study, Act (PDSA) cycle, which underpins many of the methods of IS, and then goes on to describe Formative Evaluation Feedback Loops (FEFLs), which is an application that links multiple PDSA cycles with Shewhart's control chart philosophy and is well suited to applying interventions in the complex, dynamic systems we see in healthcare today. Carayon continues the foundation concepts of methodology with an overview of the application of human factors principles to intervention design and implementation. Ogden talks about how to differentiate the core and variation components of an intervention, and Aron and Leykum round off our introduction to methodology with a discussion of the critical contribution of sensemaking and identifying patterns in complexity to developing and implementing successful change.

We then begin a series of essays on applying some of the key IS tools that were introduced in Part I. Rapport and Zurynski warm us to the essays that follow on methodology and methods of IS with an essay on the value of methodological diversity to address the messy problems we see in healthcare and how it can furnish a richness to our understanding of the healthcare system. Lorencatto then begins a deeper dive into specific methodologies with a discussion on the use and limitations of the Theoretical Domains Framework (TDF). Waring and Clarke present an introduction to ethnography and its uses in IS, and then Rapport returns to talk about a variation on ethnography involving the movement of the observer through the environment, or "mobile methods". Hollnagel and Clay-Williams introduce the Functional Resonance Analysis Method (FRAM), in this case a tool for process mapping and identifying variation in complex processes. Pivoting again, there are long talks about the application of Social Network Analysis (SNA) to understanding the complex interplay of interactions between clinicians, consumers, and other healthcare stakeholders. J. Smith introduces the method of sentiment analysis, followed by Palinkas, who rounds off this group

DOI: 10.4324/9781003109945-21

of essays with a discussion on how to combine tools using mixed method quantitative and qualitative approaches.

Following the essays on some of the key methodologies of IS, we then turn to a range of methods that are gaining traction as innovative and useful ways of understanding and improving everyday work in healthcare and hospitals. Patterson and Deutsch introduce patient simulation and discuss its contribution to patient safety. Nakamura and Nakajima continue the conversation with two illustrative examples of how in situ simulation contributes to clinician learning and to improved team functioning in a hospital. Following on from these practical exemplars, Øvretveit introduces the concept of "emergency" implementation science, where fast change is required to address emerging situations. A. Smith and Hutchinson delve further into the practical aspects of implementation with a discussion on the importance of planning and how to do it successfully. Moving further into the practical application of the tools that have become so central to IS, Susskind discusses the importance of consensus building and bringing everyone along on the journey to shared understanding, and Lamprell introduces readers to "nudge" as a way to get this process started. Staying with the practicalities of IS, Ludlow and Westbrook provide an introduction to dashboards, both as a way to monitor improvement associated with an intervention and as an intervention in itself to improve health system functioning. Leykum then returns, asking us to pay attention to stories as a way of sensemaking when instituting change. Finally, we finish Part II with an essay from von Thiele Schwarz, Hasson, and Aarons on the need for, and implications of, adaptation. Together, these essays offer a comprehensive understanding and intriguing insight into the range, scope, and power of the right methodologies to underpin methods that drive rigorous research in the IS space.

19 Application

Nick Sevdalis and Louise Hull

This essay focuses on the question, "How applied is implementation science?" On the one hand, this is an oxymoron for a science that focuses on accelerating the transition of evidence into practice. On the other hand, there is a potential disconnect, we believe, between healthcare staff whose role is to implement interventions, programs, and policies and implementation scientists who study implementation processes, strategies, and measures.

Implementation science can only be a very applied health science. Early conceptualizations situated implementation science at the right-hand side of the translational pathway (Thornicroft, Lempp, and Tansella 2011). It is a science aiming to apply concepts and measures often derived from broader psychological, social, and organizational sciences to the process of introducing newly developed clinical evidence and innovation into practice, hence identifying behavioural, cultural, and organizational bottlenecks and addressing them (Boulton, Sandall, and Sevdalis 2020).

However, perusal of peer-reviewed journals suggests that our scientific community is focused on theory development and applications of implementation concepts and measures within the context of large-scale, often lengthy, clinical trials. For the purposes of this essay, we consider 2006 as an arbitrary starting point for the formal *inception* of the field – this is when the first specialist peer-reviewed journal was launched (Eccles and Mittman 2006). In the 15 years since, there has been a burgeoning literature on implementation theories and frameworks – several dozen of them have been developed and are currently in use in a rather short space of time (Damschroder 2020, Nilsen 2015). An optimistic appraisal of this state of affairs is that the field remains intellectually curious and very productive; a pessimistic view of it is that the field is rapidly becoming a conceptual Tower of Babel, in which even when theories are used, they are superficially or inconsistently applied (Birken et al. 2017).

There are interesting parallels here between implementation science and related fields of scientific enquiry similarly aimed at improving practice. One such field is improvement science, where similar debates have been taking place over at least two decades (Davidoff et al. 2015, The Health Foundation 2011). The tension there is found between the development of the science of improvement (with a focus on measurement and theory, not dissimilar to that found in implementation science) and the (larger) body of quality improvement specialists typically found in most healthcare organizations globally, whose roles revolve around fast-paced, practical improvement solutions to everyday pressing clinical problems. Mirroring recent debates within the field of implementation, improvement scientists have commented on poor application of even flagship improvement techniques, such as the Plan, Do, Study, Act technique (Taylor et al. 2014). Another field where similar tensions have been identified is organizational psychology. Organizational psychologists have long been reflecting on what is described as an "academic-practitioner divide" (Church 2011). They have found

DOI: 10.4324/9781003109945-22

that organizational psychology practitioners face significant barriers, including their relationship with their business partners or clients, in applying evidence from their own field into their practice (Bartlett and Francis-Smythe 2016). A useful conceptualization of the divide places organizational psychology research on "high/low relevance × high/low rigour" 2 × 2 framework and articulates researchers versus organizational or business clients as different stakeholders, with different needs, interested in different deliverables (Anderson, Herriot, and Hodgkinson 2001).

There are several indications that implementation scientists have started to acknowledge such tensions and are attempting to address them. First, substantial efforts have been made to map and synthesize competencies for implementation researchers and practitioners (Moore and Khan 2020, Tabak et al. 2017, Albers, Metz, and Burke 2020). Establishing these subsequently allows training programs to be developed, targeting either or both groups (Davis and D'Lima 2020, Davis et al. 2020, Moore et al. 2018). Second, capacity development efforts are further supported by novel toolkits developed with the aim to guide researchers and practitioners through the ever-expansive frameworks and taxonomies of the field and assist them in setting up high-quality implementation projects. The recently developed Implementation Science Research Development (ImpRes) tool offers such a facilitated application of the methods and concepts of the field to users with less exposure to them (Hull et al. 2019). Lastly, the COVID-19 pandemic has brought to the fore the need for implementation science to engage proactively with practical and urgent implementation challenges forced upon health systems globally (Wensing et al. 2020). The pandemic represents a substantial opportunity for implementation science to reaffirm its orientation towards clinical practice and policy applications. Many implementation science centres and groups are precisely undertaking this role. In our own centre, the Centre for Implementation Science at King's College, the response to the pandemic included the rapid development of an "implementation and evaluation resource", to be used as a quick reference guide for rapid health service reconfigurations due to the pandemic (e.g., shift from face-to-face to virtual clinics) and subsequent pragmatic evaluations to determine sustainability (see Box 19.1 for the development process and for the resource).

We have briefly highlighted a potential tension between implementation science and its application, contextualized it through comparisons with similar applied fields of science, and pointed towards current directions which we feel are fruitful for the future. We hope the essay will spark further analysis and debate.

Box 19.1   The "Implementation and Evaluation Resource" developed by the Centre for Implementation Science at King's College for use during COVID-19 rapid service reconfigurations and innovations

The interactive resource to support rapid implementation and evaluation of health and social care innovations, interventions, and new services during the COVID-19 pandemic was developed as a direct result of the support requests we received from our partner organizations, as well as our direct involvement in COVID-19-related implementation projects during the early stages of the pandemic (March–May 2020).

Given the need to rapidly respond to these requests, a pragmatic approach to the development of the resource was taken. We aimed to create a digestible and practical resource to support implementation efforts. An obvious starting point was to review the Implementation Science Research Development (ImpRes) tool and guide, which supports users in the design of implementation research. We sought to identify which ImpRes domains were of particular importance and relevance to implementing change rapidly and under crisis conditions.

A small team of academics with implementation and improvement science expertise initiated the development process. The content of the resource was drafted and shared with a wider team of applied health scientists, program directors of the regional Academic Heath Science Network (Health Innovation Network, which focuses on spread and adoption of healthcare innovations across all of South London, UK: https:// healthinnovationnetwork.com/), and other stakeholders through a "snowball" approach (frontline healthcare professionals, service managers, clinical service leads). Communication experts were consulted to optimize the wording and design of the resource. Through this process, we gathered rapid feedback and suggested improvements, as a result of which the content of the resource was refined. Significant amendments were made to the wording of key implementation science concepts and associated terminology. For example, amendments were made to how implementation strategies were described, to ensure that the resource was accessible to a wide audience.

This pragmatic and collaborative effort resulted in the inclusion of six implementation and evaluation domains that those involved in implementing change should consider to 1) identify factors likely to affect successful implementation, 2) identify strategies to facilitate rapid and successful implementation, 3) understand early adoption, 4) support ongoing implementation, 5) keep things going or decide to stop, and 6) be mindful of unintended consequences and widening health and social inequities. Upon finalization of the content, we commissioned a design company to develop and create the resource, which was launched in July 2020 and has been in use since (see Appendix for the full resource).

Source: Created by author

References

Albers, B., A. Metz, and K. Burke. 2020. "Implementation support practitioners – a proposal for consolidating a diverse evidence base." *BMC Health Services Research* 20 (1):368. doi: 10.1186/s12913-020-05145-1.

Anderson, N., P. Herriot, and G. P. Hodgkinson. 2001. "The practitioner-researcher divide in Industrial, Work and Organizational (IWO) psychology: Where are we now, and where do we go from here?" *Journal of Occupational and Organizational Psychology* 74 (4):391–411. doi: 10.1348/096317901167451.

Bartlett, D., and J. Francis-Smythe. 2016. "Bridging the divide in work and organizational psychology: Evidence from practice." *European Journal of Work and Organizational Psychology* 25 (5): 615–630. doi: 10.1080/1359432X.2016.1156672.

Birken, S. A., B. J. Powell, C. M. Shea, E. R. Haines, M. Alexis Kirk, J. Leeman, C. Rohweder, L. J. Damschroder, and J. Presseau. 2017. "Criteria for selecting implementation science theories and frameworks: Results from an international survey." *Implementation Science* 12 (1):124. doi: 10.1186/s13012-017-0656-y.

Boulton, R., J. Sandall, and N. Sevdalis. 2020. "The cultural politics of 'Implementation Science'." *Journal of Medical Humanities* 41 (3):379–394. doi: 10.1007/s10912-020-09607-9.

Church, A. H. 2011 "Bridging the gap between the science and practice of psychology in organizations: State of the practice reflections." *Journal of Business and Psychology* 26 (2):125–128. doi: 10.1007/s10869-011-9229-2.

Damschroder, L. J. 2020. "Clarity out of chaos: Use of theory in implementation research." *Psychiatry Research* 283:112461. doi: 10.1016/j.psychres.2019.06.036.

Davidoff, F., M. Dixon-Woods, L. Leviton, and S. Michie. 2015. "Demystifying theory and its use in improvement." *BMJ Quality and Safety* 24 (3):228–238. doi: 10.1136/bmjqs-2014-003627 %J BMJ Quality & Safety.

Davis, R., and D. D'Lima. 2020. "Building capacity in dissemination and implementation science: A systematic review of the academic literature on teaching and training initiatives." *Implementation Science* 15 (1):97. doi: 10.1186/s13012-020-01051-6.

Davis, R., B. Mittman, M. Boyton, A. Keohane, L. Goulding, J. Sandall, G. Thornicroft, and N. Sevdalis. 2020. "Developing implementation research capacity: Longitudinal evaluation of the King's College London Implementation Science Masterclass, 2014–2019." *Implementation Science Communications* 1:74. doi: 10.1186/s43058-020-00066-w.

Eccles, M. P., and B. S. Mittman. 2006. "Welcome to Implementation Science." *Implementation Science* 1 (1):1. doi: 10.1186/1748-5908-1-1.

Hull, L., L. Goulding, Z. Khadjesari, R. Davis, A. Healey, I. Bakolis, and N. Sevdalis. 2019. "Designing high-quality implementation research: Development, application, feasibility and preliminary evaluation of the implementation science research development (ImpRes) tool and guide." *Implementation Science* 14 (1):80. doi: 10.1186/s13012-019-0897-z.

Moore, J., and S. Khan. 2020. *Core Competencies for Implementation Science*. Toronto, Canada: The Center for Implementation and Health Canada.

Moore, J. E., S. Rashid, J. S. Park, S. Khan, and S. E. Straus. 2018. "Longitudinal evaluation of a course to build core competencies in implementation practice." *Implementation Science* 13 (1):106. doi: 10.1186/s13012-018-0800-3.

Nilsen, P. 2015. "Making sense of implementation theories, models and frameworks." *Implementation Science* 10 (1):53. doi: 10.1186/s13012-015-0242-0.

Tabak, R. G., M. M. Padek, J. F. Kerner, K. C. Stange, E. K. Proctor, M. J. Dobbins, G. A. Colditz, D. A. Chambers, and R. C. Brownson. 2017. "Dissemination and implementation science training needs: Insights from practitioners and researchers." *American Journal of Preventive Medicine* 52 (3 Suppl 3):S322–S329. doi: 10.1016/j.amepre.2016.10.005.

Taylor, M. J., C. McNicholas, C. Nicolay, A. Darzi, D. Bell, and J. E. Reed. 2014. "Systematic review of the application of the plan – do – study – act method to improve quality in healthcare." *BMJ Quality & Safety* 23 (4):290–298. doi: 10.1136/bmjqs-2013-001862 %J BMJ Quality & Safety.

The Health Foundation. 2011. "Evidence scan: Improvement science." www.health.org.uk/publications/improvement-science

Thornicroft, G., H. Lempp, and M. Tansella. 2011. "The place of implementation science in the translational medicine continuum." *Psychological Medicine* 41 (10):2015–2021. doi: 10.1017/s0033291711000109.

Wensing, M., A. Sales, R. Armstrong, and P. Wilson. 2020. "Implementation science in times of Covid-19." *Implementation Science* 15 (1):42. doi: 10.1186/s13012-020-01006-x.

20 Plan, Do, Study, Act (PDSA)

Jeffrey Braithwaite

The Plan, Do, Study, Act (PDSA) activity cycle originated a century ago, in the 1920s, with one of the early gurus of quality control. Walter A. Shewhart was a polymath-type character who was often labelled as a physicist, engineer, mathematician, production scientist, management consultant, statistician, or some combination of these. He became interested in variation in data sets while he was working at Bell Telephone in New York in the United States and had the very bright idea that we should use control charts to make sure that business and manufacturing processes were able to be tracked and managed ("controlled") (see Figure 20.1) (Best and Neuhauser 2006).

The essential idea is that any data set can be mapped across time and by setting upper and lower limits to its variation, compared to its own average. In contrast to a control group versus an intervention group, data act as their own control. Tracking data this way can help us understand whether the data bounce around or are relatively stable and can provide signals for us to make predictions and take action. The versatility of control charts, which are often considered to be one of the seven tools of quality improvement, is immense. For any data which are plotted over time, a clear indication is given for when to intervene and what to do next.

It is not too difficult to make the link from a control chart to a PDSA cycle, which is exactly what Shewhart did. He worked collaboratively, having had these insights, with another giant of the improvement enterprise, W Edwards Deming. In point of fact, PDSA cycles are also known as Deming Cycles (Best and Neuhauser 2006).

If the control chart is monitored over time and the data tell us about variation from average performance, then we can start to think about how to improve that performance. We can in fact *plan* for improvement (P), *do* some improvement in a test (D), *study* and hence learn about the extent to which improvement is accomplished (S), and then *act* to determine what changes should be made to create further improvement (A) (see Figure 20.2) (Best and Neuhauser 2006).

PDSA cycles have become very widespread across healthcare and are represented in the academic literature. A search in PubMed, a bibliographic database, found 1,349 citations to the PDSA cycle in July 2021. PDSA has been used by quality and safety scholars and professionals to underpin improvements in all sorts of projects and programs of activity. Their importance in implementation science has also become clear over time: getting evidence into practice can be guided by a PDSA cycle. So, for example, an implementation science advocate can plan for the adoption or take-up of new evidence, do an intervention or improvement activity in support of adoption or take-up, study progress and discover how and to what extent evidence-based practice has changed, and act to improve things further by applying additional measures needed to further enhance evidence-based practice.

DOI: 10.4324/9781003109945-23

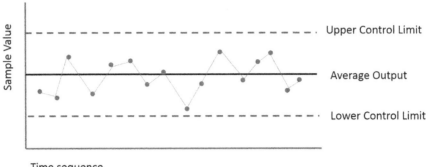

Figure 20.1 Simple control chart

Source: Reprinted from KaiNexus

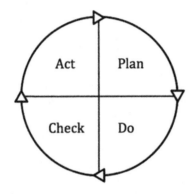

Figure 20.2 PDSA cycle

Source: Adapted from Taylor et al. 2014

References

Best, M., and D. Neuhauser. 2006. "Walter A Shewhart, 1924, and the Hawthorne factory." *BMJ Quality & Safety* 15 (2):142–143.

Taylor, M. J., C. McNicholas, C. Nicolay, A. Darzi, D. Bell, and J. E. Reed. 2014. "Systematic review of the application of the plan–do–study–act method to improve quality in healthcare." *BMJ Quality & Safety* 23 (4):290–298.

21 Formative Evaluation Feedback Loops

Jeffrey Braithwaite

The core idea of Formative Evaluation Feedback Loops (FEFLs) builds on the Plan, Do, Study, Act (PDSA) model or cycle, which was first developed a century ago, in the 1920s, with one of the early gurus of quality control, Walter A. Shewhart. That work conceptualized change as a cycle of activity and introduced PDSA and control charts so that change could be guided and monitored during each improvement project.

These days, everywhere you look in organizations and settings where quality improvement is taken seriously, people use control charts and PDSA cycles. One of the things that Shewhart and W Edwards Deming, another giant in the field of quality improvement no doubt thought about, but did not push far enough in their time, is to also create feedback loops in the system and add the idea of ongoing or formative evaluation so that the system's improvers can create impetus for further change. Dating from 2007, and published in 2012 (Braithwaite et al. 2012), we sought to bring all these concepts together in a model we called FEFLs (see Figure 21.1 and Table 21.1) (Braithwaite, Glasziou, and Westbrook 2020).

Feedback is a potentially powerful model for creating momentum for change. We know that it is often difficult to operationalize PDSA cycles over time and to continue the efforts after the initial excitement at the inception of an improvement program (Braithwaite, Marks, and Taylor 2014). Examples of feedback are to elicit information from patients about their progress post-surgery, providing 360-degree information to managers, and furnishing clinicians with data about their patients' length of stay and treatment outcomes benchmarked against clinicians with similar caseloads. Similarly, the idea of formative evaluation is to take a sounding of where a change process is at a point in time and use the information taken during the snapshot evaluation point to promote further change. This is also a potentially powerful mechanism for improvement.

These ideas are combined in the FEFLs model depicted in Figure 21.1. It is predicated on the core idea that we would like to change behaviour in a system by promoting ongoing improvement over time. In implementation science terms, this is about getting more evidence into practice with insight that this is not a one-off event, and nor is it achieved by one PDSA cycle of activity but by ongoing, longitudinal change over time.

FEFLs essentially bring together multiple PDSA cycles and build in such longitudinal progress. This is in contrast to what typically happens in healthcare organizations and other types of institutions where change is short-lived and things stumble from one improvement project to another – what has been labelled "projectitis" (Gaddis 1959).

In the FEFLs model, there are several factors which are important in promoting the long-term improvement we are seeking. These include adequately preparing for change in the first place, before initiating it; thinking through the capacity that is available within the organizational setting for the implementation being considered, such as the people involved and

DOI: 10.4324/9781003109945-24

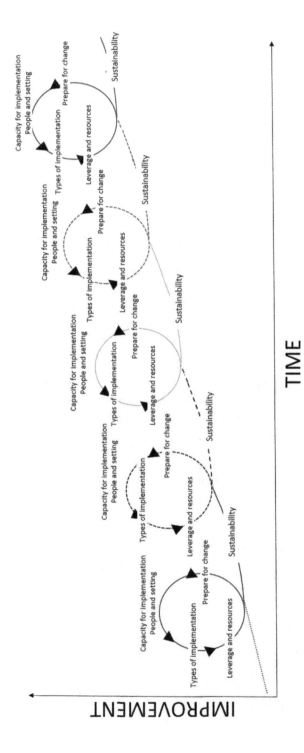

Figure 21.1 FEFLs diagram

Source: Originally published in Braithwaite, Glasziou, and Westbrook 2020. Adapted from Braithwaite, Marks, and Taylor 2014 and Braithwaite et al. 2007, with permission from Oxford University Press

Table 21.1 Glossary of terms

Control chart	A method for depicting data over time, also known as Statistical Process Monitoring. Data are tracked with reference to upper and lower control levels (UCL and LCL); if data fall outside of these levels, it signals that a formal examination of the situation depicted by the data is needed.
Feedback, feedback loop	A recursive mechanism creating reciprocal behaviours which reverberate back in on themselves. A positive (self-reinforcing) feedback loop increases the rate of change of a factor, creating more of its own output. In a negative (self-correcting) feedback loop, the output responses dampen the change or modulate its direction.
FEFLs	Formative Evaluation Feedback Loops
Path dependence	Current events and circumstances are influenced by, and can be determined by, prior events and circumstances, harking back to the origins of the entity or system; path dependence underpins the point that "history matters".
PDSA	Plan, Do, Study, Act; a cycle of activity used in quality improvement.
Perturbation	An internal or external disruption or unexpected event which affects normal patterned behaviours, structures, or processes; often thought of as an external disturbance or interruption to the current state of affairs.
System dynamics	An analytical modelling methodology used for problem-solving, which combines qualitative and quantitative data and identifies the fundamental elements of a system, and how they influence one another, over time.
Tipping point	A critical point in a system in which a kind of radical, potentially irreversible change may occur, resulting in a different state of system behaviour which can settle into a new equilibrium.

Source: Modified from Braithwaite et al. (2018)

the characteristic of the setting; choosing the type of implementation we want; seeking an optimal, fit-for-purpose design; and securing sufficient leverage and resources to continue the momentum (Braithwaite, Glasziou, and Westbrook 2020). The goal is then to build in sustainability, meaning that the change that has been produced in one cycle is sufficiently anchored in and sufficiently sustained until the next cycle of the change journey.

Applied to implementation science more squarely, it is clear that if implementation science is about getting evidence into practice, or creating an evidence base for implementation and improvement as discussed across the pages of this book, then control charts and PDSA cycles, conjoined with powerful concepts such as feedback and formative evaluation, encoded in a FEFLs design, offer a very attractive model for ongoing change and improvement.

FEFLs offer three important additional design features to the standard PDSA template. They focus the attention of users on the fact that most change is longitudinal rather than bound to one particular event, that ongoing evaluation of the change is important, and that the introduction of feedback provides a mechanism for building momentum and making further performance gains.

References

Braithwaite, J., K. Churruca, J. C. Long, L. A. Ellis, and J. Herkes. 2018. "When complexity science meets implementation science: A theoretical and empirical analysis of systems change." *BMC Medicine* 16 (1):63. doi: 10.1186/s12916-018-1057-z.

Braithwaite, J., P. Glasziou, and J. Westbrook. 2020. "The three numbers you need to know about healthcare: The 60–30–10 Challenge." *BMC Medicine* 18:1–8.

Braithwaite, J., D. Marks, and N. Taylor. 2014. "Harnessing implementation science to improve care quality and patient safety: A systematic review of targeted literature." *International Journal of Quality in Health Care* 26 (3):321–329. doi: 10.1093/intqhc/mzu047.

Braithwaite, J., J. Westbrook, A. Foxwell, R. Boyce, T. Devinney, M. Budge, K. Murphy, M. Ryall, J. Beutel, R. Vanderheide, E. Renton, J. Travaglia, J. Stone, A. Barnard, D. Greenfield, A. Corbett, P. Nugus, and R. Clay-Williams. 2007. "An action research protocol to strengthen system-wide inter-professional learning and practice." *BMC Health Services Research* 7 (144):1–10. doi: 10.1186/1472-6963-7-144.

Braithwaite, J., M. Westbrook, P. Nugus, D. Greenfield, J. Travaglia, W. Runciman, A. R. Foxwell, R. A. Boyce, T. Devinney, and J. Westbrook. 2012. "A four-year, systems-wide intervention promoting interprofessional collaboration." *BMC Health Services Research* 12 (1):99.

Gaddis, P. O. 1959. *The Project Manager*. Boston, MA: Harvard University.

22 Implementation or continuous design? The contribution of human factors and engineering to healthcare quality and patient safety

Pascale Carayon

Implementation of healthcare interventions such as cancer screening, rapid response systems, and clinical guidelines can involve many changes in how healthcare work is performed and organized, both individually and collectively. Therefore, implementation is about intervening on activities (or work) performed by healthcare workers, patients, and caregivers and the context or system in which they perform these activities. Implementation science focuses on understanding, evaluating, and improving the change process of getting evidence into practice. This change process is also a *work system design process*: the intervention should be designed to fit within the work system in which it is implemented. Designing a work system that produces positive outcomes for people and organizations is the key objective of the human factors (and ergonomics) discipline (Dul et al. 2012). We propose that implementation of healthcare interventions should incorporate methods and approaches of the human factors engineering (HFE)[1] scientific discipline, which "is concerned with the understanding of interactions among humans and other elements of a system" and uses this knowledge to improve the design of work systems "in order to optimise human well-being and overall system performance" (International Ergonomics Association 2000).

HFE is about *designing useful and usable interventions*, such as technologies, processes, and physical environments. HFE methods and principles can be used to improve the physical, cognitive, and organizational design of healthcare interventions. HFE emphasizes the need to understand the *actual work*[2] *performed* by physicians, nurses, patients, caregivers, and other people involved in healthcare; this work system analysis is an important step of the human-centred design process advocated by HFE and relies on a range of well-documented HFE methods and approaches. For instance, an extensive body of HFE knowledge is about usability of devices and health information technologies and includes multiple methods, such as task and process analysis, heuristic evaluation and user testing, and design principles, such as consistency and workflow integration. Such HFE methods and approaches have helped to improve the design of technologies, such as clinical decision support tools (Carayon et al. 2020) and code cart (Rousek and Hallbeck 2011). When healthcare interventions are "well-designed", that is, designed according to HFE methods and principles, they are more likely to be accepted; therefore, their implementation will be facilitated.

HFE is a large discipline with multiple approaches and perspectives; some target micro-level interactions, such as the physical design of infusion devices and patient rooms, and cognitive design of alarms and decision support tools. Increasingly, HFE has emphasized macro-level approaches, also known as macroergonomics or "systems ergonomics" (Wilson 2014). The macroergonomic Systems Engineering Initiative for Patient Safety (SEIPS) model of work system and patient safety conceptualizes a healthcare work system as composed of elements (i.e., person, task, tools and technologies, as well as physical environment

DOI: 10.4324/9781003109945-25

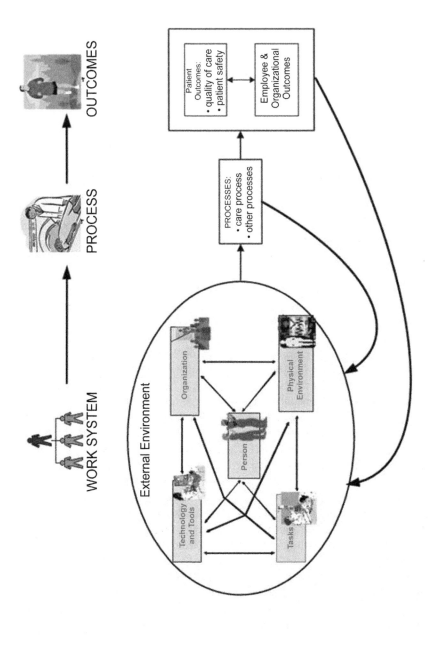

Figure 22.1 SEIPS model of work system and patient safety

Source: Adapted from Carayon et al. 2006, with permission from Elsevier

and organization) and emphasizes interactions between system elements, which in turn can influence care process, patient outcomes, and employee/organizational outcomes (see Figure 22.1) (Carayon et al. 2006, 2014). This HFE systems model can be used to improve the design of healthcare interventions as it draws attention to *all elements of the work system and their interactions*. Professionals and researchers involved in implementing a healthcare intervention need to think about the intervention's influence on all elements of the work system and their interactions. Identifying work system barriers and facilitators of an intervention can help to improve its design and its integration in the care process. This has been done for a range of healthcare interventions, such as infection prevention practices (Musuuza et al. 2017).

When an intervention is implemented in a complex healthcare work system, system elements and their interactions change and evolve over time; some of the changes may have been anticipated, but many changes will *emerge* and be surprises. We need to do our best to anticipate some of the negative consequences, for example, via an HFE proactive risk assessment method (Carayon et al. 2011). We need to apply HFE methods and approaches and invest in a human-centred design process to create an intervention that is as well-designed as possible. But we should also expect to be surprised. Therefore, we need mechanisms to understand and assess these emergent changes and engage in a process of *continuous work system design*; these are the feedback loops in the SEIPS model (see Figure 22.1). Implementation is often thought as a one-shot activity or a project; we advocate for a conceptualization of implementation as a continuous improvement process where changes will emerge over time. This implies that designing a healthcare intervention, and the work system in which it is embedded, should rely on a continuous design process (Carayon et al. 2008).

As outlined above, in order to improve the design, implementation, acceptance, and impact of healthcare interventions, HFE advocates for a deep understanding of the actual work and work system. Therefore, the continuous design process requires involvement of the people who are at the centre of the work system. HFE has developed a range of participatory design approaches, also known as *participatory ergonomics*. In healthcare, participatory ergonomics has been applied to improve the physical design of work (Driessen et al. 2010), the design of the bedside rounding process in a paediatric hospital (Xie et al. 2015), and the safety of inpatient medication management (Ibrahim Shire, Jun, and Robinson 2020).

Implementation science is increasingly paying attention to the complexity of interventions, the context in which interventions are implemented, and the process by which transformation occurs (or does not occur) (Braithwaite et al. 2018). This discussion has been enriched by other disciplines and approaches, such as complexity science. The HFE discipline provides an additional perspective for implementation science: its human-centred design methods and approaches can be used to continuously improve the design of healthcare interventions and make them more useful and usable. This will go a long way in supporting healthcare quality and patient safety.

Notes

1 In this essay I use the term "human factors engineering" to emphasize the engineering perspective of my approach to the continuous design of work systems.
2 In the French ergonomics literature, the actual work is referred to as "activity", in contrast to the prescribed task.(Leplat 1989, Daniellou 2005) This has been recently called as the difference between "Work-as-Done" and "Work-as-Imagined".

References

Braithwaite, J., K. Churruca, J. C. Long, L. A. Ellis, and J. Herkes. 2018. "When complexity science meets implementation science: A theoretical and empirical analysis of systems change." *BMC Medicine* 16 (1):63. doi: 10.1186/s12916-018-1057-z.

Carayon, P., H. Faye, A. S. Hundt, B.-T. Karsh, and T. Wetterneck. 2011. "Patient safety and proactive risk assessment." In *Handbook of Healthcare Delivery Systems*, edited by Y. Yuehwern, 12–1/12–15. Boca Raton, FL: Taylor & Francis.

Carayon, P., P. Hoonakker, A. S. Hundt, M. Salwei, D. Wiegmann, R. L. Brown, P. Kleinschmidt, C. Novak, M. Pulia, Y. Wang, E. Wirkus, and B. Patterson. 2020. "Application of human factors to improve usability of clinical decision support for diagnostic decision-making: A scenario-based simulation study." *BMJ Quality & Safety* 29:329–340. doi: 10.1136/bmjqs-2019-009857.

Carayon, P., A. S. Hundt, B.-T. Karsh, A. P. Gurses, C. J. Alvarado, M. Smith, and P. F. Brennan. 2006. "Work system design for patient safety: The SEIPS model." *Quality & Safety in Health Care* 15 (Suppl I):i50–i58.

Carayon, P., T. B. Wetterneck, A. S. Hundt, S. Rough, and M. Schroeder. 2008. "Continuous technology implementation in health care: The case of advanced IV infusion pump technology." In *Corporate Sustainability as a Challenge for Comprehensive Management*, edited by K. Zink, 139–151. New York: Springer.

Carayon, P., T. B. Wetterneck, A. J. Rivera-Rodriguez, A. S. Hundt, P. Hoonakker, R. Holden, and A. P. Gurses. 2014. "Human factors systems approach to healthcare quality and patient safety." *Applied Ergonomics* 45 (1):14–25.

Daniellou, F. 2005. "The French-speaking ergonomists' approach to work activity: Cross-influences of field intervention and conceptual models." *Theoretical Issues in Ergonomics Science* 6 (5):409–427.

Driessen, M. T., K. I. Proper, J. R. Anema, P. M. Bongers, and A. J. van der Beek. 2010. "Process evaluation of a participatory ergonomics programme to prevent low back pain and neck pain among workers." *Implementation Science* 5:65. doi: 10.1186/1748-5908-5-65.

Dul, J., R. Bruder, P. Buckle, P. Carayon, P. Falzon, W. S. Marras, J. R. Wilson, and B. van der Doelen. 2012. "A strategy for human factors/ergonomics: Developing the discipline and profession." *Ergonomics* 55 (4):377–395.

Ibrahim Shire, M., G. T. Jun, and S. Robinson. 2020. "Healthcare workers' perspectives on participatory system dynamics modelling and simulation: Designing safe and efficient hospital pharmacy dispensing systems together." *Ergonomics* 63 (8):1044–1056. doi: 10.1080/00140139.2020.1783459.

International Ergonomics Association. 2000. "The discipline of ergonomics." Accessed August 22, 2004. https://iea.cc/what-is-ergonomics/.

Leplat, J. 1989. "Error analysis, instrument and object of task analysis." *Ergonomics* 32 (7):813–822.

Musuuza, J. S., T. J. Roberts, P. Carayon, and N. Safdar. 2017. "Assessing the sustainability of daily chlorhexidine bathing in the intensive care unit of a Veteran's Hospital by examining nurses' perspectives and experiences." *BMC Infectious Diseases* 17 (1):75. doi: 10.1186/s12879-017-2180-8.

Rousek, J. B., and M. S. Hallbeck. 2011. "Improving medication management through the redesign of the hospital code cart medication drawer." *Human Factors* 53 (6):626–636. doi: 10.1177/0018720811426427.

Wilson, J. R. 2014. "Fundamentals of systems ergonomics/human factors." *Applied Ergonomics* 45 (1):5–13.

Xie, A., P. Carayon, E. D. Cox, R. Cartmill, Y. Li, T. B. Wetterneck, and M. M. Kelly. 2015. "Application of participatory ergonomics to the redesign of the family-centred rounds process." *Ergonomics*:1–19. doi: 10.1080/00140139.2015.1029534.

23 Core and variation components

Terje Ogden

Core components are the active ingredients that actually make an intervention work and benefit the user (Humphrey et al. 2016). Variation components, on the other hand, are additional components that can add to the effectiveness of the intervention or act as adaptation alternatives. *Core intervention components* are the most essential and effective ingredients that make an intervention work, while *core implementation components* are the most critical components for the successful implementation of an intervention (Fixsen et al. 2009). Core components also include contextual factors, such as the particular setting in which the intervention occurs (at home or at a treatment centre); structural elements, such as the obligatory number; and/or sequence of sessions and specific practices, such as techniques used to reinforce appropriate behaviour in a behaviour management intervention. Core intervention components that have been shown to produce reliable effects can be used separately or in combination to form more complex interventions or programs. *Intervention kernels* are single components assumed to produce change in human behaviour, for instance, the use of "praise" and "timeout" in parenting. But most core components are parts of a comprehensive program or intervention, and it is not clear how much their effectiveness is reliant on the other elements, processes, and the context of the intervention.

Based on their synthesis of the research literature on implementation, Fixsen et al. (2009) identified the following implementation components which they named *core implementation drivers*: careful staff selection, ongoing training and coaching, performance and program evaluation, facilitative administrative support, and systems interventions. Even if these are considered to be core components, they are also integrated and compensatory, that is, integrated in order to maximize their influence on staff behaviour and the organizational culture. They may compensate for each other so that weakness in one component can be overcome by strengths in other components. A major implementation effort has been underway in medicine in order to reduce research findings and best practices to "clinical guidelines" that can be used by medical staff to eliminate errors, reduce variability, and improve consumer outcomes. But research has shown that modifying practitioners' behaviour to conform more closely to practice guidelines and manuals has proven to be a difficult task in medicine as it has in other disciplines (Bellg et al. 2004, Luciano, Aloia, and Brett 2019).

Most complex interventions or intervention programs consist not only of core components but also of variation components that are alternatives that maintain the function of the core elements if these are not available or appropriate. Children may not have parents available, but close relations with grandparents or older siblings may be a viable substitute in a parenting intervention. Families that are reluctant to show up in outpatient clinics can be offered home visits. Variation components may also be important but not vital in relation to outcomes as when school homework is carried out at school rather than at home.

DOI: 10.4324/9781003109945-26

Interventionists may, based on their generic competence and familiarity with the intervention and the local context, add or subtract from the original manual in order to improve outcomes. Because of geographical and cultural variation in locations and services, intervention models have to be adapted to local conditions in order to be implemented and produce positive outcomes. Variation may be considered as a way of eliminating quality problems by adapting a standard treatment or practice to the different needs or characteristics of clients but without compromising the core components of the intervention as described in a research protocol (Langley et al. 2009).

In Norway, core components have been central to the process of testing and implementing research-based treatment programs for children and youth with serious conduct problems and their families. These are Parent Management Training, the Oregon model (PMTO) (Ogden et al. 2018) and Multisystemic Therapy (MST) (Henggeler et al. 2009). Research on the core components of PMTO has identified the following core components: 1) positive reinforcement to promote prosocial behaviour, 2) effective limit setting to decrease deviant behaviour, 3) monitoring to ensure that behaviour stays on track, 4) family problem-solving to provide skills to prevent and manage stress and conflict, and 5) positive involvement to emphasize the importance of spending time together in pleasant activity (Forgatch, Patterson, and Gewirtz 2013). In PMTO, the core components are monitored with a Fidelity of Implementation measure (Knutson, Forgatch, and Rains 2003) in which therapist behaviour and client interaction are assessed and rated based on video recordings.

MST is an adolescent-oriented program in which the core intervention components are formulated as nine theoretical principles, and adherence to these is measured on a monthly basis with the Therapist Adherence Measure-Revised (TAM-R) (Multisystemic Therapy Institute 2018). Each family undergoing treatment receives a monthly phone call by a non-clinical employee and is asked 25 questions related to the nine principles. The therapists and teams are evaluated according to the fidelity scores they receive from families, and a cut-off score indicates the level of implementation quality. Variation components include meetings with the family or the adolescent at their home, or at another place in the local community, variations in the number and length of meetings, and matching the structure of the treatment to the travel distance between therapist and client.

The challenge of implementing evidence-based practices is to strike a good balance between fidelity and adaptation to the local context. Fidelity to the core components of an evidence-based intervention is usually required in order to obtain optimal outcomes. But variation components are equally important in order to adapt the intervention to the local context, including staff variations (training, profession, and experience), culture, and attitudes.

References

Bellg, A. J., B. Borrelli, B. Resnick, J. Hecht, D. S. Minicucci, M. Ory, G. Ogedegbe, D. Orwig, D. Ernst, and S. Czajkowski. 2004. "Enhancing treatment fidelity in health behavior change studies: Best practices and recommendations from the NIH Behavior Change Consortium." *Health Psychology* 23 (5):443.

Fixsen, D. L., K. A. Blase, S. F. Naoom, and F. Wallace. 2009. "Core implementation components." *Research on Social Work Practice* 19 (5):531–540.

Forgatch, M. S., G. R. Patterson, and A. H. Gewirtz. 2013. "Looking forward: The promise of widespread implementation of parent training programs." *Perspectives on Psychological Science* 8 (6):682–694.

Henggeler, S. W., S. K. Schoenwald, C. M. Borduin, M. D. Rowland, and P. B. Cunningham. 2009. *Multisystemic Therapy for Antisocial Behavior in Children and Adolescents*. New York: Guilford Press.

Humphrey, N., A. Lendrum, E. Ashworth, K. Frearson, R. Buck, and K. Kerr. 2016. *Implementation and Process Evaluation (IPE) for Interventions in Education Settings: An Introductory Handbook*. Edited by Education Endowment Foundation (Ed.). London: Education Endowment Foundation.

Knutson, N. M., M. S. Forgatch, and L. A. Rains. 2003. "Fidelity of implementation rating system (FIMP): The training manual for PMTO." Eugene: Oregon Social Learning Center.

Langley, G. J., R. D. Moen, K. M. Nolan, T. W. Nolan, C. L. Norman, and L. P. Provost. 2009. *The Improvement Guide: A Practical Approach to Enhancing Organizational Performance*. Hoboken, NJ: John Wiley & Sons.

Luciano, M., T. Aloia, and J. Brett. 2019. "4 ways to make evidence-based practice the norm in health care." *Harvard Business Review*.

Multisystemic Therapy Institute. 2018. "The therapist adherence measure-revised (TAM-R)." MST Institute. https://msti.org/mstinstitute/qa_program/tam.html.

Ogden, T., E. Askeland, B. Christensen, T. Christiansen, and J. Kjøbli. 2018. "Crossing national, cultural, and language barriers: Implementing and testing evidence-based practices in Norway." In *Evidence Based Psychotherapies with Children and Adolescents*, edited by J. Weisz and A. Kazdin. New York, NY: The Guilford Press.

24 Sensemaking

Appreciating patterns and coherence in complexity

David C. Aron and Luci K. Leykum

People alone or in groups have been making sense of things (or not) since time immemorial and certainly longer than academics have used the term "sensemaking" and exhaustively parsed its meanings from the perspectives of different academic disciplines (Weick 1995, Maitlis and Christianson 2014, Klein, Moon, and Hoffman 2006, Kolko 2010). At its core, sensemaking is the process by which individuals and collectives give meaning to an experience that is somehow at odds with expectations so as to enable action. It is about giving structure to the unknown (Ancona 2012). Sensemaking is a dynamic process which involves identification of salient cues, making connections between them, creating a rational account, and then acting upon it. The cues (people, artefacts, events) are found in the context which has been defined as "the circumstances that form the setting for an event, statement, or idea, and in terms of which it can be fully understood and assessed" (Oxford Dictionaries). Things are experienced in a context, that is to say, the circumstances, conditions, surroundings, factors, state of affairs, frame of reference, situation, environment, or milieu in which they occur.

So, what about sensemaking in the way described and implementation? In implementation practice, context is critical, and effective implementation of an intervention can be said to reflect (and depend on) how the intervention interacts with the context (i.e., the intervention by context interaction). Let's examine context in a little more detail. When aspects of the context are at odds with expectations, one's mental model no longer fits, and a new mental model needs to be created that better accounts for the observed reality. Effective sensemaking is built on a foundation of several abilities. When faced with a mass of sensory experience, we have to pick out the important things, select the right or salient "dots", and connect them. How we connect them is the structure that gives meaning to them. Cognitive flexibility, defined as "the readiness with which the person's concept system changes selectively in response to appropriate environmental stimuli" (Scott 1962), enables us to identify particular aspects as dots whether they appear in one dimension of concepts or another. Analogical reasoning provides a means to identify the dots by application of knowledge of a similarly acting system to the problem at hand. Systems thinking – focusing on structures and patterns in the environment – provides a way of connecting the dots, but with creativity, it also provides a means for identifying where dots should be even if you can't see them.

Take a weaving analogy. From a weaver's perspective, the cues make up the threads and the combination of systems thinking, analogical thinking, and cognitive flexibility make up the loom from which a pattern emerges from seeming disarray, making it possible for us to act upon it. It is not only a matter of weaving a tapestry, but rather visualizing and revisualizing it as the tapestry is made and modifying it along the way. Hence, sensemaking is dynamic and in its iterations uses different types of reasoning: fast and slow, heuristic and algorithmic

DOI: 10.4324/9781003109945-27

(Kahneman 2011). Each mode of thinking has its limitations. Heuristics or "rules of thumb" reduce the mental effort needed to make decisions and simplify complex issues, but they are subject to cognitive biases. For example, the availability bias refers to the ease with which something is brought to mind, and the representative bias involves comparing the present situation to the most representative mental model. These can lead to overlooking more relevant information, in short, oversimplifying the situation. Algorithms are linear step-by-step logical instructions for a computation, diagnosis, or decision, but they tend to break down in the non-linear world of people. When Earnest Rutherford said, "The only possible conclusion that social sciences can draw is some do, some don't," it was probably not meant as a compliment. Yet, it is that world of people and interactions in which sensemaking happens and in which change has to be made.

Sensemaking, whether an individual cognitive exercise or a social process (Jordan et al. 2009), is critical in implementation (Castillo 2020, Luig et al. 2018). Sensemaking is inherent in the variety of methods used in making changes in situations which are partially structured and partially predictable. These approaches include the Plan, Do, Study, Act cycle of Deming in which the Study phase involves making sense, that is to say, abstracting from the findings of the test of change (Moen 2009). Similarly, the Orient phase of Observe, Orient, Decide, Act (Boy's OODA loop) (Richards 2012) is one of sensemaking as is the Sense phase of the Sense, Respond, Probe of the Cynefin process of Snowden (Fietz 2013). Whether joining the process as consultant (internal or external) or being an integral part of the initial team, it is necessary to know the rules of the game and how the game is played – and this involves sensemaking. The most effective leaders and implementors can do this well and do it while they are playing the game (Arthur 1996, Jaworski and Scharmer 2000). In summary, sensemaking is an essential process in enabling us to negotiate our way in the world by identifying patterns and creating a coherent picture that can guide our actions.

References

Ancona, D. 2012. "Sensemaking: Framing and acting in the unknown." In *The Handbook for Teaching Leadership*, edited by S. Snook, N. Nohria and R. Khurana, 3–19. Thousand Oaks, CA: Sage Publishing.

Arthur, W. 1996. "Increasing returns and the new world of business." *Harvard Business Review* July–August:100–109.

Castillo, J. 2020. "The intersection between systems change, implementation science, and human beings: A call to investigate people and context in future systems-level consultation research." *Journal of Educational and Psychological Consultation* February 22:1–10.

Fietz, M. 2013. *Approaches to Adaptive Iteration: A Comparative Review*.

Jaworski, J., and C. Scharmer. 2000. *Leadership in the New Economy: Sensing and Actualizing Emerging Futures*. Houston, TX: Generon Consulting.

Jordan, M., H. Lanham, B. Crabtree, P. Nutting, W. Miller, K. Stange, and R. McDaniel. 2009. "The role of conversation in health care interventions: Enabling sensemaking and learning." *Implementation Science* 4 (1):15.

Kahneman, D. 2011. *Thinking, Fast and Slow*. 1st ed. ed. New York: Farrar, Straus and Giroux.

Klein, G., B. Moon, and R. Hoffman. 2006. "Making sense of sensemaking 1: Alternative perspectives." *IEEE Intelligent Systems* 21 (4):70–73.

Kolko, J. 2010. *Sensemaking and Framing: A Theoretical Reflection on Perspective in Design Synthesis*. Design Research Society (DRS) International Conference 2010, 7–9 July, Montreal, Canada.

Luig, T., J. Asselin, A. Sharma, and D. Campbell-Scherer. 2018. "Understanding implementation of complex interventions in primary care teams." *The Journal of the American Board of Family Medicine* 31 (3):431–444.

Maitlis, S., and M. Christianson. 2014. "Sensemaking in organizations: Taking stock and moving forward." *Academy of Management Annals* 8 (1):57–125.

Moen, R. 2009. "Foundation and history of the PDSA cycle." Asian Network for Quality Conference, Tokyo.

Oxford Dictionaries. "Context | Definition of context." Accessed August 25, 2020. www.lexico.com/en/definition/context.

Richards, C. 2012. *Boyd's OODA Loop*. Atlanta, GA: J. Addams & Partners Inc.

Scott, W. 1962. "Cognitive complexity and cognitive flexibility." *Sociometry* December 1:405–414.

Weick, K. 1995. *Sensemaking in Organizations*. Thousand Oaks, CA: Sage Publications.

25 Methodological diversity

Frances Rapport and Yvonne Zurynski

Implementation science is currently experiencing a novel shift of focus regarding how research is conducted (Rapport and Braithwaite 2018, Braithwaite and Rapport 2020). In health and medical research contexts, this includes novel approaches to data collection and analysis and the mixing of methodologies and methods to more successfully assess service provision and patient care (Rapport and Braithwaite 2018). The resultant methodologies and their associated methods are diverse, yet can be coherent and flexible, and are able to be mobilized to make a sustained impact on healthcare systems and services (Rapport and Braithwaite 2018), with outcomes that recognize and may offer solutions to seemingly intractable system problems. In essence, methodological diversity, when at its most effective, can provide evidential, person-focused, and theoretically informed data to fashion evidence-based implementation.

The drive for methodological diversity is propelled by the desire for clear, appropriate translational pathways (Rapport et al. 2018a, 2018b), and when theory, design, and intent come together, this can lead to profoundly important research findings, well-considered actions, and new ways to implement system change. Indeed, we argue that methodological diversity is the hallmark of good implementation science. Just as our healthcare systems are widely varied and constantly adapting, so our research methods must adapt to the complexity and messiness of the real world, where a multitude of factors can stand in the way of clear implementation (Greenhalgh and Papoutsi 2018). Contextual factors define that messiness and may include local workforce characteristics, normative and cultural influences, new ways of working, characteristics of local populations, available resources, local policies, and governance structures.

Traditionally, randomized controlled trials (RCTs) have been the mainstay (the gold standard) of assessing the efficacy of interventions, but their applicability has been found to be limited when studying the implementation of interventions in the ever-evolving healthcare ecosystem (Schliep, Alonzo, and Morris 2017). Pragmatic trials and their linked methods are increasingly applied to intervention implementation (Haff and Choudhry 2018). In fact, the success of change interventions is as dependent on a pragmatic implementation process as it is on the evidence showing interventional effectiveness. When it comes to considering diverse methods for assessing adaptive healthcare systems, therefore, mixed methods, drawn from both quantitative and qualitative research paradigms, can be useful. Mixed methods enable researchers to study factors that help or hinder implementation from the viewpoint of the patient, the healthcare provider, and the healthcare system, while mixed methods data can be assessed through the application of, for example, the Consolidated Framework for Implementation Research (CFIR) to provide a guide and structure to data analysis (Kirk et al. 2015).

DOI: 10.4324/9781003109945-28

As part of the researcher's methodological portfolio, there may also be opportunities to embed economic evaluations into assessments of system adaptation. This includes not only the cost of system functioning but also the comparative economic evaluation of the implementation process (Eisman et al. 2020). In addition, longitudinal methods, which enable the measurement of an intervention's sustainability across time, are increasingly being used to determine how new interventions "normalize". "Normalize" refers to how complex interventions are operationalized and become part of the routine or norm, often according to processes outlined in Normalization Process Theory (NPT) (Agreli et al. 2019), with interventions examined as they translate (or fail to translate) into practice (Braithwaite et al. 2020, May et al. 2009). If longitudinal methods are adopted to measure intervention normalization and sustainability, it may also be important to consider how networks or communities of practice coalesce around adaptations. Social Network Analysis can help with this (see *Social Network Analysis* essays 1 and 30), supporting the evaluation of the evolution of such networks or communities of practice (Pomare et al. 2019). Methodological diversity applied to formative evaluation (a way of evaluating an intervention's potential for translation and impact) is also important (Stetler et al. 2006), if we want to develop a deeper understanding of the context of care and apply that understanding to change-implementation in healthcare systems (Nilsen and Bernhardsson 2019, Moullin et al. 2020). Figure 25.1 summarizes the main methodological approaches and

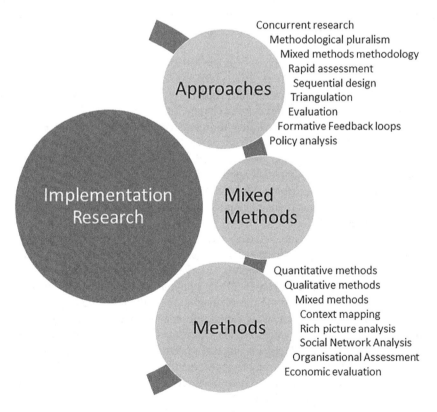

Figure 25.1 Methodological diversity for implementation science

Source: Created by authors

research methods that may be applied in different combinations, or adapted, depending on the research question and context.

Whether there is the need for a greater understanding of the world of messy healthcare systems, the inclusion of economic evaluation alongside longitudinal interventional assessment, or the clarification of multiple factors influencing implementation, methodological diversity will commonly call for responsive data triangulation (this refers to the use of multiple methods or data sources to examine a proposition from many angles and verify research findings more rigorously) as a result. Triangulation is a concept that predominates in qualitative research and was originally developed by Patton (1999). Triangulation has its own challenges, however, including yielding conflicting results (Rapport et al. 2020). But when conducted sensitively, mixed methods data triangulation can lead to "richer, more comprehensive findings, while posing the opportunity for a deeper understanding of the data and consideration of further research questions" (Rapport et al. 2020, 39). Having synthesized mixed methods data effectively, more rigorous evidence can then be translated into practice, while understanding the implications of mixed methods data can lead to a more considered approach to problem-solving, and hence implementation, in the complex world of healthcare delivery.

References

Agreli, H., F. Barry, A. Burton, S. Creedon, J. Drennan, D. Gould, C. R. May, M. P. Smiddy, M. Murphy, and S. Murphy. 2019. "Ethnographic study using Normalization Process Theory to understand the implementation process of infection prevention and control guidelines in Ireland." *BMJ Open* 9 (8):e029514.

Braithwaite, J., K. Ludlow, L. Testa, J. Herkes, H. Augustsson, G. Lamprell, E. McPherson, and Y. Zurynski. 2020. "Built to last? The sustainability of healthcare system improvements, programmes and interventions: A systematic integrative review." *BMJ Open* 10 (6):e036453.

Braithwaite, J., and F. Rapport. 2020. "Conclusion: On progress, directions and signposts to a transformed healthcare system." In *Transforming Healthcare with Qualitative Research*, edited by Frances Rapport and Jeffrey Braithwaite. Oxford: Routledge.

Eisman, A. B., A. M. Kilbourne, A. R. Dopp, L. Saldana, and D. Eisenberg. 2020. "Economic evaluation in implementation science: Making the business case for implementation strategies." *Psychiatry Research* 283:112433.

Greenhalgh, T., and C. Papoutsi. 2018. "Studying complexity in health services research: Desperately seeking an overdue paradigm shift." *BMC Medicine* 16 (1):1–6.

Haff, N., and N. K. Choudhry. 2018. "The promise and pitfalls of pragmatic clinical trials for improving health care quality." *JAMA Network Open* 1 (6):e183376–e183376.

Kirk, M. A., C. Kelley, N. Yankey, S. A. Birken, B. Abadie, and L. Damschroder. 2015. "A systematic review of the use of the consolidated framework for implementation research." *Implementation Science* 11 (1):1–13.

May, C. R., F. Mair, T. Finch, A. MacFarlane, C. Dowrick, S. Treweek, T. Rapley, L. Ballini, B. N. Ong, A. Rogers, E. Murray, G. Elwyn, F. Légaré, J. Gunn, and V. M. Montori. 2009. "Development of a theory of implementation and integration: Normalization Process Theory." *Implementation Science* 4 (1):29. doi: 10.1186/1748-5908-4-29.

Moullin, J. C., K. S. Dickson, N. A. Stadnick, B. Albers, P. Nilsen, S. Broder-Fingert, B. Mukasa, and G. A. Aarons. 2020. "Ten recommendations for using implementation frameworks in research and practice." *Implementation Science Communications* 1:1–12.

Nilsen, P., and S. Bernhardsson. 2019. "Context matters in implementation science: A scoping review of determinant frameworks that describe contextual determinants for implementation outcomes." *BMC Health Services Research* 19 (1):1–21.

Patton, M. Q. 1999. "Enhancing the quality and credibility of qualitative analysis." *Health Services Research* 34 (5 Pt 2):1189.

Pomare, C., J. C. Long, K. Churruca, L. A. Ellis, and J. Braithwaite. 2019. "Social network research in health care settings: Design and data collection." *Social Networks*. (In press)

Rapport, F., and J. Braithwaite. 2018. "Are we on the cusp of a fourth research paradigm? Predicting the future for a new approach to methods-use in medical and health services research." *BMC Medical Research Methodology* 18 (1):1–7.

Rapport, F., R. Clay-Williams, K. Churruca, P. Shih, A. Hogden, and J. Braithwaite. 2018a. "The struggle of translating science into action: Foundational concepts of implementation science." *Journal of Evaluation in Clinical Practice* 24 (1):117–126.

Rapport, F., A. Hogden, M. Faris, M. Bierbaum, R. Clay-Williams, J. Long, P. Shih, L. M. R. Seah, and J. Braithwaite. 2018b. *Qualitative Research in Healthcare: Modern Methods, Clear Translation: A White Paper*. Sydney: Macquarie University.

Rapport, F., J. Smith, T. A. O'Brien, V. J. Tyrrell, E. V. A. Mould, J. C. Long, H. Gul, and J. Braithwaite. 2020. "Development of an implementation and evaluation strategy for the Australian 'Zero Childhood Cancer' (Zero) Program: A study protocol." *BMJ Open* 10 (6):e034522.

Schliep, M. E., C. N. Alonzo, and M. A. Morris. 2017. "Beyond RCTs: Innovations in research design and methods to advance implementation science." *Evidence-Based Communication Assessment and Intervention* 11 (3–4):82–98.

Stetler, C. B., M. W. Legro, C. M. Wallace, C. Bowman, M. Guihan, H. Hagedorn, B. Kimmel, N. D. Sharp, and J. L. Smith. 2006. "The role of formative evaluation in implementation research and the QUERI experience." *Journal of General Internal Medicine* 21 (2):S1.

26 Applying the Theoretical Domains Framework

Its uses and limitations

Fabiana Lorencatto

The Theoretical Domains Framework (TDF) integrates various behavioural theories into an overarching framework of 14 theoretical domains representing individual, sociocultural, and environmental influences on behaviour, thereby providing a comprehensive theoretical basis for investigating implementation problems and designing implementation interventions. The TDF has been applied to numerous implementation problems and contexts to date, reflecting progress made towards achieving its original aims of making theory more accessible and useful to interdisciplinary researchers in implementation science and beyond and towards improving our understanding of behaviour-change processes in implementation.

Specifically, the TDF has been applied to investigate diverse implementation problems. Examples are listed in a thematic series on the TDF published in the journal *Implementation Science* (Francis, O'Connor, and Curran 2012). Applications of the TDF to date have primarily focused on improving quality of healthcare, given the TDF was initially developed to explore influences on healthcare professional behaviours (Atkins et al. 2017). For example, Fleming and colleagues (Fleming et al. 2014) applied the TDF to conduct semi-structured interviews with 37 healthcare providers to identify barriers/enablers of antibiotic prescribing in long-term care facilities. Key influences on antibiotic use in this setting fell within the domains of "knowledge" (e.g., variable knowledge of antibiotic guidelines), "environmental context and resources" (e.g., lack of diagnostic equipment and interpretation of microbiology results), "social influences" (e.g., pressure from nurses on doctors to prescribe antibiotics), "beliefs about consequences" (e.g., concern over potential harm and hospitalization of vulnerable patients), "memory attention and decision-making" (e.g., balancing risk/benefits of letting a patient go without antibiotics), and "behavioural regulation" (e.g., lack of surveillance and reviewing of antibiotic practices). Similarly, Kenny et al. (Kenny et al. 2020) conducted a TDF-based survey to investigate barriers and enablers to seasonal influenza vaccine uptake among 327 healthcare workers. Significant predictors of vaccine uptake fell within the domains: "goals" (e.g., having clear plan for when/where they will get vaccine), "social influences" (e.g., encouragement and approval from colleagues, colleagues also being vaccinated), and "reinforcement" (e.g., feeling as though they are making a difference by being vaccinated). However, the TDF has also been applied to patient and public behaviours (e.g., increasing physical activity in stroke survivors (Nicholson et al. 2014)) and in contexts beyond health, such as sustainability (e.g., recycling behaviours (Gainforth et al. 2016)).

The most useful frameworks also link determinants to behaviour change strategies so that interventions can be developed to address barriers and enablers to implementation. A key strength of the TDF is that it has been mapped to two associated behavioural science frameworks which specify different types of intervention strategies. First, the Behaviour Change Wheel (Michie, Atkins, and West 2014), which specifies nine broad intervention types (e.g.,

DOI: 10.4324/9781003109945-29

education, incentivisation, modelling, environmental restructuring). Second, the Behaviour Change Technique Taxonomy (Michie et al. 2013), which specifies 93 more granular techniques for changing behaviour (e.g., goal setting, self-monitoring, feedback on behaviour). There are published matrices pairing domains of the TDF with the intervention types and techniques in the aforementioned frameworks, in order to suggest types of behaviour change strategies that are likely to be effective in targeting barriers and enablers within each domain (Cane et al. 2015, Johnston et al. 2020). These tools can guide decision-making during intervention design and support more systematic, transparent, and theory-based development of behaviour change and implementation interventions (Michie, Atkins, and West 2014).

Regarding limitations, some argue that using the TDF to structure interview questions and analysis restricts findings to those that fit within the framework, thereby limiting opportunities for identifying barriers/enablers outside the 14 domains (McGowan, Powell, and French 2020). However, a study comparing results of interviews using the TDF versus atheoretical approaches identified that while the findings from both approaches overlapped, the TDF-based studies elicited a greater number of influences that were not mentioned in the atheoretical studies, particularly around emotional factors influencing behaviour (Dyson et al. 2011). Another critique is that the TDF domains are too focused on individual behaviour and thus not applicable to investigating implementation problems at organizational levels (Francis, O'Connor, and Curran 2012). Organizational theories were among the 33 theories contributing to the development of the TDF. Organizational influences on behaviour are represented in the domains' "environmental context and resources", "social influences", and "social professional role and identity"; however, some may feel these are not sufficiently elaborated. For this reason, many studies have applied the TDF concurrently alongside other determinant frameworks such as the Consolidated Framework for Implementation Research (CFIR), which contains domains relating to outer contextual influences on implementation (Damschroder et al. 2009, Birken et al. 2017). Lastly, each domain does not exist in a vacuum, and barriers and enablers identified within each domain will likely interact with those in other domains (e.g., fear within the domain "emotions" may result from negative beliefs about consequences). However, most TDF-based studies do not discuss relationships between domains. Future TDF-based studies should move beyond generating descriptive lists of barriers/enablers, towards investigating and theorizing how domains interact for the behaviour of interest. A recent example of such an approach includes a qualitative study of influences on opioid prescribing among family physicians (Desveaux et al. 2019).

References

Atkins, L., J. Francis, R. Islam, D. O'Connor, A. Patey, N. Ivers, R. Foy, E. M. Duncan, H. Colquhoun, and J. M. Grimshaw. 2017. "A guide to using the Theoretical Domains Framework of behaviour change to investigate implementation problems." *Implementation Science* 12 (1):77.

Birken, S. A., B. J. Powell, J. Presseau, M. A. Kirk, F. Lorencatto, N. J. Gould, C. M. Shea, B. J. Weiner, J. J. Francis, and Y. Yu. 2017. "Combined use of the Consolidated Framework for Implementation Research (CFIR) and the Theoretical Domains Framework (TDF): A systematic review." *Implementation science* 12 (1):2.

Cane, J., M. Richardson, M. Johnston, R. Ladha, and S. Michie. 2015. "From lists of behaviour change techniques (BCT s) to structured hierarchies: Comparison of two methods of developing a hierarchy of BCT s." *British Journal of Health Psychology* 20 (1):130–150.

Damschroder, L. J., D. C. Aron, R. E. Keith, S. R. Kirsh, J. A. Alexander, and J. C. Lowery. 2009. "Fostering implementation of health services research findings into practice: A consolidated framework for advancing implementation science." *Implementation Science* 4 (1):1–15.

Desveaux, L., M. Saragosa, N. Kithulegoda, and N. Ivers. 2019. "Understanding the behavioural determinants of opioid prescribing among family physicians: A qualitative study." *BMC Family Practice* 20 (1):1–12.

Dyson, J., R. Lawton, C. Jackson, and F. Cheater. 2011. "Does the use of a theoretical approach tell us more about hand hygiene behaviour? The barriers and levers to hand hygiene." *Journal of Infection Prevention* 12 (1):17–24.

Fleming, A., C. Bradley, S. Cullinan, and S. Byrne. 2014. "Antibiotic prescribing in long-term care facilities: A qualitative, multidisciplinary investigation." *BMJ Open* 4 (11).

Francis, J. J., D. O'Connor, and J. Curran. 2012. "Theories of behaviour change synthesised into a set of theoretical groupings: Introducing a thematic series on the theoretical domains framework." *Implementation Science* 7 (1):35.

Gainforth, H. L., K. Sheals, L. Atkins, R. Jackson, and S. Michie. 2016. "Developing interventions to change recycling behaviors: A case study of applying behavioral science." *Applied Environmental Education and Communication* 15 (4):325–339.

Johnston, M., R. N. Carey, L. E. Connell Bohlen, D. W. Johnston, A. J. Rothman, M. de Bruin, M. P. Kelly, H. Groarke, and S. Michie. 2020. "Development of an online tool for linking behavior change techniques and mechanisms of action based on triangulation of findings from literature synthesis and expert consensus." *Translational Behavioral Medicine* 11 (5):1049–1065.

Kenny, E., Á. McNamara, C. Noone, and M. Byrne. 2020. "Barriers to seasonal influenza vaccine uptake among health care workers in long-term care facilities: A cross-sectional analysis." *British Journal of Health Psychology* 25 (3):519–539.

McGowan, L. J., R. Powell, and D. P. French. 2020. "How can use of the Theoretical Domains Framework be optimized in qualitative research? A rapid systematic review." *British Journal of Health Psychology* 25 (3):677–694.

Michie, S., L. Atkins, and R. West. 2014. "The behaviour change wheel." In *A Guide to Designing Interventions*. 1st ed., 1003–1010. Great Britain: Silverback Publishing.

Michie, S., M. Richardson, M. Johnston, C. Abraham, J. Francis, W. Hardeman, M. P. Eccles, J. Cane, and C. E. Wood. 2013. "The behavior change technique taxonomy (v1) of 93 hierarchically clustered techniques: Building an international consensus for the reporting of behavior change interventions." *Annals of Behavioral Medicine* 46 (1):81–95.

Nicholson, S. L., M. Donaghy, M. Johnston, F. F. Sniehotta, F. Van Wijck, D. Johnston, C. Greig, M. E. McMurdo, and G. Mead. 2014. "A qualitative theory guided analysis of stroke survivors' perceived barriers and facilitators to physical activity." *Disability and Rehabilitation* 36 (22):1857–1868.

27 Ethnography

Justin Waring and Jenelle Clarke

The implementation of change in health and care services is inherently a social endeavour. It may be attractive to treat new interventions, therapies, and technologies as somehow independent from the social milieu in which they are put to use, but it is important to recognize that all stages of their development, testing, application, and embedding involve people "doing things" in particular social "contexts". These people do not manifest in some experimental vacuum; rather they exist within complex sociocultural systems made up of shared meanings, beliefs, and identities; customs, routines, and rituals; institutionalized roles and rules; and underlying structures of status and inequality. It is often the case within implementation research that these diverse aspects of the social world are bundled together under the amorphous label of "context", but this can oversimplify the rich combination of influences that condition and enable how people engage in change processes (Leslie et al. 2014). How then can implementation research better account for the way people do things in their sociocultural context?

One answer to this question is through ethnography, an approach to social research that involves, in its broadest sense, first-hand engagement and experience with a social or cultural setting (Atkinson 2015, Fetterman 2010). The intention is to develop a rich description and interpretative understanding of the meaningful practices and patterns of social organization that distinguish a given social setting, or possibly virtual community (Wolcott 1999). Ethnography can be thought of as a methodology, a method, and an account (Waring and Jones 2016). It is premised on certain assumptions about the nature of the social world and how it can be understood, it is associated with a corresponding set of research methods for studying the social world, and it results in a particular form of descriptive and interpretative account of the social world.

Ethnography typically seeks a naturalistic, holistic, and emic understanding of how people make sense of and organize their social lives. It is perhaps best defined by the methods used to acquire this first-hand understanding: "participant observations". Through immersion in the lives and "doings" of participants, researchers use themselves as an instrument of data collection to directly see and share the lived experiences of a given community from which deeper insight and understanding can be developed, such as how people implement a change initiative. Other methods are often used during ethnographic fieldwork including non-participant observations, semi-structured interviews, documentary research, and even quantitative approaches, but all are directed towards developing a rich insider understanding of a given social setting (Fetterman 2010).

Ethnographies are often characterized by "rich" or "thick" description, in which social activities, events, and situations are recounted in such a way to elaborate and explain the underlying meanings, beliefs, rules, expectations, rituals, and other elements that order these

DOI: 10.4324/9781003109945-30

social activities and hence illuminate what is going on in the target community (Atkinson 2015). Key to an ethnographic approach is the idea of inductive and interpretative understanding; first-hand empirical insights drive analytical and conceptual understanding. Such empirical accounts afford detailed understanding of a given community and can also provide the basis for more conceptual and theoretical understanding that, in some instance, may have applications beyond the given setting. The test is often thought to be one of credibility of the rendering rather than generalizability.

It is important to recognize that ethnography remains the focus of controversy and disagreement (Hammersley 2013). As well as subtle disciplinary differences in how ethnography is understood and used, there are also divergent expectations around the role of social theory in sensitizing research, ethical controversies around the role of the ethnographer within a given community, the time and resource commitments for developing ethnographic insights, and variations in the political commitment of ethnography towards social justice (Pachirat 2018). Although many implementation studies report being "ethnographies" or using "ethnographic methods" (Vindrola-Padros and Vindrola-Padros 2018), it is important to stress that simply undertaking observational research does not necessarily qualify a study as ethnographic, nor does the exclusive use of qualitative interviewing (Waring and Jones 2016). Rather, ethnography is about the methodological commitment to developing a holistic and insider's perspective of the social milieu of implementation through direct and participatory experience of change processes. Ethnographic implementation research, therefore, involves directly observing the processes through which health and care innovations are developed, experienced, and embedded in different services settings. It involves focusing, for example, on the meaningful practices of social actors and groups as they work together, or against each other, to make sense or engage in change processes while also seeking to explain these actions as framed by wider cultural influences and social structures.

References

Atkinson, P. 2015. *For Ethnography, Ethnography*. London: Sage Publications.

Fetterman, D. M. 2010. *Ethnography: Step-by-step*. 3rd ed. ed. Vol. 17, *Applied Social Research Methods Series*. Los Angeles: Sage Publications.

Hammersley, M. 2013. *What's Wrong with Ethnography?* London: Taylor and Francis.

Leslie, M., E. Paradis, M. A. Gropper, S. Reeves, and S. Kitto. 2014. "Applying ethnography to the study of context in healthcare quality and safety." *BMJ Qual Safety* 23 (2):99–105. doi: 10.1136/bmjqs-2013-002335 %J BMJ Quality & Safety.

Pachirat, T. 2018. *Among Wolves: Ethnography and the Immersive Study of Power*. 1 ed. Vol. 6, *Routledge series on interpretive methods*. Florence: Routledge.

Vindrola-Padros, C., and B. Vindrola-Padros. 2018. "Quick and dirty? A systematic review of the use of rapid ethnographies in healthcare organisation and delivery." *BMJ Qual Safety* 27 (4):321–330. doi: 10.1136/bmjqs-2017-007226 %J BMJ Quality & Safety.

Waring, J., and L. Jones. 2016. "Maintaining the link between methodology and method in ethnographic health research." 25 (7):556–557. doi: 10.1136/bmjqs-2016-005325 %J BMJ Quality & Safety.

Wolcott, H. F. 1999. *Ethnography: A Way of Seeing*. Walnut Creek, CA: AltaMira.

28 Walking methods

Frances Rapport

Walking Methods, also known as mobile methods (Braithwaite and Rapport 2020, Rapport and Braithwaite 2020), necessitate the active joining together of researcher and participant in a shared reflection on a range of issues while moving together through the world. Temporarily on an equal footing, Walking Methods usually take place in a research setting (such as a hospital ward) with researcher and participant sharing an experience in time and space. Discussions during a Walking Methods encounter can be informal or formal, recorded or remembered, notated word-for-word or abbreviated. Irrespective of the data recording technique, however, Walking Methods often lead to the collection of clarificatory and detailed information with greater variety that can be achieved using more static techniques. Furthermore, data interpretation as part of an implementation process can help underpin the translation of research findings into changes in policy or practice (Rapport et al. 2018).

It is as if the activity of moving together stimulates both information exchange and introspection and, at the same time, rewards the researcher with rich outward expression. Conversations provide information with a degree of clarity and openness rarely seen using other kinds of narrative techniques. In effect, Walking Methods are data collection "on the hoof" (Rapport and Braithwaite 2018). Talking can stimulate "trigger points" (also known as "eureka moments"). Trigger points allude to when "a new thought occurs, something important is said or done, or something impactful is experienced" (Rapport and Braithwaite 2020). They can lead to intense reflection, often providing insights that indicate depth and truthfulness. In effect, the very act of walking encourages memories to surface (both old and new), while moving alongside someone places the researcher in a very central position to observe the world as the participant sees it, in vivid technicolour. Sensory and emotively invested, Walking Methods offer personalized, individual thoughts and experiences, while moving around a setting with someone adds a level of depth to information retrieval.

There are times when Walking Methods might jar and, for example, highlight some unusual, even unethical practices, including situations where people may be at risk, implicated in unprofessional behaviour, or seen as uncaring. In these circumstances, the researcher may need to make choices about how to manage data, whether all data should be included, and in all circumstances, and what messages might inadvertently be carried forward. When others are involved, there are also considerations around the proximity of data, its content, and quality and what constitutes ethical data appropriation. However, despite inherent challenges, Walking Methods herald a new wave of research, with data that are raw and realistic, and which provide extensive opportunity for new insights into people's lives. This can help researchers understand not only what goes right most of the time in healthcare delivery and across space and time (Hollnagel, Braithwaite, and Wears 2013, Hollnagel, Wears, and Braithwaite 2015) but also how problems are circumvented or overcome (also known as

DOI: 10.4324/9781003109945-31

"work arounds"). Understanding how people manage challenges on a daily basis indicates the adjustments that may be needed to ensure that high-quality healthcare continues to be provided while highlighting people's embodied and emergent knowledge, at the coalface of care delivery.

References

Braithwaite, J., and F. Rapport. 2020. "Conclusion: On progress, directions and signposts to a transformed healthcare system." In *Transforming Healthcare with Qualitative Research*, edited by Frances Rapport and Jeffrey Braithwaite. Oxford: Routledge.

Hollnagel, E., J. Braithwaite, and R. L. Wears. 2013. *Resilient Health Care*. Farnham: Ashgate Publishing, Ltd.

Hollnagel, E., R. L. Wears, and J. Braithwaite. 2015. "From safety-I to safety-II: A white paper." In *The Resilient Health Care Net*. Sydney: University of Southern Denmark, University of Florida, USA, and Macquarie University, Australia.

Rapport, F., and J. Braithwaite. 2018. "Are we on the cusp of a fourth research paradigm? Predicting the future for a new approach to methods-use in medical and health services research." *BMC Medical Research Methodology* 18 (1):1–7.

Rapport, F., and J. Braithwaite. 2020. "The Fourth Research Paradigm: Activating researchers for real world need." In *Transforming Healthcare with Qualitative Research*, edited by Frances Rapport and Jeffrey Braithwaite. Oxford: Routledge.

Rapport, F., R. Clay-Williams, K. Churruca, P. Shih, A. Hogden, and J. Braithwaite. 2018. "The struggle of translating science into action: Foundational concepts of implementation science." *Journal of Evaluation in Clinical Practice* 24 (1):117–126.

29 Modelling complex socio-technical systems

The Functional Resonance Analysis Method (FRAM)

Erik Hollnagel and Robyn Clay-Williams

Despite the absence of a generally accepted definition of what a complex socio-technical system is, the adjective *complex* signals that it is difficult to understand how the system works and therefore also how to analyse, manage, or improve it. It may even be difficult to talk to others about it. A common solution to overcome this difficulty is to construct a model – an informative representation – of the system. Models are ubiquitous in the scientific literature and are also used in many other places, for instance, to support a political or financial decision. Most researchers also find it irresistible to propose models as part of their work although mostly as intricate diagrams of components and their interconnections. A model should, however, be more than a diagram of components with lines or arrows between them. The real purpose of a model is to represent the essential characteristics of something in a way that is amenable to analysis and manipulation. "The basic defining characteristics of all models is the representation of some aspects of the world by a more abstract system. In applying a model, the investigator identifies objects and relations in the world with some elements and relations in the formal system" (Coombs, Dawes, and Tversky 1970). A model is thus a deliberate simplification of the important features or characteristics of an object that make it possible to investigate issues of interest. Yet it is not enough to want to model something. It is also necessary to provide a concise way of doing it. The simplification must therefore be based on a well-defined set of principles that can represent the "objects and relations in the world" that are being investigated. The principles that are used to build a model essentially represent the assumptions about "the world", about what lies behind the phenomena being studied or analysed. Without them, a model in practice becomes meaningless.

Models of socio-technical systems: parts or functions?

A system, whether simple or complex, is often defined as a set of parts together with relationships between the parts and their attributes. The parts are usually physical entities, such as humans and machines, but can also be factors or other elements that are assumed to have an effect on how the system performs. Indeed, in socio-technical theory, it is the interaction of social and technical factors that creates the conditions for successful (and unsuccessful) performance. The interaction is habitually described as tasks that in turn are modelled as sequences of steps or actions.

When a socio-technical system is described in terms of constituent parts, the result is a structural model. The model describes how the system works in terms of how the parts are ordered temporally or hierarchically or in terms of exchanges of information, energy, or matter. The graphical representation is typically a diagram of boxes and lines representing nodes and connections. A structural model describes what a socio-technical system is,

DOI: 10.4324/9781003109945-32

in terms of its parts and how they are organized. It is, however, also possible to describe a socio-technical system in terms of what it does, (i.e., the functions that are needed to bring about a specific outcome and how these functions depend on each other). This mapping of the dependencies or couplings among the functions is necessary to understand what actually goes on. The analysis can, for instance, begin by what the system does or should do – the goals – and then proceeds to describe how it can be done – the means.

In healthcare, work is done by large or small interdependent patient care teams, and a functional model can show how each team member contributes to the overall performance. Creating this shared insight can improve team understanding of the process they are part of and facilitate interdisciplinary collaboration and learning. The model describes how work usually takes place by showing how the everyday variability of functions affects how work is carried out. Without a sensible model of what actually goes on, it is impossible both to plan changes and effectively to implement them.

The Functional Resonance Analysis Method (FRAM)

Currently, the leading method to develop a functional model is the Functional Resonance Analysis Method (FRAM) (Hollnagel 2012). This method is based on the following principles: 1) work that goes well and work that doesn't happen in essentially the same way, 2) performance on all levels of an organization is variable because it must be adjusted to existing conditions (resources and demands), 3) acceptable and unacceptable outcomes both emerge from variability due to the everyday adjustments, which 4) can lead to functional resonance and non-linear (disproportionate) consequences.

The FRAM provides a way to describe functions that can be used to develop a model of how a system performs. The basic component of a FRAM model is a function which represents an act or activity – simple or complicated – that is needed to produce a certain result. Functions can be further characterized by aspects that define essential conditions for their realization: Input, Output, Preconditions, Resources, Time, and Control.

Example of a FRAM model

To illustrate what a FRAM model may look like, consider the case of taking a blood sample in preparation for a transfusion. Figure 29.1 shows a step-by-step description of the actions to be taken:

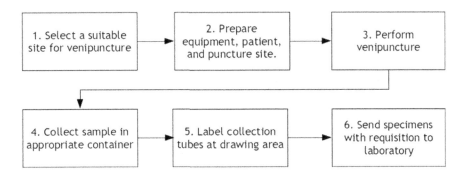

Figure 29.1 Blood sample as a simple task

Source: Created by authors

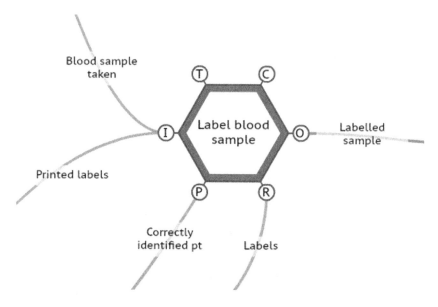

Figure 29.2 Blood sample (detail) by FRAM
Source: Created by authors

In reality, taking a blood sample is not as straightforward as the structural model in Figure 29.1 suggests. There are preparations and checks to be made; hence, many non-trivial dependencies. Figure 29.2 shows the fifth step (labelling) described as a function using the FRAM. In this figure we can see that, in addition to input and output, preconditions and resources are important aspects to be considered. Changes and improvements that are based on simple structural models without acknowledging these dependencies are likely to be unsuccessful.

Improvements to how something is done should never be undertaken without a good understanding of how work is accomplished on the frontlines of patient care. This understanding must, at a minimum, include a description or model of how the activities of individual team members interlace to complete the task and how this makes functions mutually dependent. Simplified assumptions about Work-as-Imagined cannot replace facts about Work-as-Done.

References

Coombs, C. H., R. M. Dawes, and A. Tversky. 1970. *Mathematical Psychology: An Elementary Introduction, Prentice-Hall Series in Mathematical Psychology*. Englewood Cliffs, NJ: Prentice-Hall.
Hollnagel, E. 2012. *FRAM: The Functional Resonance Analysis Method: Modelling Complex Sociotechnical Systems*. 1st ed. Farnham, UK: Routledge.

30 Getting a handle on the social processes of implementation

Social network research

Janet C. Long

Healthcare is a highly social process. It involves a complex interplay between teams of clinicians, non-clinical staff, the patients, and their family or carers. Social processes such as communication, sensemaking, negotiation, group problem-solving, and decision-making predominate. Social interactions may be formal (e.g., a GP referring a patient to a cardiologist) or informal (e.g., nurses on ward 5 decide to introduce bedside handovers after seeing how well it works in ward 6). Implementing new interventions into this complex system can, in a broad sense, be understood as fostering social processes that will help the diffusion, dissemination, and adoption of the new practice. Acceptability and appropriateness of an intervention are largely defined by socially constructed understandings (Sekhon, Cartwright, and Francis 2017) and adoption, as shown in Rogers' study of the Diffusion of Innovation (Rogers 2003), which is driven by a mixture of social comparison (keeping up with the Jones') and persuasion ("I'm convinced now that it works").

Social network research provides a unique methodology and a valuable theoretical framework to quantify and understand this web of social interactions. It can provide valuable insights to assist the implementer to understand "How things work around here" and who is doing what. At its most basic, a social network is defined as a group of individuals who interact in some way. The sum of these interactions makes up the network. Sociograms are graphs or maps of these interactions. They show each entity – person, or group – in the network as a node and the ties between them as lines.

Figure 30.1 shows before and after the implementation of a community-based suicide prevention program, showing how collaborative links between a diverse range of stakeholders grew. This increase in collaboration and coordination was a major outcome of the project, allowing interventions to be more widely spread and accepted in the community, and increasing the communication pathways so that the interventions could be delivered in a timely, coordinated way.

There are two types of key players essential to implementation. Central actors are usually easy to identify and are highly visible; they are the ones with the most interaction with others, the ones who wield the most power, or who take the lead. Implementation without the buy-in and support of central actors is unlikely to succeed (Braithwaite, Marks, and Taylor 2014).

Case example

We studied a new translational research network being implemented to drive more collaboration between university-based researchers, hospital-based clinicians, and consumers with lived experience of cancer (Long et al. 2013a, 2013b). When members were asked who they thought were most powerful and influential in the network, the network manager and the

DOI: 10.4324/9781003109945-33

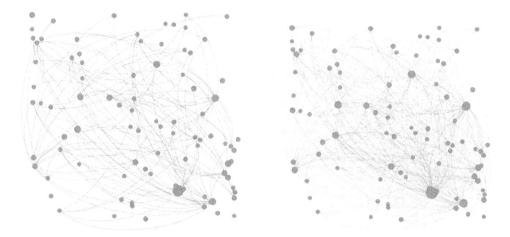

Figure 30.1 Collaborative ties before and after implementation of a community-based suicide prevention program

Source: Created by author

network director were nominated most often. The success of the implementation in driving
cross-silo collaboration could be tracked directly to their efforts (confirmed by longitudinal
data (Long, Hibbert, and Braithwaite 2015) and interview data (Long et al. 2013b)).

Other key players may be less visible yet no less important for the success of an implementation, and this is where a formal Social Network Analysis is so useful. Brokers go by
a number of names, reflecting the type of role they play: bridge, go-between, knowledge
broker, and boundary spanner are just a few (Long et al. 2013a). These people are the ones
who hold a position between different subgroups in the network. Like a bridge, they may be
the only path for communication to pass from one group to another. This is very important
where multiple stakeholders are involved in an implementation and coordination of effort is
needed. Healthcare is often called tribal (Braithwaite 2006) with each discipline, department,
or institution focusing introspectively on their own siloed team and activities. Bridges can
bring these groups together. Knowledge brokers may have a foot in two separate groups and
knowledge of both making them a useful source of knowledge to members of both groups.
Brokers may be the person who "knows everyone" and who can direct you to the right person
or resource. In the translational research cancer network, for example, brokers were shown to
be invisible yet crucial to the efficient functioning of the network (Long et al. 2013a, 2013b,
2014, Long, Hibbert, and Braithwaite 2015).

Social network research can be done by everything from sketching on the back of an envelope
for groups up to 10 to clarify communication flows through to giant networks, such as traffic
on the internet requiring specialist software. In healthcare settings where the numbers of stakeholders are less than 100, an online survey works well to collect data. Network data can also be
extracted from documents where ties, such as communication, collaboration, or referrals, can be
tracked and counted. Pomare et al. (2019) have written a useful summary of the strengths and
limitations of the methods, especially when used in healthcare. Unless the implementation team
understands how work gets done in a healthcare setting and who the key players are, however,
implementation processes of diffusion, dissemination, and adoption will be hampered.

References

Braithwaite, J. 2006. "An empirical assessment of social structural and cultural change in clinical directorates." *Health Care Analysis* 14 (4):185–193. doi: 10.1007/s10728-006-0025-5.

Braithwaite, J., D. Marks, and N. Taylor. 2014. "Harnessing implementation science to improve care quality and patient safety: A systematic review of targeted literature." *International Journal for Quality in Health Care* 26 (3):321–329. doi: 10.1093/intqhc/mzu047.

Long, J. C., F. C. Cunningham, P. Carswell, and J. Braithwaite. 2013a. "Who are the key players in a new translational research network?" *BMC Health Services Research* 13 (1):1–11.

Long, J. C., F. C. Cunningham, P. Carswell, and J. Braithwaite. 2014. "Patterns of collaboration in complex networks: The example of a translational research network." *BMC Health Services Research* 14 (1):1–10.

Long, J. C., F. C. Cunningham, J. Wiley, P. Carswell, and J. Braithwaite. 2013b. "Leadership in complex networks: The importance of network position and strategic action in a translational cancer research network." *Implementation Science* 8 (1):1–11.

Long, J. C., P. Hibbert, and J. Braithwaite. 2015. "Structuring successful collaboration: A longitudinal social network analysis of a translational research network." *Implementation Science* 11 (1):1–14.

Pomare, C., J. C. Long, K. Churruca, L. A. Ellis, and J. Braithwaite. 2019. "Social network research in health care settings: Design and data collection." *Social Networks*. doi: 10.1016/j.socnet.2019.11.004.

Rogers, E. M. 2003. *Diffusion of Innovations*. 5th ed. ed. New York, NY: Free Press.

Sekhon, M., M. Cartwright, and J. J. Francis. 2017. "Acceptability of healthcare interventions: An overview of reviews and development of a theoretical framework." *BMC Health Services Research* 17 (1):88. doi: 10.1186/s12913-017-2031-8.

31 Sentiment analysis for use within rapid implementation research

How far and fast can we go?

James Smith

What is Sentiment Analysis?

Sentiment Analysis helps us to rapidly detect the positive or negative opinions in a piece of text. We can use Sentiment Analysis, a machine learning technique, considered to be a subfield of Natural Language Processing (NLP: a field at the intersection of computer science, artificial intelligence, and linguistics), to detect sentiment polarity (e.g., very positive, positive, neutral, negative, very negative opinions) within any piece of text. Text data can be drawn from transcripts, fieldnotes (Smith et al. in review), or data from microblogging websites, such as Twitter (McMullen et al. 2011). Twitter is a treasure trove of sentiment. Sentiment Analysis can rapidly convert data from unstructured Twitter data to structured text data. Examples include opinions of health interventions, such as vaccination (Zhou et al. 2015), and the delivery of outcomes such as those relating to seasonal affective disorder and obesity (Gore, Diallo, and Padilla 2015, Golder and Macy 2011, Coppersmith et al. 2015).

How Sentiment Analysis can contribute to rapid implementation research

An example of the application of Sentiment Analysis can be found in the work of Smith et al. (in review), in which ethnographic fieldnotes for an implementation science–driven early-phase clinical trial, PRecISion Medicine for Children with Cancer (PRISM), were analysed. This study analysed the positive and negative views of healthcare professionals to detect the divergence and convergence of opinions around the implementation of a precision medicine model of care (Smith et al. in review). Sentiment Analysis was found to be a rigorous scientific method for speeding up the qualitative analytic inquiry and providing timely evaluation, identification, and dissemination of critical intervention components in a dynamic environment. Implementation science studies can and should be designed to address the need for cost-effective and timely results in rapidly changing situations (Rapport et al. 2020). To achieve this requires rapid qualitative analytic methods (Gale et al. 2019, Smith et al. 2020). Sentiment Analysis with its characteristically speedy processing can make sense of large qualitative data sets in very little time. Sentiment Analysis is therefore a promising way to automate the extraction of vital insights from vast unstructured data, thus reducing this time resource-intensive activity (Table 31.1).

Conclusion

Despite its potential, Sentiment Analysis has not been taken up to the extent that it might. Consideration over the method of Sentiment Analysis for use within the rapid implementation and evaluation assessment of interventions is long overdue. There are many potential

DOI: 10.4324/9781003109945-34

Table 31.1 Advantages of Sentiment Analysis for use within rapid implementation research

Applications of Sentiment Analysis	How Sentiment Analysis does it
Rapid analysis of qualitative data	Rapidly sorts large amounts of data, a process that could otherwise be resource intensive
Rapid-cycle Formative Evaluation Feedback Loop	Quickly produces information to disseminate findings in a short time frame to provide sponsors with useful feedback in a short amount of time
Intervention optimization	Can help easily identify actionable feedback for enhancing intervention optimization
Trial outcomes	Can help in interpreting "how" and "why" an intervention may or may not be successful through opinion mining text of transcripts or fieldnotes, and so forth

Source: Created by author

advantages of Sentiment Analysis that include producing rapid actionable information to sponsors, planners, and decision-makers when an intervention takes place in a rapidly changing context. These advantages offer a rapid approach to those who need it.

References

Coppersmith, G., M. Dredze, C. Harman, and K. Hollingshead. 2015. "From ADHD to SAD: Analyzing the language of mental health on Twitter through self-reported diagnoses." *NAACL HLT 2015*1:1–10.

Gale, R. C., J. Wu, T. Erhardt, M. Bounthavong, C. M. Reardon, L. J. Damschroder, and A. M. Midboe. 2019. "Comparison of rapid vs in-depth qualitative analytic methods from a process evaluation of academic detailing in the Veterans Health Administration." *Implementation Science* 14 (1):11. doi: 10.1186/s13012-019-0853-y.

Golder, S. A., and M. W. Macy. 2011. "Diurnal and seasonal mood vary with work, sleep, and daylength across diverse cultures." *Science* 333 (6051):1878–1881.

Gore, R. J., S. Diallo, and J. Padilla. 2015. "You are what you tweet: Connecting the geographic variation in America's obesity rate to Twitter content." *PLoS One* 10 (9):e0133505.

McMullen, C. K., J. S. Ash, D. F. Sittig, A. Bunce, K. Guappone, R. Dykstra, J. Carpenter, J. Richardson, and A. Wright. 2011. "Rapid assessment of clinical information systems in the healthcare setting: An efficient method for time-pressed evaluation." *Methods of Information in Medicine* 50 (4):299–307. doi: 10.3414/me10-01-0042.

Rapport, F., J. Smith, T. A. O'Brien, V. J. Tyrrell, E. V. Mould, J. C. Long, H. Gul, and J. Braithwaite. 2020. "Development of an implementation and evaluation strategy for the Australian 'Zero Childhood Cancer' (Zero) Program: A study protocol." *BMJ Open* 10 (6):e034522. doi: 10.1136/bmjopen-2019-034522.

Smith, J., J. Braithwaite, T. A. O'Brien, S. Smith, V. J. Tyrrell, E. V. A. Mould, J. C. Long, and F. Rapport. In Review. "Barriers and enablers to a complex tailored intervention: The Zero Childhood Cancer Personalised Medicine Program (The Zero Program) – results of an evaluation, and methods development "*International Journal of Qualitative Methods*.

Smith, J., F. Rapport, T. A. O'Brien, S. Smith, V. J. Tyrrell, E. V. A. Mould, J. C. Long, H. Gul, J. Cullis, and J. Braithwaite. 2020. "The rise of rapid implementation: A worked example of solving an existing problem with a new method by combining concept analysis with a systematic integrative review." *BMC Health Services Research* 20:449. doi: 10.1186/s12913-020-05289-0.

Zhou, X., E. Coiera, G. Tsafnat, D. Arachi, M.-S. Ong, and A. G. Dunn. 2015. "Using social connection information to improve opinion mining: Identifying negative sentiment about HPV vaccines on Twitter." *Studies in Health Technology and Informatics*:761–765.

32 Mixed method designs

Lawrence A. Palinkas

Mixed methods are methodologies that focus on collecting, analysing, and mixing quantitative and qualitative data in a single study or series of studies. Its central premise is that the combined use of quantitative and qualitative approaches provides a better understanding of research problems than either approach alone (Creswell and Plano Clark 2018). The key feature of mixed methods designs is the integration of qualitative and quantitative approaches into the methodology of a single study or multi-phased study where both sets of methods are used to answer the same question or each method to answer a related set of questions. For instance, the approach can be used to simultaneously answer exploratory and confirmatory questions and therefore generate and verify theory in the same study (Teddlie and Tashakkori 2003).

Mixed methods have increasingly become the standard design for implementation research (Palinkas et al. 2011). In hybrid designs, qualitative methods provide a depth of understanding of intervention and implementation processes and outcomes, while quantitative methods provide a breadth of understanding of outcomes, thereby enabling a simultaneous assessment of their construct and external validity. Quantitative methods have been used to examine implementation fidelity, and qualitative methods, to assist in adapting interventions during their implementation. Quantitative methods can reflect the perspective of the researcher, while qualitative methods might reflect consumer perspectives in implementation research. Finally, qualitative methods are occasionally used to corroborate statistically nonsignificant trends observed with quantitative data in studies lacking sufficient power.

Integration of *mixing* of qualitative and quantitative methods in an implementation study requires making several important decisions. For instance, when deciding who will be doing the mixing, it should be remembered that as with implementation research, mixed methods are team activities, involving one or more individuals with expertise in quantitative methods and one or more individuals with expertise in qualitative methods. Each team member should be sufficiently familiar with both sets of methods to facilitate communication and collaboration with each other and members possessing a different expertise (Palinkas and Soydan 2012).

A mixed method design typically involves the collection of both quantitative and qualitative data. However, there may be circumstances where the data are transformed such that qualitative data may be *quantitized* for quantitative analysis, as in concept mapping (Waltz et al. 2015), or quantitative data may be grouped into broad qualitative categories (e.g., better versus worse, expected versus unexpected). In an implementation study, quantitative methods may be used to assess intervention effectiveness and implementation determinants and outcomes, while qualitative methods such as semi-structured interviews, focus groups,

DOI: 10.4324/9781003109945-35

participant observation, and assessment of documents or texts may be used to understand implementation process and context (Palinkas, Mendon, and Hamilton 2019)

The amount of effort devoted to collecting quantitative and qualitative data may also be dependent upon the priority or weight assigned to each method. Using the terminology of mixed methods, the priority given to one method is signified by abbreviating the method in upper case (QUAN or QUAL), with the other method assigned a secondary role in the study signified by abbreviating the method in lower case (quan or qual). In some studies, equal priority can be assigned to both methods (QUAN + QUAL) (Palinkas et al. 2011).

The next decision to be made in designing mixed method studies is the timing of when data collection and analysis take place. Quantitative and qualitative data may be collected simultaneously (e.g., qual + QUAN, QUAL + quan) or sequentially (e.g., qual $\rightarrow$ QUAN, QUAL $\rightarrow$ quan). When viewed in the context of data collection and analysis, the process may be iterative such that each instance of data analysis (da) may precipitate another instance of data collection (dc) as in the following example where the analysis of quantitative data obtained from a large survey may generate some unanswered questions that necessitate the collection and analysis of qualitative data from survey participants, the results of which may lead to a subsequent survey (QUAN$_{dc/da}$ $\rightarrow$ qual$_{da}$ $\rightarrow$ QUAN2$_{dc/da}$). Another decision to be made is determining the function of each method and the rationale for integrating the two methods (the why of mixing). Palinkas et al. (2011) identified five distinct functions of mixed methods in implementation research as illustrated in Table 32.1.

Table 32.1 Five distinct functions of mixed methods in implementation research

Design type	Purpose
Convergence	• Corroboration of findings (data + interpretation) generated through quantitative methods with findings generated through qualitative designs (Triangulation). • Conversion of one type of data into another (quantitizing/qualitizing).
Complementarity	• Findings generated through qualitative methods answer exploratory questions, while findings generated through quantitative methods answer confirmatory questions. • Qualitative methods provide depth of understanding to complement breadth of understanding afforded by quantitative methods. • Qualitative methods used to study process and context and quantitative methods to study outcomes.
Expansion	• Findings from a qualitative study used to expand the depth of understanding of issues addressed in a quantitative study. • Findings from a quantitative study used to expand the breadth of understanding of issues addressed in a qualitative study.
Exploratory/ Development	• Findings from a qualitative study used to develop questions or items for a quantitative survey or instrument, develop or modify a conceptual framework used to generate hypotheses for quantitative analyses, or develop an intervention or program that can be evaluated quantitatively.
Sampling	• Use of one set of methods to identify participants who will provide data using the other set of methods (e.g., purposeful sampling of research participants for semi-structured interviews based on information collected from a quantitative survey; random sampling of a subpopulation of participants identified from interviews or participant observation as being of particular interest).

Source: Adapted from Palinkas et al. 2011

The function of mixed methods is "convergence" when seeking answers to the same question, "complementarity" when seeking answers to related questions, "expansion" or "explanation" when findings based on one method raise questions that can be answered by use of the other method, "development" when findings based on one method are a prerequisite to use of the other method, and "sampling" when one method can help to define or identify the participant sample for collection and analysis of data representing the other type of method.

In deciding how to mix the methods, one can select between three options: merging the data, connecting the data, and embedding the data. When merging the data, qualitative and quantitative data are brought together in the analysis phase to answer the same question through "triangulation" or related questions through "complementarity". When connecting the data, the insights gained from one type of method are connected to a different type of method to answer related questions sequentially through "complementarity", "expansion", "development", or "sampling". Perhaps the most common design, however, is when a qualitative study is embedded within a larger quantitative randomized controlled trial so that each method aims to seek answers to related questions simultaneously (e.g., using quantitative methods to assess intervention effectiveness and implementation outcomes and using qualitative methods to assess intervention and implementation process as well as implementation outcomes).

Any single implementation study may incorporate more than one type of design element with respect to data type, structure, timing, function, and mixing. As an illustration, a recent effort to develop a system for measuring the sustainment of prevention programs and initiatives that could, in turn, be used as an audit and feedback strategy for enhancing successful sustainment adopted a mixed method design in three distinct phases (see Box 32.1).

Box 32.1   Use of mixed methods in development of a sustainment measurement system

Phase 1: Three sets of qualitative data were collected simultaneously from 45 individuals representing ten prevention programs and initiatives and nine program officers (Palinkas et al. 2020b).

1   A series of semi-structured questions relating to experience with implementing and sustaining the grantee's program.
2   A free list exercise (Weller and Romney 1988) asking participants to respond to whatever came to mind when asked what was meant by the term "sustainment" or "sustainability", what components of their programs they most wanted to sustain, and what it would take to sustain those components.
3   A template of Consolidated Framework for Implementation Research (CFIR) domains and components (Damschroder et al. 2009) in which participants were asked to rate each of the domains and elements as being unimportant, somewhat important, important, or very important to sustainability of their program and to explain the basis for their assessment of each component to sustainability.

Phase 2: Free list exercise and CFIR construct endorsement data were transformed into quantitative data and then merged together to determine which sustainment constructs were identified by each method (*convergence*) (Palinkas et al. 2020b). Constructs identified by more than one method were then used to create a quantitative scale for measuring sustainability determinants and sustainment outcomes ("development"). The scale was then administered to a sample of 184 representatives of 145 programs to assess its validity and reliability (Palinkas et al. 2020a).

Phase 3: Fuzzy-set Qualitative Comparative Analysis (FsQCA) (Rihoux et al. 2009) was used to sequentially connect qualitative and quantitative data collected in Phase 2 to elaborate on associations between sustainability determinants and sustainment outcomes and identify causal pathways sufficient for producing sustainment ("expansion"). Sustainment was assessed by the extent to which grantees 1) continued to operate as described in the original application, 2) continued to deliver preventive services to the intended population, 3) continued to deliver evidence-based services, and 4) periodically measured fidelity of services delivered. Sustainability determinants included seven constructs identified in Phases 1 and 2 that were grouped into five CFIR construct domains: 1) financial stability ("outer setting"); 2) responsiveness to community needs and values characteristics of intervention; 3) coalitions, partnerships, and networks ("inner setting"); 4) organizational capacity (inner setting) and staff capability ("individual characteristics"); and 5) implementation leadership and monitoring, evaluation, and program outcomes ("implementation process"). Standard analysis found two configurational pathways sufficient to produce sustainment: 1) community responsiveness and organizational capacity when combined with process and 2) community responsiveness and organizational capacity when combined with coalitions, networks, and partnerships (Mendon et al. 2020).

Source: Created by author

Conclusion

Although mixed methods may be employed in any form of scientific inquiry, they are especially appropriate for use in implementation science due to the complexity of the phenomena under investigation and the opportunity to examine different aspects of these phenomena either in sequence or simultaneously.

References

Creswell, J. W., and V. L. Plano Clark. 2018. *Designing and Conducting Mixed Methods Research*. 3rd edition. ed. Thousand Oaks, CA: Sage Publications.

Damschroder, L. J., D. C. Aron, R. E. Keith, S. R. Kirsh, J. A. Alexander, and J. C. Lowery. 2009. "Fostering implementation of health services research findings into practice: A consolidated framework for advancing implementation science." *Implementation Science* 4 (1):1–15.

Mendon, S. J., L. Palinkas, M. Hurlburt, and R. Beidas. 2020. "Advancing our understanding of organizational constructs influencing the delivery of evidence-based practice across publicly-funded mental health agencies: A secondary data." In *12th Annual Conference on the Science of Dissemination and Implementation*. Academy Health.

Palinkas, L. A., G. A. Aarons, S. Horwitz, P. Chamberlain, M. Hurlburt, and J. Landsverk. 2011. "Mixed method designs in implementation research." *Administration and Policy in Mental Health* 38 (1):44–53. doi: 10.1007/s10488-010-0314-z.

Palinkas, L. A., C. P. Chou, S. E. Spear, S. J. Mendon, J. Villamar, and C. H. Brown. 2020a. "Measurement of sustainment of prevention programs and initiatives: The sustainment measurement system scale." *Implementation Science* 15 (1):1–15.

Palinkas, L. A., S. J. Mendon, and A. B. Hamilton. 2019. "Innovations in mixed methods evaluations." *Annual Review of Public Health* 40:423–442. doi: 10.1146/annurev-publhealth-040218-044215.

Palinkas, L. A., and H. Soydan. 2012. *Translation and Implementation of Evidence-Based Practice.* New York: Oxford University Press.

Palinkas, L. A., S. E. Spear, S. J. Mendon, J. Villamar, C. Reynolds, C. D. Green, C. Olson, A. Adade, and C. H. Brown. 2020b. "Conceptualizing and measuring sustainability of prevention programs, policies, and practices." *Translational Behavioral Medicine* 10 (1):136–145.

Rihoux, B., C. C. Ragin, S. Yamasaki, and D. Bol. 2009. "Conclusions – The way (s) ahead. Configurational comparative methods." *Qualitative Comparative Analysis (QCA) and Related Techniques*:167–178. doi: 10.4135/9781452226569.

Teddlie, C., and A. Tashakkori. 2003. *Major Issues and Controversies in the Use of Mixed Methods in the Social and Behavioral Sciences. Handbook of Mixed Methods in Social & Behavioral Research.* Thousand Oaks, CA: Sage Publications.

Waltz, T. J., B. J. Powell, M. M. Matthieu, L. J. Damschroder, M. J. Chinman, J. L. Smith, E. K. Proctor, and J. E. Kirchner. 2015. "Use of concept mapping to characterize relationships among implementation strategies and assess their feasibility and importance: Results from the Expert Recommendations for Implementing Change (ERIC) study." *Implementation Science* 10 (1):109. doi: 10.1186/s13012-015-0295-0.

Weller, S. C., and A. K. Romney. 1988. *Systematic Data Collection.* London: Sage Publications.

33 Simulation to improve patient care

Mary D. Patterson and Ellen S. Deutsch

Implementation science addresses processes to integrate "best practices" into healthcare delivery (Bauer et al. 2015). As discussed throughout this book, healthcare delivery is so complex and adaptive as to be incompletely knowable, and implementing interventions that improve patient care has proved challenging (Brady 2016). Simulation provides a powerful tool to advance implementation processes because it helps inform our understanding of healthcare delivery work as actually done. In particular, simulation can improve our understanding of the challenges and obstacles associated with new practices, thereby improving the likelihood of successful implementation. The term "simulation" encompasses a broad range of activities which incorporate participation in an event that replicates or represents a healthcare situation or environment. Simulations can address the skills and knowledge of individuals and teams or be used to understand or improve healthcare delivery systems.

SimulaTIONS use simulaTORS, which range from biologic or fabricated body parts to whole-body manikins, virtual or augmented reality representations of patients, or people trained to represent patients. Simulators with electronic enhancements can sense the participants' activities or demonstrate physiologic responses to interventions. Simulations can represent common or uncommon patient care events at the relative convenience of the participants, avoiding direct risks to patients (Deutsch 2011).

Simulation has been demonstrated to enhance healthcare provider confidence, knowledge, skills, and behaviours in both simulation and patient care (Barsuk et al. 2011, Fried et al. 2010, Wiet et al. 2012). Simulation has been shown to improve patient outcomes (Draycott et al. 2008) and not need to be expensive to be effective (Msemo et al. 2013).

System improvement using implementation science is a newer frontier for simulation. Simulated patient care can help bridge the gap between evidence-based practice, or Work-as-Imagined, and Work-as-Done (Hollnagel, Wears, and Braithwaite 2015), particularly when simulations are conducted in situ, involving actual patient care providers in patient care locations using patient care equipment. In situ simulation can contextualize and potentially improve efficacious processes to achieve real-world effectiveness (Learning Collaborative for Implementation Science in Global Brain Disorders). Debriefing, an essential component of learning from simulations, can explore the interactions between participants and their work systems. Recently, simulations have been conducted to understand adaptations of best practices needed to care for patients infected with COVID-19 (Daly Guris et al. 2020). The COVID-19 pandemic provided a "crash course" in the value of in situ simulation to test and implement a bewildering variety of protocols and processes. Because in situ simulation engages frontline workers and seeks their perspectives during debriefing, a more accurate understanding of the obstacles and adaptations required to adopt new processes is achieved.

DOI: 10.4324/9781003109945-36

Simulations can be conducted in response to an adverse event and may reveal actions or resources (or resource limitations), such as workarounds, that do not always surface in interviews or focus groups. Simulations conducted as components of process change planning can reveal previously unidentified hazards (Geis et al. 2011). Simulations may also be embedded as iterative process improvement activities to sustain improvement. Simulation aligned with Safety-II principles (Hollnagel, Wears, and Braithwaite 2015) can be used to explore what processes and resources are in place that contribute to patient care improvements.

In summary, simulation is a flexible and powerful tool that is currently underutilized in implementation work but that can be integrated throughout implementation processes to improve and support better patient care.

References

Barsuk, J. H., E. R. Cohen, J. Feinglass, W. C. McGaghie, and D. B. Wayne. 2011. "Unexpected collateral effects of simulation-based medical education." *Academic Medicine* 86 (12):1513–1517. doi: 10.1097/ACM.0b013e318234c493.

Bauer, M. S., L. Damschroder, H. Hagedorn, J. Smith, and A. M. Kilbourne. 2015. "An introduction to implementation science for the non-specialist." *BMC Psychology* 3 (1):32. doi: 10.1186/s40359-015-0089-9.

Brady, J. 2016. "Bridging efforts to improve patient safety and public health." *Agency for Healthcare Research and Quality*. https://archive.ahrq.gov/news/blog/ahrqviews/bridging-efforts-to-improve-patient-safety.html.

Daly Guris, R. J., E. M. Elliott, A. Doshi, D. Singh, K. Widmeier, E. S. Deutsch, V. M. Nadkarni, K. R. Jackson, R. Subramanyam, J. E. Fiadjoe, and H. G. Gurnaney. 2020. "Systems-focused simulation to prepare for COVID-19 intraoperative emergencies." *Paediatric Anaesthesia* 30 (8):947–950. doi: 10.1111/pan.13971.

Deutsch, E. S. 2011. "Simulation in otolaryngology: Smart dummies and more." *Otolaryngology Head and Neck Surgery* 145 (6):899–903. doi: 10.1177/0194599811424862.

Draycott, T. J., J. F. Crofts, J. P. Ash, L. V. Wilson, E. Yard, T. Sibanda, and A. Whitelaw. 2008. "Improving neonatal outcome through practical shoulder dystocia training." *Obstetrics and Gynecology* 112 (1):14–20. doi: 10.1097/AOG.0b013e31817bbc61.

Fogarty International Center. n.d. "Learning collaborative for implementation science in global brain disorders." In *Toolkit Part 1: Implementation Science Methodologies and Frameworks*. https://www.fic.nih.gov/About/center-global-health-studies/neuroscience-implementation-toolkit/Pages/methodologies-frameworks.aspx

Fried, M. P., B. Sadoughi, M. J. Gibber, J. B. Jacobs, R. A. Lebowitz, D. A. Ross, J. P. Bent, 3rd, S. R. Parikh, C. T. Sasaki, and S. D. Schaefer. 2010. "From virtual reality to the operating room: The endoscopic sinus surgery simulator experiment." *Otolaryngology Head and Neck Surgery* 142 (2):202–207. doi: 10.1016/j.otohns.2009.11.023.

Geis, G. L., B. Pio, T. L. Pendergrass, M. R. Moyer, and M. D. Patterson. 2011. "Simulation to assess the safety of new healthcare teams and new facilities." *Simulation in Healthcare* 6 (3):125–133. doi: 10.1097/SIH.0b013e31820dff30.

Hollnagel, E., R. L. Wears, and J. Braithwaite. 2015. *From Safety-I to Safety-II: A White Paper*. Published simultaneously by the University of Southern Denmark, University of Florida, USA, and Macquarie University, Australia. The Resilient Health Care Net.

Msemo, G., A. Massawe, D. Mmbando, N. Rusibamayila, K. Manji, H. L. Kidanto, D. Mwizamuholya, P. Ringia, H. L. Ersdal, and J. Perlman. 2013. "Newborn mortality and fresh stillbirth rates in Tanzania after helping babies breathe training." *Pediatrics* 131 (2):e353–e360. doi: 10.1542/peds.2012-1795.

Wiet, G. J., D. Stredney, T. Kerwin, B. Hittle, S. A. Fernandez, M. Abdel-Rasoul, and D. B. Welling. 2012. "Virtual temporal bone dissection system: OSU virtual temporal bone system: Development and testing." *Laryngoscope* 122 Suppl 1 (Suppl 1):S1–S12. doi: 10.1002/lary.22499.

34 In situ simulation

Kyota Nakamura and Kazue Nakajima

In situ simulation refers to simulation in actual clinical settings, with actual staff, equipment, and systems (Lockman, Ambardekar, and Deutsch 2014). It can provide an opportunity for clinicians to have more realistic experiences than simulation training in a laboratory setting. It also allows team members to review and reinforce their skills for solving problems in actual work (Patterson, Blike, and Nadkarni 2008). Thus, in situ simulation can be useful to understand how people work in given systems and assist implementation of new processes or tools for improvement. Two cases illustrate how in situ simulation using simple scenarios can help identify small barriers to interprofessional collaboration and lead to better team performance.

Scenario 1: patient collapses in the chemotherapy room

A patient safety concern in a teaching hospital is a situation when a patient suddenly collapses. This has happened in Japan, in the chemotherapy department, which was recently opened in one Japanese hospital's outpatient area. One aim of the in situ simulation in the chemotherapy department in question is to verify the current clinical response plan for patient deterioration, along with training in resuscitation skills. At the beginning of the scenario, clinical members of the chemotherapy department witnessed the patient's collapse and immediately requested the hospital resuscitation team to come to the chemotherapy room, according to the standard operating procedure that related to such a situation arising, but the team did not appear. In fact, the resuscitation team could not find the chemotherapy room. This simulation provided an opportunity to recognize that clinicians need to specify their location when asking for help, such as stating "the chemotherapy room next to the outpatient clinic", which can lead to systemic improvements, such as speedier responses, when requesting help.

Scenario 2: unexpected massive intraoperative bleeding

Another safety concern we have noted from in situ simulation in the case hospital is the stress that can be induced in anaesthesiologists who experience lengthy waiting times for the delivery of blood products in operating rooms, particularly when massive blood transfusions are urgently needed. An in situ simulation in the central operation department of the case hospital aimed to train relevant healthcare professionals to respond immediately to unexpected massive patient bleeds. Following training, during debriefing, some transfusion technicians proposed delivering blood products directly to the operating room instead of following the current practice of waiting for a circulating nurse to hand over the blood products. Everyone

DOI: 10.4324/9781003109945-37

on the team agreed with this proposal. The technicians had never expected to be able to enter an operating room, and the surgical team had never imagined that the technicians had thought this way. After the simulation, the technicians delivered blood products directly to each operating room, which consequently improved the work efficiency of the surgical team.

In situ simulations allow clinicians and others to experience actual or possible cognitive, psychological, and physical experiences, both positive and negative, that they cannot envisage in laboratory environments. Such recognition of real-world obstacles, which are sometimes trivial but at other times important, can lead to improvements in the overall quality of team performance. In situ simulations with multiple professional groups in different departments can also provide more potential solutions to difficulties through collaboration, which can then lead to an increase in the team's adaptive capacity. Since there is no harm if things do not go well in a simulation situation, it is possible to turn adversity into opportunity. Sharing constructive learning experiences among different professionals can also facilitate psychological safety at work and strengthen teamwork across workforce-imposed boundaries.

References

Lockman, J., A. Ambardekar, and E. Deutsch. 2014. "Optimizing education with in situ simulation." In *Defining Excellence in Simulation Programs*, edited by J. C. Palaganas, J. C. Maxworthy, C. A. Epps and M. E. Mancini. Society for Simulation in Healthcare. Philadelphia, PA: Wolters Kluwer.

Patterson, M., G. Blike, and V. Nadkarni. 2008. "In situ simulation: Challenges and results." In *Advances in Patient Safety: New Directions and Alternative Approaches*, edited by K. Henriksen, J. B. Battles, M. A. Keyes and M. L. Grady. Rockville, MD: Agency for Healthcare Research and Quality.

35 Emergency Implementation Science

John Øvretveit

Emergency Implementation Science (EIS) is a rapidly growing sub-discipline of implementation science. EIS is a body of knowledge about rapid change and methods and tools for making and researching changes to behaviours, organizations, and systems. Examples are knowledge about rapid implementation of virtual learning for schools, of correct use of personal protective equipment, and of plans to respond to an emergency situation, such as an earthquake or terrorist attack. EIS covers a broad range of sectors, subjects, and changes at the individual, service unit, organization, or whole system levels. It includes multilevel changes that need coordination, such as a community response to a pandemic, as well as rapid changes to computer systems, including linking databases, providing simulation models, and applying machine learning and artificial intelligence learning and feedback. This overview considers one growing field of EIS, which applies and develops implementation science to enable more effective and rapid change in healthcare responses to emergencies.

Features of emergency implementation of changes are that 1) decision-makers need to act without certain information; 2) the changes are often not tested or based on strong evidence of effectiveness; and 3) to be immediately useful, researchers need quickly to find and provide evidence about effective rapidly implementable changes for decision-makers, or monitor the change and give feedback during the change, as well as after.

One such recent emergency was the COVID-19 pandemic, which differed from other emergency responses to single events, like earthquake, flood, or a large fire, which are easier to plan and practice for and are more time limited. Other scientific disciplines, such as disaster medicine and public health, include health services as part of their knowledge base about emergency responses to crises. However, the application of behaviour and organizational change is limited, and no use is made of recent implementation science (Koenig 2016).

A number of implementation science studies are using implementation science concepts with traditional observational and mixed method designs to document and evaluate how service delivery units and systems responded to the pandemic. This research will be useful for future infectious disease outbreaks. Our EIS action evaluation of the response of Stockholm healthcare to the COVID-19 pandemic illustrates some aspects of this sub-discipline and an action evaluation partnership approach (Ovretveit 2002). This is suited to emergency implementation and, in some ways, is similar to Learning Health System approaches and some quality improvement in its research and feedback to decision-makers using data collected by the health system (Etheredge 2007, Institute of Medicine 2007, Langly et al. 1997).

In Stockholm, our study documented many changes to practice, organization, data systems, and policies rapidly made by primary and secondary care services at different times, and most were not based on strong evidence. The action evaluation approach that we used documented these changes and, where possible, gave feedback on the effects, drawing on

DOI: 10.4324/9781003109945-38

data we collected from a weekly survey of all managers and the different data systems in the Stockholm region (see Figure 35.1) (Ohrling et al. 2020). One challenge was to decide which change to study in order to be of most use to decision-making during the crisis and for future disease outbreaks.

We used the implementation science conceptual distinction between intervention-change and implementation-actions to specify the intervention as the emergency management system that healthcare established. The implementation-actions to establish this system included changes in management structures and authorities, decentralization and coordination, and changes to data systems to provide more timely data (Ohrling et al. 2020). To understand why some units were successful in their rapid change implementation, we found it useful to apply the specification of inner and other contexts in the consolidated framework for implementation (Damschroder et al. 2009). Our pre-study data gathering plan had guided data collection about this, and we were able to use the data about unit base and region and national contexts to learn how some units were hindered by policies around staffing and others by payment systems for virtual consultations. For the vaccination program and vaccination hesitancy changes, we were able to use the Capability, Opportunity, Motivation, Behaviour (COM-B) model to design and evaluate the different services and the outreach activities for refugee, migrant, and immigrant populations (Michie, Van Stralen, and West 2011, Ovretveit 2021).

Overall, the research provided timely feedback to the management team about the effect of changes and important knowledge for future emergency implementation response. We

Overview time-plan of research

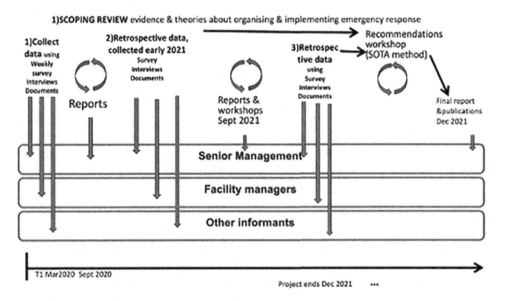

Figure 35.1 Design and data collection in an emergency implementation action evaluation of Stockholm healthcare response to COVID-19 pandemic

Source: Created by authors

discovered ways to improve action for an emergent response in a constantly evolving crisis. This was characterized by new information about effective change and new high-level policies and regulations, daily and weekly, that the healthcare system needed to implement.

For researchers, EIS provides important and exciting opportunities to work at the frontier of implementation science with new real-world research designs and action evaluation methods, digital research techniques, and in partnership with stakeholders (Øvretveit 2020). Doing so gives a "shop window" to decision-makers about the contribution that implementation science can make when shaped to provide rapid, actionable, and credible information about how to implement decisions quickly. Most importantly, this science directly and quickly can contribute to saving lives and reducing unnecessary suffering.

References

Damschroder, L., D. Aron, R. Keith, S. Kirsh, J. Alexander, and J. Lowery. 2009. "Fostering implementation of health services research findings into practice: A consolidated framework for advancing implementation science." *Implementation Science* 4 (1):1–15.

Etheredge, L. M. 2007. "A rapid-learning health system: What would a rapid-learning health system look like, and how might we get there?" *Health Affairs* 26 (Suppl 1):w107–w118.

Institute of Medicine. 2007. *The Learning Healthcare System: Workshop Summary*. Washington, DC: The National Academic Press.

Koenig, K. 2016. *Koenig and Schultz's Disaster Medicine: Comprehensive Principles and Practices*. 2nd ed. New York: Cambridge University Press.

Langly, G., K. Nolan, T. Nolan, C. Norman, and L. Provost. 1997. *The Improvement Guide*. San Francisco: Jossey Bass.

Michie, S., M. M. Van Stralen, and R. West. 2011. "The behaviour change wheel: A new method for characterising and designing behaviour change interventions." *Implementation Science* 6 (1):1–12.

Ohrling, M., J. Øvretveit, U. Lockowandt, M. Brommels, and V. Sparring. 2020. "Management of the emergency response to the SARS-CoV-2 (COVID-19) outbreak in Stockholm, Sweden, and winter preparations." *Journal of Primary Health Care* 12 (3):207–214.

Ovretveit, J. 2002. "Action evaluation: What is it and why evaluate?" In *Action Evaluation of Health Programmes and Changes: A Handbook for a User-focused Approach*. Abingdon, Oxfordshire: Radcliffe Medical Press.

Øvretveit, J. 2020. "Implementation researchers can improve the responses of services to the COVID-19 pandemic." *Implementation Research and Practice* 1:2633489520949151.

Ovretveit, J. 2021. *Vaccination Engagement and Evidence Updates: Vaccination Hesitancy and Equity Improving Vaccination Take-up in Under-vaccinated Groups and Evidence Update Briefing 6, 4th March 2021*. Stockholm: Karolinska Institute.

36 Planning for implementation

Why, who, and how

Andrea Smith and Karen Hutchinson

Implementation planning is the crucial work done in advance and throughout to maximize intervention uptake and reduce risk of failure. Effective planning for implementation takes a team. Implementation planning is relevant not only to the healthcare professionals, health promotion practitioners, policymakers, and administrators who are tasked with the adoption of programs or policies but also to the epidemiologists and public health and healthcare researchers responsible for designing, testing, and comparing interventions and programs for efficacy and effectiveness (Rankin et al. 2019, Neta, Brownson, and Chambers 2018, Bauer et al. 2015).

Why is planning for implementation relevant to effectiveness researchers?

In the past 20 years, attention in healthcare research and delivery has moved from a preoccupation with effectiveness research ("Does it work?") to asking whether an intervention will work in the real world, with real patients and real clinicians working within a real organization (Greenhalgh 2018). This is because the vast majority of the research on evidence-based interventions does not translate into policy and practice and fails to improve health outcomes (Glasgow and Emmons 2007, Neta, Brownson, and Chambers 2018). Much of the intervention research undertaken is not clinically useful and will not change clinical practice, is not feasible and fails to answer a real and important problem (Riley et al. 2013, Greenhalgh 2018), or is not pragmatic and generates results that are not generalizable to real-world patients and settings (Brownson, Fielding, and Green 2018). If effectiveness researchers want to get their evidence-based interventions into practice, to make a difference, then they need to think beyond "Does it work?" and start to think about the challenges implementation practitioners face and ask "Will it work here?" This means thinking beyond the carefully controlled research setting to consider how conditions, resources, and policies might impact the delivery of their intervention in the real world of public health and healthcare delivery and to engage and clarify roles with key stakeholders early in the implementation process (Box 36.1). Unless this is done, it is highly unlikely that their evidence-based interventions will ever be adopted or, if adopted, will be implemented appropriately or sustainably (Greenhalgh 2018).

Box 36.1 Planning for implementation of evidence-based interventions in healthcare: key points for healthcare effectiveness researchers

- Successful implementation of evidence-based healthcare interventions into routine clinical practice is not automatic. Carefully consider the complex, contextual

---

DOI: 10.4324/9781003109945-39

factors operating at the levels of the healthcare system (local, regional, or national), organization (e.g., hospital, clinic), and individual (e.g., clinician, patient, carer) that support or impede adoption of an intervention into routine clinical care.

- Engage early with stakeholders to ensure that the research is clinically useful and that it addresses a problem of genuine importance to clinicians and patients (Greenhalgh 2018).
- Pay attention to external validity by considering pragmatic study designs that more closely reflect real-world patients and settings (Brown et al. 2017).
- Consider the three types of hybrid effectiveness-implementation study designs which focus on clinical effectiveness and implementation and allow for the collection of pilot acceptability and feasibility data that can be used to inform and can hasten future implementation planning (Curran et al. 2012).
- Draw on implementation science's growing knowledge base to better understand why an effective intervention may or may not be implemented, for instance, factors that influence the decision to adopt an intervention, the resources that will be needed to deliver an intervention, and the need to change clinician and patient behaviour to deliver the intervention with fidelity and sustainability (Nilsen 2015).

Source: Created by authors

How should implementation practitioners plan for implementation?

Implementation has been described as an art and a science, but in reality, it is more than both of these. It is a *complex practice that requires skill and situational judgement* (Greenhalgh 2018, Brownson, Fielding, and Green 2018). Fortunately, policymakers and implementation practitioners, that is, those involved in selecting and making decisions about real-world use of interventions, programs, and guidelines, now have considerable resources available to help them select the most appropriate evidence-based intervention and plan for implementation within a particular setting (Box 36.2).

Box 36.2 Planning for implementation of evidence-based interventions in healthcare: key points for implementation practitioners

- Draw on implementation science's growing theoretical base (Nilsen 2015) and online tools and resources to help you identify an appropriate evidence-based intervention and to plan the implementation process.
- Ask yourself these key questions about the proposed intervention: "Does the innovation fit?" "Should we do it here?" "Can we do it here?" and then "How will we do it here?"(RTI International Agency for Healthcare Research and Quality 2008).
- Use a planning tool such as Exploration, Preparation, Implementation, Sustainment (EPIS) framework (Aarons, Hurlburt, and Horwitz 2011) to understand the different stages of the implementation process; are you at the exploratory, planning, implementation, or sustainment phase?

- Engage with relevant stakeholders, build trust, and ensure you have the right people on your team (e.g., clinicians, decision-makers, consumers, health services researchers, health economists, specialists with knowledge of sociology, organizational, behavioural, and managerial science) (Rankin et al. 2019).
- Establish roles and responsibilities; be clear about who is doing what on the implementation team and communicate routinely; this is particularly relevant when researchers and practitioners work together (as they should) and resources are limited (Wandersman et al. 2008).
- Identify and prepare effective champions to support implementation of change: success is based on "What they do" and "Who they are" (Bonawitz et al. 2020).
- Be clear about the effectiveness outcomes and implementation outcomes that you want to evaluate; determine which measures you will use to assess these outcomes (Proctor et al. 2009).

Source: Created by authors

Implementation science's growing theoretical base comprises numerous "tools" that can be used heuristically or systematically to help practitioners plan for implementation (Nilsen 2015). First, process models (also known as "research-to-practice" or "knowledge-to-action" models), such as the Knowledge-to Action (KTA) model (Graham et al. 2006), and the EPIS framework (Aarons, Hurlburt, and Horwitz 2011), are useful at the conceptual level to map out the key stages in a project. Many practitioners find more linear "how-to-implement" process models such as the Quality Implementation Framework (Meyers, Durlak, and Wandersman 2012) and Intervention Mapping (Bartholomew, Parcel, and Kok 1998), the ImpRes tool (Hull et al. 2019), and the model by Pronovost and colleagues (Pronovost, Berenholtz, and Needham 2008) particularly useful as they focus on providing step-by-step, practical guidance and support for planning and managing collaborative implementation projects. Second, determinant frameworks, such as the Diffusion of Innovations in Service Organizations model (Greenhalgh et al. 2004), the Consolidated Framework for Implementation Research (CFIR) (Damschroder et al. 2009), and Theoretical Domains Framework (TDF)(Michie et al. 2005) can help to identify factors operating at the level of the intervention, individual, organization, or system that might support or hinder successful implementation. Third, compilations of implementation strategies (Powell et al. 2015) and behavioural change techniques (Michie et al. 2013) can help guide the selection of strategies and techniques that are most likely to address the identified barriers to implementation. And finally, there are evaluation frameworks, such as the Reach, Efficacy, Adoption, Implementation, and Maintenance (RE-AIM) model (Glasgow, Vogt, and Boles 1999) that can be used to determine how successful implementation has been.

Despite the plethora of tools, they all draw attention to a number of elements that are important to successful implementation. These elements demonstrate the importance of change and the characterization of the nature of that change, the significance of context, the recognition that change requires active and deliberate action, and that particular barriers to implementation exist across different settings and sites.

Will planning for implementation ensure success?

A word of caution. Healthcare is a Complex Adaptive System, meaning it is inherently unpredictable and subject to continual change (Braithwaite et al. 2018). It is probabilistic and stochastic rather than deterministic and causal (Braithwaite et al. 2018). Although planning will increase the chances of successful implementation of an intervention within a given healthcare setting, it must always be understood that implementation can never be mechanistic or procedural. Instead, it requires an approach that is agile and adaptable and that allows for the monitoring of the implementation process and continual adjustments based on carefully collected data before, during, and after the implementation process (Greenhalgh 2018).

At times, implementation science's multitude of frameworks, models and theories, outcomes, strategies, and measures can seem overwhelming; however, it is important not to lose sight of the fact that at the end of the day, most decisions to adopt rest on whether or not the clinician, manager, policymaker, or patient is persuaded by the evidence and if they believe that change is necessary or possible (Greenhalgh 2018). If the clinician does not believe that adherence to a recommendation would be in the best interests of the patient, or that it is not practical to follow the recommendations, they will almost certainly not even attempt to follow them (Greenhalgh 2018, Smith et al. 2020).

References

Aarons, G. A., M. Hurlburt, and S. M. Horwitz. 2011. "Advancing a conceptual model of evidence-based practice implementation in public service sectors." *Administration and Policy in Mental Health and Mental Health Services Research* 38 (1):4–23. doi: 10.1007/s10488-010-0327-7.

Bartholomew, L. K., G. S. Parcel, and G. Kok. 1998. "Intervention mapping: A process for developing theory and evidence-based health education programs." *Health Education & Behavior* 25 (5):545–563.

Bauer, M. S., L. Damschroder, H. Hagedorn, J. Smith, and A. M. Kilbourne. 2015. "An introduction to implementation science for the non-specialist." *BMC Psychology* 3 (1):32. doi: 10.1186/s40359-015-0089-9.

Bonawitz, K., M. Wetmore, M. Heisler, V. K. Dalton, L. J. Damschroder, J. Forman, K. R. Allan, and M. H. Moniz. 2020. "Champions in context: Which attributes matter for change efforts in healthcare?" *Implementation Science* 15 (1):1–10.

Braithwaite, J., K. Churruca, J. C. Long, L. A. Ellis, and J. Herkes. 2018. "When complexity science meets implementation science: A theoretical and empirical analysis of systems change." *BMC Medicine* 16 (1). doi: 10.1186/s12916-018-1057-z.

Brown, C. H., G. Curran, L. A. Palinkas, G. A. Aarons, K. B. Wells, L. Jones, L. M. Collins, N. Duan, B. S. Mittman, A. Wallace, R. G. Tabak, L. Ducharme, D. A. Chambers, G. Neta, T. Wiley, J. Landsverk, K. Cheung, and G. Cruden. 2017. "An overview of research and evaluation designs for dissemination and implementation." *Annual Review of Public Health* 38:1–22. doi: 10.1146/annurev-publhealth-031816-044215.

Brownson, R. C., J. E. Fielding, and L. W. Green. 2018. "Building capacity for evidence-based public health: Reconciling the pulls of practice and the push of research." *Annual Review of Public Health* 39 (1):27–53. doi: 10.1146/annurev-publhealth-040617-014746.

Curran, G. M., M. Bauer, B. Mittman, J. M. Pyne, and C. Stetler. 2012. "Effectiveness-implementation hybrid designs: Combining elements of clinical effectiveness and implementation research to enhance public health impact." *Medical Care* 50 (3):217.

Damschroder, L. J., D. C. Aron, R. E. Keith, S. R. Kirsh, J. A. Alexander, and J. C. Lowery. 2009. "Fostering implementation of health services research findings into practice: A consolidated framework for advancing implementation science." *Implementation Science* 4 (1):50. doi: 10.1186/1748-5908-4-50.

Glasgow, R. E., and K. M. Emmons. 2007. "How can we increase translation of research into practice? Types of evidence needed." *Annual Review of Public Health* 28:413–433.

Glasgow, R. E., T. M. Vogt, and S. M. Boles. 1999. "Evaluating the public health impact of health promotion interventions: The RE-AIM framework." *American Journal of Public Health* 89 (9):1322–1327.

Graham, I. D., J. Logan, M. B. Harrison, S. E. Straus, J. Tetroe, W. Caswell, and N. Robinson. 2006. "Lost in knowledge translation: Time for a map?" *Journal of Continuing Education in the Health Professions* 26 (1):13–24.

Greenhalgh, T. 2018. *How to Implement Evidence-based Healthcare.* 1st ed. London: John Wiley & Sons Ltd.

Greenhalgh, T., G. Robert, F. Macfarlane, P. Bate, and O. Kyriakidou. 2004. "Diffusion of innovations in service organizations: Systematic review and recommendations." *The Milbank Quarterly* 82 (4):581–629.

Hull, L., L. Goulding, Z. Khadjesari, R. Davis, A. Healey, I. Bakolis, and N. Sevdalis. 2019. "Designing high-quality implementation research: Development, application, feasibility and preliminary evaluation of the implementation science research development (ImpRes) tool and guide." *Implementation Science* 14 (1):80. doi: 10.1186/s13012-019-0897-z.

Meyers, D. C., J. A. Durlak, and A. Wandersman. 2012. "The quality implementation framework: A synthesis of critical steps in the implementation process." *American Journal of Community Psychology* 50 (3–4):462–480.

Michie, S., M. Johnston, C. Abraham, R. Lawton, D. Parker, and A. Walker. 2005. "Making psychological theory useful for implementing evidence based practice: A consensus approach." *BMJ Quality & Safety* 14 (1):26–33.

Michie, S., M. Richardson, M. Johnston, C. Abraham, J. Francis, W. Hardeman, M. P. Eccles, J. Cane, and C. E. Wood. 2013. "The behavior change technique taxonomy (v1) of 93 hierarchically clustered techniques: Building an international consensus for the reporting of behavior change interventions." *Annals of Behavioral Medicine* 46 (1):81–95. doi: 10.1007/s12160-013-9486-6.

Neta, G., R. C. Brownson, and D. A. Chambers. 2018. "Opportunities for epidemiologists in implementation science: A primer." *American Journal of Epidemiology* 187 (5):899–910.

Nilsen, P. 2015. "Making sense of implementation theories, models and frameworks." *Implementation Science* 10 (1):53. doi: 10.1186/s13012-015-0242-0.

Powell, B. J., T. J. Waltz, M. J. Chinman, L. J. Damschroder, J. L. Smith, M. M. Matthieu, E. K. Proctor, and J. E. Kirchner. 2015. "A refined compilation of implementation strategies: Results from the Expert Recommendations for Implementing Change (ERIC) project." *Implementation Science* 10:21. doi: 10.1186/s13012-015-0209-1.

Proctor, E. K., J. Landsverk, G. Aarons, D. Chambers, C. Glisson, and B. Mittman. 2009. "Implementation research in mental health services: An emerging science with conceptual, methodological, and training challenges." *Administration and Policy in Mental Health and Mental Health Services Research* 36 (1):24–34.

Pronovost, P. J., S. M. Berenholtz, and D. M. Needham. 2008. "Translating evidence into practice: A model for large scale knowledge translation." *BMJ* 337.

Rankin, N. M., P. N. Butow, T. F. Hack, J. M. Shaw, H. L. Shepherd, A. Ugalde, and A. E. Sales. 2019. "An implementation science primer for psycho-oncology: Translating robust evidence into practice." *Journal of Psychosocial Oncology Research and Practice* 1 (3):e14.

Riley, W. T., R. E. Glasgow, L. Etheredge, and A. P. Abernethy. 2013. "Rapid, responsive, relevant (R3) research: A call for a rapid learning health research enterprise." *Clinical and Translational Medicine* 2 (1):1–6.

RTI International Agency for Healthcare Research Quality. 2008. *Will It Work Here? A Decisionmaker's Guide to Adopting Innovations.* Rockville, MD: Agency for Healthcare Research and Quality. Accessed February 2021. https://www.ahrq.gov/innovations/will-work/index.html.

Smith, A. L., C. G. Watts, S. Robinson, H. Schmid, C. Goumas, V. J. Mar, J. F. Thompson, F. Rapport, A. M. C. o. R. E. S. Group, and A. E. Cust. 2020. "Knowledge and attitudes of Australian dermatologists towards sentinel lymph node biopsy for melanoma: A mixed methods study." *Australasian Journal of Dermatology* 62 (2):168–176.

Wandersman, A., J. Duffy, P. Flaspohler, R. Noonan, K. Lubell, L. Stillman, M. Blachman, R. Dunville, and J. Saul. 2008. "Bridging the gap between prevention research and practice: The interactive systems framework for dissemination and implementation." *American Journal of Community Psychology* 41 (3–4):171–181. doi: 10.1007/s10464-008-9174-z.

37 Consensus building

A key concept in implementation science

Lawrence Susskind

Consensus building (CB) requires the successful completion of a series of steps. First, the sponsors of a CB process must identify the relevant participants – including individuals who can speak for self-appointed and hard-to-represent stakeholder groups. These individuals must agree to participate and, often, approve the ground rules and procedures that will govern their joint problem-solving efforts. Next, the parties must agree on 1) the selection or appointment of someone with the skills and standing to manage a multiparty negotiation and 2) a timetable and format for whatever process is being put in place. In a democratic context, CB can be used as an alternative to winner-take-all, majority rule, decision-making. It can also be added as an informal step preceding a winner-take-all vote. In the latter case, a negotiated agreement can be injected into a formal debate or deliberation, if it is timely and prepared with the permission of those in authority. Usually, ad hoc CB efforts of the former variety are used when most of the relevant stakeholders recognize that a formal governmental decision will not have a clear path forward, even if a decision is pushed from the "top".

According to negotiation theory, CB works best when the parties focus "on the merits of each other's arguments", incorporating objective evidence and seeking to create value rather than merely engaging in political horse-trading (i.e., "I'll do this for you, if you do that for me.") (Fisher and Ury 1981). CB seeks unanimity but settles for overwhelming agreement as long as outliers are given an opportunity to express the reasons for their dissent and the rest of the group makes a good-faith effort to address the concerns of the outliers (Susskind, McKearnen, and Thomas-Lamar 1999). Indeed, it is a mistake to think of consensus in terms of unanimity (even though some dictionaries define the word that way). Requiring unanimity gives a single, politically motivated actor veto power. Seeking unanimity, but settling for overwhelming agreement, does not give a dedicated blackmailer power over the group or the process.

CB is essential in formulation and implementation of international policies, programs, designs, and technology sharing agreements (i.e., treaties) where no votes are taken (and a majority does not rule) because each country's sovereignty is guaranteed. In such situations, negotiated agreement through CB is the only way disagreements in the full group can be resolved. In domestic democratic contexts, where majority rule is usually the basis for governmental decision-making, parties often proceed to decisions prior to a CB effort. If all it takes is a bare majority to act unilaterally, the group that is sure it can "win" sees no need to accommodate the interests of its opponents. We know, though, that CB can work (and is often valuable), even in these contexts – regardless of the level of contention or hostility among the parties – because unhappy parties (left out of policymaking) may mobilize in opposition. CB can help in these contexts as long as two conditions are met. First, a non-partisan facilitator must be available to assist or referee the exchange among the parties.

DOI: 10.4324/9781003109945-40

Second, this N + 1st party (i.e., where N is the number of parties in the agreement-seeking interaction) must be accepted by all the parties (Susskind and Cruikshank 1989, Susskind and Ali 2014). So, the reason a potential winning majority should seek to add a CB step to its deliberations is that implementation of its decisions can be thwarted by those who have been left out of the process.

Emerging theories of governance (Ansell and Torfing 2016) suggest that all stakeholders ought to be involved in political decision-making and public policymaking efforts (even when this is not required by law). First, it is fairer to give everyone affected by a decision a more direct role in shaping that decision. Second, a clear willingness to consult can generate political legitimacy even among those who oppose a decision. Sometimes calls for widespread engagement in governance only lead to superficial dialogue (for show) but not to real involvement in decision-making. It is possible, however, to provide opportunities for unofficial representatives to participate in meaningful CB efforts that lead to substantive proposals (and not merely to a summary of conflicting beliefs). These can then be acted on by formally elected or appointed decision-makers. Those with formal decision-making authority need to invite stakeholders to participate in an informal problem-solving "step" that ends with a proposal, not a decision. The formal decision-making body then starts its deliberations by focusing on that proposal, retaining the right to reject it, build on but revise it, or accept it as is.

Implementation of public decision-making, at every scale, usually requires continuous or ongoing support by citizens concerned about decisions that affect them. In situations where the rule of law prevails, even if a majority supports a policy or a decision, an unhappy minority can block action by appealing to the courts. CB prior to decision-making, as described previously, can eliminate the emergence of an unhappy minority and even build a broader coalition willing to make sure that decisions are implemented properly. There are numerous well-documented accounts of successful CB in a great many different cultural and cross-cultural contexts (Susskind and Crump 2009). The most general model of CB is described in Figure 37.1.

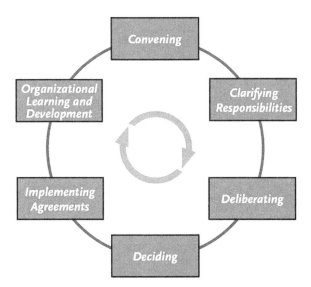

Figure 37.1 Six steps to building consensus

Source: Reprinted from Susskind, McKearnen and Thomas-Lamar 1999, with permission from the Consensus Building Institute (CBI.org)

CB is a process than can strengthen democracy. In the context of local decision-making, public participation and public engagement are often used by elected officials to legitimize the administrative actions that officials take. But, merely giving voice to the concerns of citizens and stakeholders does not really include them. Only a commitment to CB ensures that those affected by decisions are truly involved in helping to formulate and implement them.

References

Ansell, C., and J. Torfing. 2016. *Handbook on Theories of Governance*. Cheltenham: Edward Elgar Publishing.

Fisher, R., and W. Ury. 1981. *Getting to Yes*. Boston, MA: Houghton-Mifflin.

Susskind, L., and J. Cruikshank. 1989. *Breaking the Impasse: Consensual Approaches to Resolving Public Disputes*. Boston, MA: Basic Books.

Susskind, L., and L. Crump. 2009. *Volume I: An Introduction to Theory and Practice, Multiparty Negotiation*. London: Sage Publications.

Susskind, L. E., and S. H. Ali. 2014. *Environmental Diplomacy: Negotiating More Effective Global Agreements*. 2nd ed. New York: Oxford University Press.

Susskind, L. E., S. McKearnen, and J. Thomas-Lamar. 1999. *The Consensus Building Handbook: A Comprehensive Guide to Reaching Agreement*. Thousand Oaks, CA: Sage Publications.

38 Nudge

Finding clues and using cues to shift clinician behaviour

Klay Lamprell

Automated surveillance of staff hand hygiene in two wards of an Australian teaching hospital found adherence rates of just over 30 per cent in the medical ward and just over 50 per cent in the surgical ward. To prompt greater protocol compliance, data from the automated surveillance dashboards were discussed at daily handover meetings (an audit and feedback and peer comparison nudge), and staff were asked to remind each other to "take a moment" for hand hygiene before entering patients' rooms (a social norm and commitment nudge). Hand hygiene adherence lifted by 1 per cent in the medical ward and 9 per cent in the surgical ward over seven months, with both dropping back to baseline when the verbal nudge was removed (Kwok, Harris, and McLaws 2017).

Implementation scientists working in healthcare face two significant challenges: medical professionals won't necessarily make the smartest choices given access to the best information, and medical decision-making occurs in highly complex environments that can differ significantly between communities of practice, even within one organization. A nudge that has impact in one context may be ineffective in another. Nudges load a choice environment with easily accessible cognitive and/or emotive gains that draw clinicians towards evidence-based practice (Keller et al. 2011). Crucially, the gains must be relevant enough, and robust enough, to shift the physical, social, and/or cultural forces driving decision-making in the existing choice environment. Computerized prescribing that defaults to evidence-based medications, for example, offers an expedient, sanctioned decision-making pathway with significant time-saving and social norm gains (Keller et al. 2011). Retaining the option to search for alternatives preserves autonomy but makes entrenched prescribing practices less reflexive (Malhotra et al. 2016, Olshan, Rareshide, and Patel 2019).

Prescribing defaults can be coupled with other kinds of nudges to make them context specific. In a time-critical setting, such as an emergency department (ED), cognitive performance is often automatic, leaning heavily on mental shortcuts to make pragmatic choices that avoid potential for regret and loss. It is a choice environment that lends itself to habitual behaviours. Implementing a computerized default order set and concurrently stocking the default preparations in the ED dispensing machine strengthen the nudge effect relevant to that setting. Bypassing the delay of pharmacy delivery augments the time-saving gains of accepting the default order set and reinforces the default selection as normative in that context (Isenberg et al. 2018).

In primary care, general practitioners (GPs) continue to treat respiratory tract infections inappropriately with antibiotics, despite widely published clinical guidelines for treatment and significant efforts at intervention, and with disregard for well-established evidence that low-value prescribing leads to antibiotic resistance (Meeker et al. 2014). A key behavioural insight into this entrenched practice is the social force of patient expectation and high patient

DOI: 10.4324/9781003109945-41

demand for antibiotics (Fletcher-Lartey et al. 2016). GPs may lack the capacity or time to explain antibiotics, have empathy for their patients' discomfort, and want to protect the patient–doctor relationship (Fletcher-Lartey et al. 2016).

Feedback comparing GPs' antibiotic prescribing behaviours to their peers can implement a status quo nudge (BETA 2018), but it does not deflect the power of patient expectation. Poster-sized "commitment letters" in consultation waiting rooms are an effective nudge for both patient and doctor (Meeker et al. 2014). Signed declarations by individual doctors pledging high-value prescribing of antibiotics have the effect of resetting patient–doctor relationships; it establishes new norms for prescribing practices and reduces the pressure on doctors by managing patients' expectations.

Interventions that are relatively simple to implement and that can rapidly shift behaviour are an exciting prospect for implementation scientists, driving emerging exploration of nudging opportunities, especially where education and dissemination of guidelines have not been effective in changing care. However, reviews of choice architecture interventions involving a nudge (Lamprell et al. 2020, Yoong et al. 2020, Szaszi et al. 2018) indicate that few studies undertake research to investigate the adaptive, heuristic, and subjective processes of decision-making in existing contexts before implementing a nudge.

The automated hand hygiene feedback and peer reminder to "take a moment" failed to have impact on hand hygiene adherence in the medical ward but nudged change in the surgical ward because of social and cultural differences between the two populations. The surgical ward was a socially cohesive unit, the nursing unit manager driving the verbal reminders was well regarded and liked, and senior doctors acted as role models. In contrast, the medical ward had no sense of community and no respected opinion leader providing guidance. The staff were distrustful of the accuracy of the mechanical audits, indignant at the claim that their adherence was poor, and extremely uncomfortable with the nudge. Staff on both wards noted that the hierarchical nature of medical care made nudging "upwards" unrealistic. Understanding the existing culture may have pre-empted barriers to the nudge or informed a different approach (Kwok, Harris, and McLaws 2017).

References

BETA. 2018. *Nudge vs Superbugs: A Behavioural Economics Trial to Reduce the Overprescribing of Antibiotics*. Canberra, Commonwealth of Australia. Canberra, Australia: Australian Government.

Fletcher-Lartey, S., M. Yee, C. Gaarslev, and R. Khan. 2016. "Why do general practitioners prescribe antibiotics for upper respiratory tract infections to meet patient expectations: A mixed methods study." *BMJ Open* 6 (10):e012244–e012244. doi: 10.1136/bmjopen-2016-012244.

Isenberg, D. L., K. M. Kissman, E. P. Salinski, M. A. Saks, and L. B. Evans. 2018. "Simple changes to emergency department workflow improve analgesia in mechanically ventilated patients." *Western Journal of Emergency Medicine* 19 (4):668–674. doi: 10.5811/westjem.2018.4.36879.

Keller, P. A., B. Harlam, G. Loewenstein, and K. G. Volpp. 2011. "Enhanced active choice: A new method to motivate behavior change." *Journal of Consumer Psychology* 21 (4):376–383. doi: 10.1016/j.jcps.2011.06.003.

Kwok, Y. L., P. Harris, and M. L. McLaws. 2017. "Social cohesion: The missing factor required for a successful hand hygiene program." *American Journal of Infection Control* 45 (3):222–227. doi: 10.1016/j.ajic.2016.10.021.

Lamprell, K., Y. Tran, G. Arnolda, and J. Braithwaite. 2020. "Nudging clinicians: A systematic scoping review of the literature." *Journal of Evaluation in Clinical Practice*. doi: 10.1111/jep.13401.

Malhotra, S., A. D. Cheriff, J. T. Gossey, C. L. Cole, R. Kaushal, and J. S. Ancker. 2016. "Effects of an e-Prescribing interface redesign on rates of generic drug prescribing: Exploiting default options."

Journal of the American Medical Informatics Association 23 (5):891–898. doi: 10.1093/jamia/ocv192.

Meeker, D., T. K. Knight, M. W. Friedberg, J. A. Linder, N. J. Goldstein, C. R. Fox, A. Rothfeld, G. Diaz, and J. N. Doctor. 2014. "Nudging guideline-concordant antibiotic prescribing: A randomized clinical trial." *JAMA Internal Medicine* 174 (3):425–431. doi: 10.1001/jamainternmed.2013.14191.

Olshan, D., C. A. L. Rareshide, and M. S. Patel. 2019. "Longer-term durability of using default options in the electronic health record to increase generic prescribing rates." *Journal of General Internal Medicine* 34 (3):349–350. doi: 10.1007/s11606-018-4719-9.

Szaszi, B., A. Palinkas, B. Palfi, A. Szollosi, and B. Aczel. 2018. "A systematic scoping review of the choice architecture movement: Toward understanding when and why nudges work." *Journal of Behavioral Decision Making* 31 (3):355–366. doi: 10.1002/bdm.2035.

Yoong, S. L., A. Hall, F. Stacey, A. Grady, R. Sutherland, R. Wyse, A. Anderson, N. Nathan, and L. Wolfenden. 2020. "Nudge strategies to improve healthcare providers' implementation of evidence-based guidelines, policies and practices: A systematic review of trials included within Cochrane systematic reviews." *Implementation Science* 15 (1):50. doi: 10.1186/s13012-020-01011-0.

39 Design and implementation of dashboards in healthcare

Kristiana Ludlow and Johanna Westbrook

Introduction to dashboards in healthcare

Healthcare organizations collect vast amounts of data about clients, work processes, and quality of care indicators. These data are often captured and stored in siloed and fragmented systems (Mehta and Pandit 2018). Dashboards are one solution for integrating data and providing a more wholistic view of what is happening within an organization. By bringing disparate data together in a meaningful way, they can be transformed into information which can support effective decision-making. Dashboards utilize colour, graphs, and symbols to communicate important information quickly and concisely to reduce cognitive burden for users (Faiola, Srinivas, and Duke 2015, Hartzler et al. 2015). In clinical settings, dashboards are digital tools that provide visual displays of key information, such as a client's diagnoses, medications, allergies, treatment/care plans, and needs (Figure 39.1). These displays provide an "at-a-glance" view of individual client profiles or can offer an aggregated summary of data trends in a defined population (Dowding et al. 2015).

Dashboards are typically categorized as either clinical dashboards or quality dashboards (Dowding et al. 2015). Clinical dashboards provide clinical indicators which assist healthcare professionals to make decisions about patient care, whereas quality dashboards provide performance indicators to inform quality improvement activities (Dowding et al. 2015). Both types of dashboards have been primarily used in acute care or primary care settings to support decision-making (Dowding et al. 2015, Khairat et al. 2018). As a form of decision support, dashboards can identify clients at potential risk of poor outcomes or harm in real time and may provide evidence-based recommendations and guidelines to address these risks. Dashboard data may also enable opportunities for benchmarking practices at the organization, unit, and health professional levels (Dowding et al. 2015).

Dashboard design and implementation issues

Key facilitators and barriers to effective dashboard implementation include the following:

- *Co-design with users*. Involving users in the design of dashboards will increase acceptance and the likely integration of the technology with work practices (Hartzler et al. 2015). This process is iterative and should include workshops with prototype testing with multiple users and other relevant stakeholders (Franklin et al. 2017, Hartzler et al. 2015).
- *User-friendly*. The degree to which a dashboard is intuitive to use can impact effective use and uptake. The incorporation of graphics, colours, and symbols

DOI: 10.4324/9781003109945-42

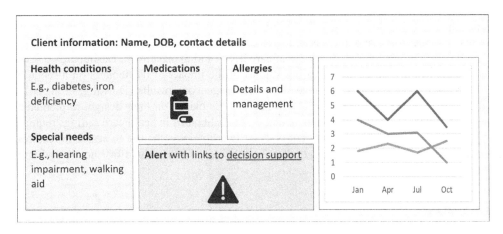

Client information: Name, DOB, contact details

Health conditions	Medications	Allergies
E.g., diabetes, iron deficiency		Details and management

Special needs	
E.g., hearing impairment, walking aid	Alert with links to decision support

Figure 39.1 Simplified example of a clinical dashboard displaying client-level information.

Source: Created by authors

(e.g., "traffic-light"-coloured alert systems) can enhance dashboard effectiveness, but these should be tailored to the user audiences (Ghazisaeidi et al. 2015, Dowding et al. 2015). It is important to consider users' digital literacy and ability to understand graphs and data displays (Dixon et al. 2017, Ghazisaeidi et al. 2015). Other aesthetic features may also facilitate or hinder dashboard use and effectiveness, for example, the simplicity of displays, the size and font of text, and the amount of information presented.

- *Accessibility.* Whether or not a dashboard is easy to access when needed has implications for the success of implementation. For example, needing to move to another location, or use a lengthy sign-in process to access a dashboard, may act as a barrier to its effective integration into routine practice. Presentation of dashboards which are continually visible or as a screensaver means that users can have constant access to information, which has shown to be associated with positive client outcomes (Dowding et al. 2015).
- *Data accuracy.* One of the defining features of dashboards is their ability to continuously capture the latest data, allowing users to make informed decisions in real time (Ghazisaeidi et al. 2015). If a dashboard has missing, inaccurate, or outdated information, healthcare professionals are unlikely to use it for decision-making.
- *Uses existing infrastructure.* Implementation of a new technology can be costly, time-consuming, and effortful, creating challenges to implementation of dashboards (Ghazisaeidi et al. 2015). Utilizing existing infrastructure can overcome these barriers by embedding, where possible, a dashboard within an organization's current information system. This also is likely to promote dashboard use with users who are familiar and experienced with the existing technology.
- *Alignment with current workflows.* Dashboard implementation can create additional burden for users as they transition to using the new technology. To facilitate implementation, dashboards should have a clear purpose and produce improvements or complement current work processes (Pickering et al. 2015). If a dashboard duplicates current workflows or adds additional workload, uptake by users is likely to be poor.

Concluding remarks

In healthcare organizations where the volume of data available about individual patients and clients continues to expand, there is an increasing need for tools that enable healthcare workers and consumers to gain an overview of care needs and management. Dashboards present one solution to this challenge. Existing studies of the impact of dashboards on a range of process and outcome indicators have shown heterogeneous results (Dowding et al. 2015, Khairat et al. 2018), and greater research needs to be placed on their design, implementation, and outcomes. Successful implementation of dashboards in healthcare settings requires consideration of users' needs, preferences, and digital literacy; the use of aesthetic features; accessibility of the program; accurate data; and the use of available infrastructure and integration with current workflows.

References

Dixon, B. E., K. Barboza, A. E. Jensen, K. J. Bennett, S. E. Sherman, and M. D. Schwartz. 2017. "Measuring practicing clinicians' information literacy. An exploratory analysis in the context of panel management." *Applied Clinical Informatics* 8 (1):149–161. doi: 10.4338/ACI-2016-06-RA-0083.

Dowding, D., R. Randell, P. Gardner, G. Fitzpatrick, P. Dykes, J. Favela, S. Hamer, Z. Whitewood-Moores, N. Hardiker, E. Borycki, and L. Currie. 2015. "Dashboards for improving patient care: Review of the literature." *International Journal of Medical Informatics* 84 (2):87–100. doi: 10.1016/j.ijmedinf.2014.10.001.

Faiola, A., P. Srinivas, and J. Duke. 2015. "Supporting clinical cognition: A human-centered approach to a novel ICU information visualization dashboard." *AMIA Annual Symposium Proceedings* 2015:560–569.

Franklin, A., S. Gantela, S. Shifarraw, T. R. Johnson, D. J. Robinson, B. R. King, A. M. Mehta, C. L. Maddow, N. R. Hoot, V. Nguyen, A. Rubio, J. Zhang, and N. G. Okafor. 2017. "Dashboard visualizations: Supporting real-time throughput decision-making." *Journal of Biomedical Informatics* 71:211–221. doi: 10.1016/j.jbi.2017.05.024.

Ghazisaeidi, M., R. Safdari, M. Torabi, M. Mirzaee, J. Farzi, and A. Goodini. 2015. "Development of performance dashboards in healthcare sector: Key practical issues." *Acta informatica medica: AIM: Journal of the Society for Medical Informatics of Bosnia & Herzegovina: Casopis Drustva za medicinsku informatiku BiH* 23 (5):317–321. doi: 10.5455/aim.2015.23.317-321.

Hartzler, A. L., S. Chaudhuri, B. C. Fey, D. R. Flum, and D. Lavallee. 2015. "Integrating patient-reported outcomes into spine surgical care through visual dashboards: Lessons learned from human-centered design." *EGEMS (Washington, DC)* 3 (2):1133–1133. doi: 10.13063/2327-9214.1133.

Khairat, S. S., A. Dukkipati, H. A. Lauria, T. Bice, D. Travers, and S. S. Carson. 2018. "The Impact of visualization dashboards on quality of care and clinician satisfaction: Integrative literature review." *JMIR Human Factors* 5 (2):e22. doi: 10.2196/humanfactors.9328.

Mehta, N., and A. Pandit. 2018. "Concurrence of big data analytics and healthcare: A systematic review." *International Journal of Medical Informatics* 114:57–65. doi: 10.1016/j.ijmedinf.2018.03.013.

Pickering, B. W., Y. Dong, A. Ahmed, J. Giri, O. Kilickaya, A. Gupta, O. Gajic, and V. Herasevich. 2015. "The implementation of clinician designed, human-centered electronic medical record viewer in the intensive care unit: A pilot step-wedge cluster randomized trial." *International Journal of Medical Informatics* 84 (5):299–307. doi: 10.1016/j.ijmedinf.2015.01.017.

40 Sensemaking

Paying attention to the stories we tell to improve our ability to act

Luci K. Leykum and David C. Aron

Interprofessional rounds

Our studies of sensemaking across a variety of healthcare settings provide insights into the ways that people make sense of what is happening and the impact that sensemaking has on implementation.

What are we here to do? This is an important question that teams must answer. This may seem obvious – we are here to take care of patients – but in reality, people are asked to do many things, and the ways they make sense of those "asks" influence how they approach implementing them (Weick 1995). For example, is the faculty member on an inpatient medicine team there to teach learners? To take care of patients? New implementation "asks" may not align with how they have made sense of what they are there to do. A lack of alignment often leads to a lack of attention.

Why are we doing this? How people make sense of why they are being asked to implement something new will impact how it is done. For example, whether clinicians see interprofessional rounds as a way to better understand their patients' needs or as an interruption they need to go to in the middle of their morning will influence not only their attendance but also what they talk about.

What are the real causes behind a problem? The degree to which clinicians believe that what they are asked to do addresses the root cause of a problem will influence what they do and how they do it. Asking clinicians to engage in a new medication reconciliation process, when they think that readmissions are related to access to specialty appointments, is unlikely to be successful. If individuals do not believe that the "real causes" are actually addressable, success is even less likely. If patients come back to the hospital because "they have home situations that we cannot fix", what is the point of giving patients a follow-up call?

How people make sense of what they are asked to do matters (Leykum et al. 2015), particularly when they are asked to do something they perceive as disrupting their usual way of doing things. What does that mean for how we approach implementation?

Make sure the nature of the solution matches the nature of the problem in the eyes of those being asked to do the work. A joint, mutual understanding of problems and solutions at all organizational levels is necessary, as it creates the foundation for sensemaking around interventions and how to accomplish them. This mutual understanding requires conversation and reflection. It has the benefit of not only making the implementation more effective but also ensuring that the intervention is the best one for the organization at that point in time.

Pay attention to the stories people tell each other. These stories reflect how people have made sense. If stories don't match the implementation goals, this mismatch must be addressed. Conversation can be a tool to change those stories and update how people make sense of implementation.

DOI: 10.4324/9781003109945-43

An illustration: a goal of discharging hospitalized patients earlier in the day was seen by frontline clinicians as just another example of administrators being completely out of touch. Clinicians didn't care about length of stay – they needed to focus on assessing their new admissions and sickest patients, not patients who were fine and ready to go home. Patients needed to wait for their family to pick them up after work anyway. Reframing this goal in terms of preventing long waits in the emergency department, and using stories of patients who had near-misses during these waits, helped to shift how clinicians made sense of the problem. Involving clinicians in the solution helped them to create workflows that made sense and helped administration to understand that frontline clinicians were not resistant to change but rather very busy with competing demands. Finally, hearing the experiences of patients and families helped clinicians understand that patients preferred earlier discharges to ensure they had everything they needed at home before the end of the workday.

References

Leykum, L., H. Chesser, H. Lanham, C. Pezzia, R. Palmer, T. Ratcliffe, H. Reisinger, M. Agar, and J. Pugh. 2015. "The association between sensemaking during physician team rounds and hospitalized patients' outcomes." *Journal of General Internal Medicine* 30 (12):1821–1827. doi: 10.1007/s11606-015-3377-4.

Weick, K. 1995. *Sensemaking in Organizations*. Thousand Oaks, CA: Sage Publications.

41 Adaptations

Ulrica von Thiele Schwarz, Henna Hasson,
and Gregory A. Aarons

Implementation research often focuses on preparing individual providers (e.g., by train-ing) and delivering organizations (e.g., by introducing follow-up systems) to accommodate evidence-based interventions (EBIs). This package entails changing the context so that the EBI can be delivered as designed in research (i.e., with high fidelity). Factors related to both the individual provider and the provider organization ("inner context") and factors related to the system where the organization operates ("outer context") may be addressed to facili-tate implementation with high fidelity (Aarons, Hurlburt, and Horwitz 2011). Thus, system factors, such as policies, funding, and directives, as well as organizational factors, such as workflows, electronic health records, and organizational climate, may be addressed to sup-port high-fidelity EBI use.

EBI fidelity is important for several reasons, in the steps preceding implementation (e.g., efficacy trials) as well as in implementation research and practice (i.e., when EBIs are adopted and used in routine care). Reasons for research and evaluation to focus on fidelity include 1) difficulties in drawing valid conclusions about causality when the EBI is inconsistently delivered, 2) difficulties in accumulating findings across studies (e.g., systematic reviews), 3) decreased transparency about what is actually delivered, diminishing true patient choice and ability to hold providers accountable for services, 4) decreased ability to determine if lack of EBI effect is because the EBI was not properly implemented or if it was implemented with fidelity, and failed nevertheless, and 5) risk of unwanted variation in implementation across patient groups, providers, and organizations (von Thiele Schwarz, Aarons, and Has-son 2019).

Thus, fidelity is a concern across the research and practice pathway. Yet, the arguments in favour of high fidelity notwithstanding, EBI adaptation is a reality. In fact, adaptations are so frequent that some have observed that "there is no implementation without adaptation" (Lyon and Bruns 2019). When EBIs are used in a certain setting, it is impossible to escape the need to ensure that the EBI fits the context (e.g., provider preference, patient needs), and sometimes, this is best achieved by *adapting the EBI* to fit the context rather than adapting the context to fit the EBI.

The fidelity-adaptation dilemma is a constant in implementation research. However, the implications of adaptation can be reconciled, when done systematically, planned, and approached thoughtfully. Benefits of adaptations can include 1) higher efficiency (e.g., EBIs optimized for specific contexts); 2) better balance of patient, professional, organization, and system outcomes; 3) possibility to implement EBIs in contexts different from contexts where they were developed; and 4) ability to fit EBIs to the needs of patients, embracing that EBIs seldom are effective for all (von Thiele Schwarz, Aarons, and Hasson 2019).

DOI: 10.4324/9781003109945-44

The Value Equation

The seemingly contradictory claims concerning the consequences of fidelity and adaptation have been described as a dilemma. In the Value Equation, we propose a way to reconcile fidelity and adaptation by focusing on implementation strategies as a way to create fit between an EBI and context so that the value of an EBI in a certain context is maximized by considering the needs and preferences of relevant stakeholders (von Thiele Schwarz, Aarons, and Hasson 2019) (Figure 41.1).

In the Value Equation, value (V) is the result of an EBI (IN = intervention), in a context (C), given how well the implementation strategies (IS) resolve the tension between EBI and context. The end product – value – is maximized when EBI and context fit. This can be achieved by adapting the context to accommodate an EBI *and* by adapting the EBI to context. Most discussion of adaptation is about the EBI. The Value Equation expands this by proposing that fidelity and adaptation determine how IN, C, and IS are mixed and, in turn, the value that is achieved.

In this conceptualization of fidelity and adaptation, the focus of implementation shifts from a myopic perspective only on getting an EBI in place to the value the implementation process can lead to, more broadly. We acknowledge that there may be many nuances to value: a multicomponent, multilevel construct that represents the combined benefit for each stakeholder group. For example, for a service system, value may be increased population health; for an organization, optimized service delivery and efficiency; and for a clinical professional, consideration of individual patient needs and the patient's better daily functioning. By making these sometimes illusive and implicit values explicitly, value conflicts can be negotiated to achieve fit between EBI and context, through thoughtful fidelity and adaptation considerations. Thus, balancing fidelity and adaptation becomes a proactive decision-making process involving value judgements.

The never-ending story of fidelity and adaptation decisions

In general, fidelity-adaptation decisions should be proactive as many problems can be solved upstream (Hasson et al. 2020). Starting *before* an EBI is taken up in practice, an EBI that has been tested for efficacy with participants from the majority population in one country might require redesign and re-evaluation to determine its relevance and effectiveness in minority groups, or for other national and cultural contexts (Sundell et al. 2015).

However, even with studies that repurpose EBIs for new contexts, fidelity and adaptation decisions are often needed when it is time to implement the EBI in practice. The Exploration, Preparation, Implementation, Sustainment (EPIS) framework (Aarons, Hurlburt, and Horwitz 2011) outlines the implementation in four phases, and decisions affecting fidelity and adaptation should begin early and continue throughout all phases. Thus, an overall fit between EBI and professional, organizational, and system factors needs to be continuously addressed, not only during the "exploration and preparation phases" but also during the early "implementation phase", as practical need for adaptation becomes more apparent, and during the "sustainment phase" to encompass continual contextual changes. During the

$$V = IN + C + IS$$

Figure 41.1 The Value Equation

Source: Created by authors

"exploration" and "preparation phases", for example, stakeholders may be able to trouble-shoot and manage misfit by purposeful decisions about adaptations, to the context or to the EBI (e.g., Frykman et al. 2014). The result of such a process can be an adapted version of the EBI, as well as an implementation plan that includes system or organizational system or organizational strategies needed to retain fidelity to EBI core elements.

Despite efforts to ensure fit during "exploration and preparation phases", adaptation and fidelity are nevertheless often still a concern during the "implementation phase". With substantive implementation support, adaptations can be made part of iterative, problem-solving, and improvement-oriented cycles (Becan et al. 2018). This requires that decisions concerning fidelity and adaption are based on data and feedback on how the EBI is *actually* used, as well as process, implementation, and end outcomes, which in turn requires measurement and feedback systems, documentation, and development of local research evidence to inform the process (Aarons et al. 2012). The data-driven approach to adaptations bridges implementation research with fields such as quality improvement and measurement-based care. All three emphasize the need for high-quality data as a basis for decisions about work processes (e.g., how EBIs are used).

In contrast to the focus on fidelity and adaptation during the "exploration, preparation and implementation phases", there has been relatively little focus on what happens in the "sustainment phase", when the EBI has become part of regular practice (i.e., institutionalized). Maybe this is because of the expectation that all knots preventing a good fit have already been untied so that those delivering the EBI can now proceed to use it as intended, forever after. In other words, consistent delivery of an EBI over time is exactly how sustainability sometimes is defined (Moore et al. 2017).

However, as the context changes and tension between EBI and context increases, negotiation to create fit between EBI and context continues. This has been acknowledged in conceptualizations such as the Dynamic Sustainability Framework (Chambers, Glasgow, and Stange 2013), which, along with other definitions of sustainment, highlight the ability to continuously deliver value over time rather than sustaining the use of a certain EBI (Moore et al. 2017). Yet, it is a very different territory for fidelity and adaptation decisions during the "sustainment phase" compared to earlier "implementation phases". Most stakeholders have moved on, believing that the EBI is institutionalized. Thus, the extra resources needed to facilitate the structured, proactive decision process that is recommended for adaptation decisions have often passed. Left are the frontline professionals who have no choice other than to continuously respond to changes that affect the fit between EBI and context.

The expectation of no change in EBI or context is a naïve assumption. It neglects the challenges that frontline practitioners face when using EBIs. For them, the fidelity-adaptation dilemma is not a philosophical or theoretical question. It entails a complicated decision process where practitioners need to weigh up their options for action based on several, sometimes conflicting, values. For them, adaptation and fidelity are a never-ending story. Ongoing consideration of the Value Equation can help structure the decision process and support successful dynamic sustainment.

In conclusion

Fidelity and adaptation decisions happen throughout the implementation process, across all EPIS phases. The Value Equation provides a theory-based and practical approach that can inform development and testing of hypotheses, moving implementation science towards a more granular understanding of the roles that context, EBIs, and implementation strategies play in the fidelity and adaptation process. For implementation practice, the Value Equation provides a way to identify, operationalize, and make decisions about fidelity, adaptation, and the impact adaptation may have on outcomes that key stakeholders value. The Value Equation proposes implementation strategies as a way to create fit between EBIs and context. It emphasizes overall value rather than limited focus on one or two outcomes and can act as a guiding light for fidelity and adaptation decisions.

References

Aarons, G., M. Hurlburt, and S. Horwitz. 2011. "Advancing a conceptual model of evidence-based practice implementation in public service sectors." *Administration and Policy in Mental Health* 38:4–23.

Aarons, G. A., A. E. Green, L. A. Palinkas, S. Self-Brown, D. J. Whitaker, J. R. Lutzker, J. F. Silovsky, D. B. Hecht, and M. J. Chaffin. 2012. "Dynamic adaptation process to implement an evidence-based child maltreatment intervention." *Implementation Science* 7 (1):32.

Becan, J. E., J. P. Bartkowski, D. K. Knight, T. R. Wiley, R. DiClemente, L. Ducharme, W. N. Welsh, D. Bowser, K. McCollister, and M. Hiller. 2018. "A model for rigorously applying the Exploration, Preparation, Implementation, Sustainment (EPIS) framework in the design and measurement of a large scale collaborative multi-site study." *Health & Justice* 6 (1):9.

Chambers, D., R. Glasgow, and K. Stange. 2013. "The dynamic sustainability framework: Addressing the paradox of sustainment amid ongoing change." *Implementation Science* 8 (1):117.

Frykman, M., H. Hasson, Å. M. Athlin, and U. von Thiele Schwarz. 2014. "Functions of behavior change interventions when implementing multi-professional teamwork at an emergency department: A comparative case study." *BMC Health Services Research* 14 (1):1–13.

Hasson, H., H. Gröndal, Å. H. Rundgren, G. Avby, H. Uvhagen, and U. von Thiele Schwarz. 2020. "How can evidence-based interventions give the best value for users in social services? Balance between adherence and adaptations: A study protocol." *Implementation Science Communications* 1 (1):1–9.

Lyon, A. R., and E. J. Bruns. 2019. "User-centered redesign of evidence-based psychosocial interventions to enhance implementation – hospitable soil or better seeds?" *JAMA Psychiatry* 76 (1):3–4.

Moore, J. E., A. Mascarenhas, J. Bain, and S. E. Straus. 2017. "Developing a comprehensive definition of sustainability." *Implementation Science* 12 (1):110.

Sundell, K., A. Beelmann, H. Hasson, and U. von Thiele Schwarz. 2015. "Novel programs, international adoptions, or contextual adaptations? Meta-analytical results from German and Swedish intervention research." *Journal of Clinical Child & Adolescent Psychology*:1–13. doi: 10.1080/15374416.2015.1020540.

von Thiele Schwarz, U., G. A. Aarons, and H. Hasson. 2019. "The value equation: Three complementary propositions for reconciling fidelity and adaptation in evidence-based practice implementation." *BMC Health Services Research* 19 (1):868.

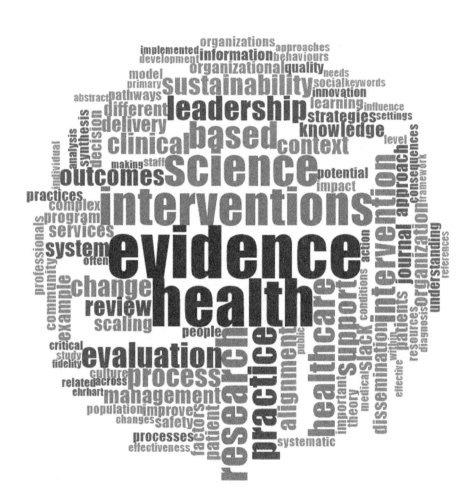

Part III

Challenges with evidence into practice

Translation, evaluation, sustainability

In this third section, Part III of the book, we take a look at an overarching idea of getting evidence into practice, divided into three ambient ideas: aspects of translation, thinking about evaluation, and features of sustainment, so that what we do to create more evidence-based practice anchors and sticks. As to translation, Hollnagel and Clay-Williams provide an outline drawn from ergonomics and much-used in resilient healthcare: the distinction between expectations of what people do and what they actually do, also known as Work-as-Imagined and Work-as-Done.

Other features of translation follow in subsequent essays. Rycroft-Malone grapples with synthesizing the evidence needed for effective translation and Nilsen and colleagues look at learning for, and about, implementation. Wensing, on the other hand, in one of his many contributions to the field focuses on the nature of interventions, specifically around patient self-management. In changing focus, Laver thinks about the agent of change, providing an example of allied healthcare professionals. Changing pace again, Schiff, who has made it a lifelong commitment to reducing diagnostic errors, discusses that topic to address the need for a higher-quality, safer health system. The final contributions in this first part of Part III look at some of the characteristics of the setting in which implementation is harnessed and translation takes place: Saurin, who discusses the need for slack or redundancy in healthcare so that there is additional capacity for changes to be made; Bridges, who looks at a specific application, in this case the aged care setting; Bates, who is interested in getting the right information technology support to clinicians who are making decisions; and Ehrhart and Aarons who consider whether there is good alignment between activities and whether "fit" is occurring sufficiently for effective implementation to be accomplished.

The second theme in this third section of the book focuses specifically on evaluation. Wensing, in a second contribution, considers process evaluation and the importance of this for understanding whether an assessment process is being created and put in place. Chen looks specifically at how evaluation, which optimally must be richly theorized, can contribute to progress in evaluating projects and programs in implementation.

The third and final part of this section is about sustainability – sustaining change, having sustainable implementation in the first place, and bedding down and securing the gains made when we have implemented something new. Straus talks about how implementation sustainability is crucial; otherwise if the gains are not embedded or anchored in, the pendulum can swing back to where it was. On that theme, Chambers looks at dissemination through this lens, realizing how dissemination is not an event but is always a work in progress and always longitudinal. Aarons and Ehrhart look at how strategic leadership is necessary for good implementation, and Clay-Williams reflects on the unintended consequences whenever implementation is in train.

DOI: 10.4324/9781003109945-45

Finally, Vanhaecht focuses on teamwork and the necessity for mobilizing a care pathway; Sklar and Aarons look at forms of scaling out for accelerating implementation; and Williams and Mannion consider almost two decades of work reflecting on de-implementation which, in many respects, is the reciprocal of implementation. All these ideas and informative pieces of advice need to be considered when trying to get as much bang for the buck as possible in implementing new evidence. Accomplishing implementation and developing the field of implementation science will both be progressed more effectively and on a long-term, sustainable basis if the wisdom of these essays is absorbed and utilized widely.

42 Evidence synthesis

Maximizing the potential

Jo Rycroft-Malone

There's nothing like a global public health crisis to bring into stark relief the critical role that evidence can play in decision-making. The timely production and use of research can be life-saving. In the context of an exponential growth in research evidence, and a persistent need to narrow gaps in quality of care, it is unsurprising that the evidence synthesis has become an increasingly useful tool in an implementation scientist's toolbox. Bringing together the findings of existing research in a rigorous and transparent way offers an evidence base for action and a valuable informant for policy and practice – a jumping off point, a catalyst, and a "crucial step" (Gough et al. 2020). However, we know that the existence of evidence, compelling or otherwise, is not usually sufficient for action. Therefore, there is a question about how to maximize the potential utility of evidence syntheses as a feature of implementation science, to increase the potential of both the method and findings to be impactful, whether that be about putting something into practice or stopping it.

Over the last decade or so, there has been a gradual shift to realize that what typically sits at the top of an evidence hierarchy in the form of meta-analyses of randomized trials is highly appropriate for answering some questions but provides limited help for many other issues. The users of reviews often want to know more than an estimate of the effect size of a single intervention. This is particularly the case when it comes to the synthesis of evidence about the effect of complex interventions, which are of typical concern to implementation scientists. Rather than being preoccupied with the estimates of effect size, there has been increasing interest in knowing about how interventions might work (or not), understanding causal mechanisms, and uncovering implementation processes. The need to better understand a broader range of issues has resulted in an interest in, and recognition of, a wider range of approaches to synthesizing evidence beyond that of the traditional systematic review. Arguably, this has led to some of the hegemonies of evidence syntheses beginning to melt away, or at least, a greater awareness of the merits of the potential contribution of different syntheses approaches, and an appreciation of the value of different types of evidence – particularly in the context of implementation science.

The growing acceptance of the highly contextualized nature of implementation practice and research has also translated into the evidence synthesis menu. As implementation science evolved from the framing of evidence-based practice, so too has the notion of individualized endeavour – the approach of skilling up individuals to be research aware leading to greater use of evidence. Many of us had argued for a broader framing of the issue and for a greater recognition that individual decision-making is situated in the context of action (Rycroft-Malone et al. 2002). Context is, therefore, a critical feature of implementation science. As such, the potential of evidence syntheses to be contextually sensitive and able to surface and

DOI: 10.4324/9781003109945-46

capture features of context that might impact implementation efforts is important; enter the realist synthesis.

"What works, for whom, why, and in what circumstances" is a seductive phrase to an implementation scientist. A realist synthesis (also referred to as realist review) goes beyond providing summative evidence about whether an intervention worked or not, by focusing on why an intervention or program might (or might not) work in what contexts and for whom in order to gain a theory-driven understanding of complex causation between implementation and outcome. A focus on context, mechanisms, theory, and impact goes to the core of the implementation science endeavour. Consequently, there has been an increasing interest in the potential of realist synthesis to implementation science. A realist synthesis is a theory-driven evidence review that uses as the starting point hypotheses about why and how particular interventions or programs might work. Drawing on a wide range of evidence through iterative searching, these hypotheses or theories are refined and tested through retroductive analysis. In an early example illustrating the approach (Rycroft-Malone et al. 2012), we suggested that while intellectually demanding and not for the faint-hearted, the process and outputs of a realist synthesis offer the potential for practical, theoretical, transferable recommendations about what might work as well as what might not. A focus on embedded stakeholder engagement and inclusion of multiple perspectives, ability to untangle (rather than control for) the implementation of complex interventions within real-world contexts, and an encouragement to take a pluralistic view of evidence align well with what we know about successful implementation.

A simple search of Google Scholar with the terms "realist review" and "realist synthesis" reveals over 400,000 hits, and a search of the PROSPERO database shows nearly 350 records for "realist". Of course, not all records relate directly to implementation science, but these numbers will likely be the tip of the iceberg. Nevertheless, while an increasingly popular approach, it has not been without critique, particularly when positioned aside characteristics of traditional "scientific" systematic review methods, resulting in questions about risks of being open to researcher prejudices and bias, because of, for example, the iterative and targeted approach to searching and selecting evidence. In contrast to some of the outputs of traditional systematic reviews, perhaps the popularity of realist syntheses is that intuitively, and in reality, they provide useful information that has the potential to influence practice – particularly as we know, interventions do work differently in different conditions and for different people.

Realist synthesis has really taken off by catching the imagination of those wishing to unpack change processes that are prone to adaptation and are contingent upon contextual conditions. However, it is perhaps surprising that there has not been greater interest in other evidence synthesis approaches that have the capacity to pay attention to context, such as meta-ethnography (France et al. 2019). Also, theory-driven, meta-ethnography involves synthesizing concepts across primary studies taking into account the contexts of those studies. Given that a meta-ethnography's potential contribution is in explaining how different interventions might have an impact in the context of their implementation, in providing a rich description of implementation contexts, and in offering fresh insights, it is interesting to note that there are few implementation science examples to date. The seductive pull of realist synthesis is perhaps leaving meta-ethnography as an untapped resource.

Increasing the potential for impact from an evidence synthesis is not just a function of the chosen method, but it is also about how we approach it. We have seen a rise in the concept and the practice of co-production in recent times, particularly in the context of implementation science (Rycroft-Malone et al. 2016) that has mirrored a move away from problematizing evidence use as a function of a gap between those who produce knowledge and those who use it. The democratization of the research ecosystem that includes the emergence of a more socially constructed and embedded view of the relationship between evidence and its use foregrounds collaboration, that is, in bringing together a plurality of knowledge sources to resolve real-world problems through engaged scholarship. Despite the typically significant amount of deskwork involved, evidence syntheses are also co-productive opportunities but are frequently not framed as such. Accumulating and synthesizing knowledge through the authentic engagement of partners as review team members bring practical wisdom and plurality of evidence (including real-world data) and provide insight into the extraction of key implementation features (e.g., acceptability, usefulness, reach, sustainability, context) as part of the review process. In this context, the synthesis has the potential to be a boundary object, objects that translate across boundaries and people by enhancing communication (Melville-Richards et al. 2020) where co-production leads to greater meaningfulness and resonance. This type of collaboration, if done well, can only enhance the relevance and usefulness of both the review process and the review outputs and therefore the potential for impact in practice and policy.

"Knowledge objects", which organize knowledge in coherent and structured ways, can be useful bridges between evidence and action. For example, guideline recommendations have played a long-standing role in implementation practice and science. The speed of evidence production, particularly in areas that are rapidly changing (such as a crisis), is leading to innovations in "rapid review approaches" and "living systematic reviews", which have the potential to be helpful in narrowing the evidence-to-practice gap. The consequence of living reviews is in the potential for "living guidelines" (Elliott et al. 2017) in which particular guideline recommendations can be rapidly updated with the arrival of new evidence. In that sense, living recommendations can offer timely advice. How much of a role living reviews and their partner "living guidelines" will play in the context of progressing implementation science remains to be seen, particularly given the resources, including infrastructure, needed to support their development, and continued updating. Intuitively, the idea of up-to-date and timely information is appealing particularly if embedded into systems that are close to decision-making and the point of care.

The potential of an evidence synthesis as a component of implementation science has to be in its relevance, timeliness, and utility. As implementation science has developed as an area of inquiry and the evidence base grows about what does and does not work and why, the methodological horizons of evidence synthesis have also necessarily expanded. The wider evidence ecosystem of which implementation science is a part is dynamic and, as such, evolving. Therefore, if evidence syntheses are to provide a trustworthy foundation or catalyst for action, there needs to be greater multidisciplinary, co-productive effort galvanized towards reciprocal learning and methodological innovation and evaluation.

References

Elliott, J. H., A. Synnot, T. Turner, M. Simmonds, E. A. Akl, S. McDonald, G. Salanti, J. Meerpohl, H. MacLehose, J. Hilton, D. Tovey, I. Shemilt, J. Thomas, and N. Living Systematic Review. 2017. "Living systematic review: 1. Introduction-the why, what, when, and how." *Journal of Clinical Epidemiology* 91:23–30. doi: 10.1016/j.jclinepi.2017.08.010.

France, E. F., I. Uny, N. Ring, R. L. Turley, M. Maxwell, E. A. S. Duncan, R. G. Jepson, R. J. Roberts, and J. Noyes. 2019. "A methodological systematic review of meta-ethnography conduct to articulate the complex analytical phases." *BMC Medical Research Methodology* 19 (1):35. doi: 10.1186/s12874-019-0670-7.

Gough, D., P. Davies, G. Jamtvedt, E. Langlois, J. Littell, T. Lotfi, E. Masset, T. Merlin, A. S. Pullin, M. Ritskes-Hoitinga, J.-A. Røttingen, E. Sena, R. Stewart, D. Tovey, H. White, J. Yost, H. Lund, and J. Grimshaw. 2020. "Evidence synthesis international (ESI): Position statement." *Systematic Reviews* 9 (1):155. doi: 10.1186/s13643-020-01415-5.

Melville-Richards, L., J. Rycroft-Malone, C. Burton, and J. Wilkinson. 2020. "Making authentic: Exploring boundary objects and bricolage in knowledge mobilisation through National Health Service-university partnerships." *Evidence and Policy: A Journal of Research, Debate and Practice* 16 (4):517–539. doi: 10.1332/174426419X15623134271106.

Rycroft-Malone, J., C. R. Burton, T. Bucknall, I. D. Graham, A. M. Hutchinson, and D. Stacey. 2016. "Collaboration and co-production of knowledge in healthcare: Opportunities and challenges." *International Journal of Health Policy and Management* 5 (4):221–223. doi: 10.15171/ijhpm.2016.08.

Rycroft-Malone, J., A. Kitson, G. Harvey, B. McCormack, K. Seers, A. Titchen, and C. Estabrooks. 2002. "Ingredients for change: Revisiting a conceptual framework." *Quality and Safety in Health Care* 11:170–180.

Rycroft-Malone, J., B. McCormack, A. M. Hutchinson, K. DeCorby, T. K. Bucknall, B. Kent, A. Schultz, E. Snelgrove-Clarke, C. B. Stetler, M. Titler, L. Wallin, and V. Wilson. 2012. "Realist synthesis: Illustrating the method for implementation research." *Implementation Science* 7 (1):33. doi: 10.1186/1748-5908-7-33.

43 Theory-driven evaluation

Huey T. Chen

The purpose of dissemination and implementation science is to facilitate the uptake of evidence-based interventions (EBIs) for regular use in communities (Estabrooks, Brownson, and Pronk 2018, Proctor et al. 2009). Since the beginning of the twenty-first century, implementation science has rapidly grown into an interdisciplinary study (Brownson, Colditz, and Proctor 2017, Glasgow et al. 2012). Despite its achievements, the literature (Aarons, Hurlburt, and Horwitz 2011, Dearing 2008) suggests that more accomplishments are possible if more attention is given to contextual factors that influence the delivery of interventions. Since theory-driven evaluation (TDE) (Chen 1990, 2005, 2013, 2015) has a long tradition of addressing contextual issues, this perspective is useful for further advancing implementation science. This can be accomplished by providing a conceptual framework for understanding the relationships between contextual factors and the intervention in a community setting, by proposing a holistic assessment of the intervention, by offering proactive evaluation approaches for assessing and diagnosing programs involving interventions, and by balancing the bottom-up and top-down approach to intervention dissemination.

Provide a conceptual framework for understanding the relationship between an intervention and its contextual factors in the implementation process

The conceptual framework proposed by TDE is called the action model/change model schema (Chen 2005, 2015) and is illustrated in Figure 43.1.

The schema consists of two related models: an action model and a change model. The change model describes causal processes for generating changes. The action model prescribes how to implement the change and consists of six components: implementing organization, implementers, associate organizations/partners, ecological context, intervention protocol/delivery platform, and target population. When implementing an EBI in a community, stakeholders should adequately address issues related to all five components to ensure a successful implementation. A sound action model is needed to drive the causal processes in the change model.

Provide a holistic assessment of the EBI as implemented in the community

Evaluators or researchers can apply the schema to holistically assess the implementation of an EBI or new intervention in a community. The assessment should provide empirical information on how the EBI and the contextual factors work together to produce desired results (Chen 2015). For example, this approach was used to assess the implementation of the national school-based drug abuse prevention program in Taiwan (Chen 1997). The Ministry

DOI: 10.4324/9781003109945-47

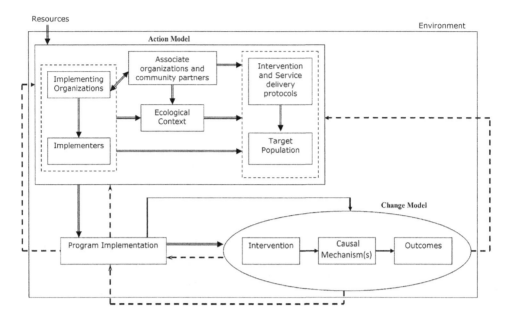

Figure 43.1 Action model/change model schema

Source: Created by author

of Education designed a new intervention based upon the literature that provided middle-school teachers with tools for counselling drug-using students. TDE was applied to holistically assess the implementation of the program. The great majority of schools only partially implemented a few key elements of the intervention. The evaluation provided empirical evidence that supported the reasons for partial implementation, such as communication barriers and mistrust between the Ministry of Education and school principals and teachers, insufficient training, insufficient resources, difficulty to secure the parents' support, and some unrealistic demands from the Ministry.

Provide the ex-ante program stress test for diagnosing weaknesses of a program plan

Many implementation problems of EBIs or new interventions can be traced back to poor program planning (Dvir, Raz, and Shenhar 2003). However, this issue has not been sufficiently addressed in the implementation literature. TDE is proposing the ex-ante program stress test (Chen and Morosuna 2020) to proactively diagnose whether an EBI-based program plan has potential implementation problems that can be anticipated. It is important to point out that it is much easier and more efficient to revise a program plan in the planning stage than it is to make changes after implementation is routinized.

Provide the ex-post program stress test to proactively assess implementation problems

Stakeholders are typically interested in following the early progress of implementation. They hope to identify problems early, to prevent them from getting worse. The traditional formative evaluation is good for troubleshooting a program's immediate implementation problems but not for detecting underlying structural and functional issues in implementation. TDE introduced the ex-post program stress test (Chen and Morosuna 2020) to meet this need. In a safe environment, participants express their views about the structural and functional resilience of the program, under simulated overload or extreme contextual conditions. The ex-post stress test was used to assess a retention program for minority nursing students (Chen and Morosuna 2020). The results were used to improve the program structure and the implementation process.

Balance the bottom-up and top-down approach to dissemination

Biomedical research has a well-established model for developing and disseminating pharmaceuticals starting from animal studies, through multiple testing phases, to final dissemination for physician's prescriptions (Shamley and Wright 2017). The entire process usually takes several years. Behavioural and social science researchers tried to replicate this model to develop a simplified version for designing and testing EBIs over a much shorter time period. This approach is a top-down approach, from researchers to practitioners (Chen and Garbe 2011), as illustrated in the left side of Figure 43.2. Under this approach, the dissemination of an EBI travels the path from design to efficacy testing, effectiveness evaluation, and community use and, sometimes, simply from efficacy evaluation directly to community use.

Despite its popularity, TDE argues that the top-down approach for disseminating behavioural EBIs has a range of limitations: the conditions for designing and testing EBIs do not

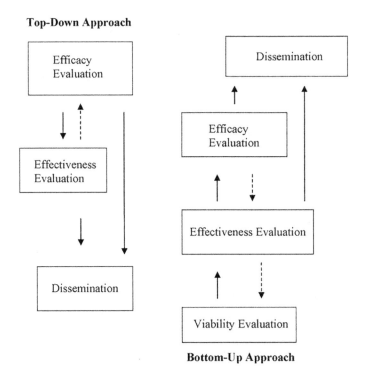

Figure 43.2 Top-down approach versus bottom-up approach

Source: Created by author

resemble real-world operation, EBIs do not address the nuts and bolts of implementation issues of interest to stakeholders, EBIs are ignorant of real-world social environments, and the EBI efficacy does not necessarily imply real-world effectiveness (Chen 2010, Chen and Garbe 2011). Because of these limitations, TDE argues that the top-down approach should be used as a discretionary option rather than as the gold standard for disseminating and implementing behavioural or social EBIs. TDE recognizes the merit of the bottom-up approach (Chen 2010, Chen and Garbe 2011) as illustrated in the right-hand side of Figure 43.2. This approach stresses that when developing and disseminating behavioural or social interventions, the initial evaluation should start with a viability evaluation to assure that a proposed intervention is practical, affordable, suitable, evaluable, and helpful for a community. If the intervention is viable, its subsequent effectiveness evaluation is likely to provide sufficient objective evidence for its merit. If necessary, an efficacy evaluation can rigorously assess causal relationships between the intervention and the outcomes. TDE argues that the bottom-up approach has several merits, including assuring that the intervention is useful to stakeholders and not the least, avoiding wasting money (Chen and Garbe 2011).

References

Aarons, G. A., M. Hurlburt, and S. M. Horwitz. 2011. "Advancing a conceptual model of evidence-based practice implementation in public service sectors." *Administration and Policy in Mental Health and Mental Health Services Research* 38 (1):4–23.

Brownson, R. C., G. A. Colditz, and E. K. Proctor. 2017. *Dissemination and Implementation Research in Health: Translating Science to Practice*. New York: Oxford University Press.

Chen, H. T. 1990. *Theory-driven Evaluations*. Thousand Oaks, CA: Sage Publications.

Chen, H.-T. 1997. "Normative evaluation of an anti-drug abuse program." *Evaluation and Program Planning* 20 (2):195–204. doi: 10.1016/S0149-7189(96)00050-X

Chen, H. T. 2005. *Practical Program Evaluation: Assessing and Improving Planning, Implementation, and Effectiveness*. Thousand Oaks, CA: Sage.

Chen, H. T. 2010. "The bottom-up approach to integrative validity: A new perspective for program evaluation." *Evaluation and Program Planning* 33 (3):205–214.

Chen, H. T. 2013. "The roots and growth of theory-driven evaluation: An integrated perspective addressing viability, effectuality, and transferability." In *The Roots and Growth of Theory-Driven Evaluation: An integrated Perspective Addressing Viability, Effectuality, and Transferability*, edited by M. C. Akin, 2nd ed. Los Angeles, CA: Sage Publications.

Chen, H. T. 2015. *Practical Program Evaluation: Theory-driven Evaluation and the Integrated Evaluation Perspective*. 2nd ed. Thousand Oaks, CA: Sage Publications.

Chen, H. T., and P. Garbe. 2011. "Assessing program outcomes from the bottom-up approach: An innovative perspective to outcome evaluation." In *Advancing Validity in Outcome Evaluation: Theory and Practice*, edited by Huey T Chen, S. I. Donaldson, and M. M. Mark. San Francisco, CA: Jossey Bass.

Chen, H. T., and Morosuna. 2020. "Proactive evaluation of program plan to improve implementation of evidence-based interventions: The theory-driven evaluation perspective." *American Evaluation 2020*.

Dearing, J. W. 2008. "Evolution of diffusion and dissemination theory." *Journal of Public Health Management and Practice* 14 (2):99–108. doi: 10.1097/01.PHH.0000311886.98627.b7.

Dvir, D., T. Raz, and A. J. Shenhar. 2003. "An empirical analysis of the relationship between project planning and project success." *International Journal of Project Management* 21 (2):89–95. doi: 10.1016/S0263-7863(02)00012-1.

Estabrooks, P. A., R. C. Brownson, and N. P. Pronk. 2018. "Dissemination and implementation science for public health professionals: An overview and call to action." *Preventing Chronic Disease* 15. doi: 10.5888/pcd15.180525.

Glasgow, R. E., C. Vinson, D. Chambers, M. J. Khoury, R. M. Kaplan, and C. Hunter. 2012. "National institutes of health approaches to dissemination and implementation science: Current and future directions." *American Journal of Public Health* 102 (7):1274–1281. doi: 10.2105/AJPH.2012.300755.

Proctor, E. K., J. Landsverk, G. Aarons, D. Chambers, C. Glisson, and B. Mittman. 2009. "Implementation research in mental health services: An emerging science with conceptual, methodological, and training challenges." *Administration and Policy in Mental Health and Mental Health Services Research* 36 (1):24–34.

Shamley, D., and B. Wright. 2017. *A Comprehensive and Practical Guide to Clinical Trials*. San Diego, CA: Academic Press.

44 Process evaluation of implementation strategies

Michel Wensing

The evaluation of interventions (including implementation strategies) can focus on outcomes (effectiveness evaluation), costs (economic evaluation), and other aspects. The latter is usually referred to as "process evaluation", which is a container for different items. Research questions for process evaluation may include the following: 1) have the targeted individuals and populations been reached? 2) Have the interventions been delivered as planned, or have these been adapted? 3) Has the targeted group been exposed to the interventions? 4) Which intervention components contribute to outcomes? 5) What contextual factors (organizational, physical, cultural) influence outcomes? 6) What are the mechanisms of change, or absence of it? 7) What are consequences of the interventions, positive or negative, beyond the anticipated outcomes? 8) What are participants' experiences with the interventions? 9) Can the interventions be sustained over time? 10) Can the interventions be transferred to other settings? Frequently used sources of data for process evaluations are surveys and interviews in the targeted policymakers, healthcare professionals, managers, and patients. Other sources of data include direct observation of practices and analysis of available documents, written communication, and administrative and clinical data. The analysis is often descriptive, but it may involve more advanced methods of analysis.

This contribution focuses specifically on process evaluation of implementation strategies, which are interventions to enhance the uptake of innovations in healthcare practice. Ideally, these innovations were evaluated before implementation and proved to have an attractive profile of benefits and harms (i.e., they are "evidence-based"). Implementation strategies may include providing information and education, engagement of patients, organizational changes, financial incentives, and regulatory measures. Here, I discuss several aspects of the process evaluation of implementation strategies.

Process evaluation should address implementation strategies

First and foremost, it is essential to plan for process evaluation that relates to interventions and implementation strategies separately, as well as in combination. Influential guidance on process evaluation does not distinguish implementation strategies from interventions that are implemented. For instance, the guidance of the UK Medical Research Council relates to "complex interventions" generally (Moore et al. 2015). However, mixed effects on outcomes may be related to issues around interventions (e.g., low fidelity of delivery), issues around implementation strategies (e.g., little participation of healthcare professionals in planned activities), or both. Only if implementation strategies are analysed separately from interventions, it is possible for such determinants of outcomes to be unravelled.

DOI: 10.4324/9781003109945-48

Fidelity of interventions is central

Measurement of the degree that interventions are delivered as planned, or adapted during their delivery, is central to any process evaluation. It is difficult to interpret outcomes, or any other result of process evaluation, if the fidelity of interventions is unknown. Intervention fidelity is typically actively optimized in clinical trials (Bellg et al. 2004), while it is a variable that is observed in implementation research. The fidelity of implementation strategies has been conceptualized in terms of 1) adherence in terms of planned content, coverage, frequency, and duration; 2) essential ingredients; and 3) moderators, including intervention complexity, facilitation strategies, quality of delivery, and participant responsiveness (Carroll et al. 2007). A review of published implementation research found that reporting on implementation fidelity was limited, suggesting a need for inclusion of this aspect in evaluation research (Slaughter, Hill, and Snelgrove-Clarke 2015). Actual measurement of these concepts requires tailormade measures; there are few, if any, standardized measures for intervention fidelity.

Process evaluation needs outcomes evaluations

As outcomes of implementation strategies tend to be mixed and, overall, moderate, insight into factors and processes related to effects is often more informative than (only) an estimate of the average effectiveness. Process evaluation is most informative if intervention outcomes are known, because the findings can then be contextualized. For instance, the journal *Implementation Science* only considers process evaluations, if the effects of implementation have been assessed, ideally in a rigorous outcomes' evaluation. Descriptions of implementation processes do not contribute much to the accumulation of scientific knowledge, if it remains unclear how these relate to outcomes of implementation.

Theorizing is needed in process evaluation

Theories, models, and frameworks help to relate a specific study to the broader body of scientific knowledge and a wider understanding of the world at large. Most relevant for process evaluation are theories of change (De Silva et al. 2014) and logic models of interventions (Rehfuess et al. 2018). For analysis of contextual factors, implementation science frameworks may be used (e.g., the Tailored Implementation in Chronic Disease framework) (Flottorp et al. 2013). While such frameworks are helpful, it is generally believed that more analytical depth is required to enhance the field of implementation science. Theorizing is required to identify potential mechanisms of change (Kislov et al. 2019). For instance, process evaluation in five randomized trials largely confirmed the relevance of previously identified determinants of implementation, which can inform the later choice of tailored interventions. In addition, new determinants emerged during actual implementation, as compared to the *a priori* analysis of barriers for implementation (Jäger et al. 2015). This confirmed the relevance of process evaluation and showed that stakeholders did not fully foresee barriers and needs for implementation before they actually were exposed to the implementation program.

Transferability should be addressed

Decision-makers frequently need to assess whether interventions with demonstrated effectiveness can be implemented with a high degree of fidelity in populations or delivery systems that are (somewhat or much) different from the one in which it was tested (Aarons et al. 2017). Such assessment can be informed by process evaluation, if it sufficiently documents and analyses the population and delivery system in which interventions were applied. Arguably, this is the least well-recognized purpose of process evaluation but highly important for decision-makers in healthcare.

Process evaluation is key to rigorous evaluation of interventions, including implementation strategies. If conducted well, it can support decision-making on the use of interventions and contribute to knowledge accumulation.

References

Aarons, G. A., M. Sklar, B. Mustanski, N. Benbow, and C. H. Brown. 2017. "'Scaling-out' evidence-based interventions to new populations or new health care delivery systems." *Implementation Science* 12 (1):111.

Bellg, A. J., B. Borrelli, B. Resnick, J. Hecht, D. S. Minicucci, M. Ory, G. Ogedegbe, D. Orwig, D. Ernst, and S. Czajkowski. 2004. "Enhancing treatment fidelity in health behavior change studies: Best practices and recommendations from the NIH Behavior Change Consortium." *Health Psychology* 23 (5):443.

Carroll, C., M. Patterson, S. Wood, A. Booth, J. Rick, and S. Balain. 2007. "A conceptual framework for implementation fidelity." *Implementation science* 2 (1):40.

De Silva, M. J., E. Breuer, L. Lee, L. Asher, N. Chowdhary, C. Lund, and V. Patel. 2014. "Theory of change: A theory-driven approach to enhance the Medical Research Council's framework for complex interventions." *Trials* 15 (1):267.

Flottorp, S. A., A. D. Oxman, J. Krause, N. R. Musila, M. Wensing, M. Godycki-Cwirko, R. Baker, and M. P. Eccles. 2013. "A checklist for identifying determinants of practice: A systematic review and synthesis of frameworks and taxonomies of factors that prevent or enable improvements in healthcare professional practice." *Implementation Science* 8 (1):1–11.

Jäger, C., J. Steinhäuser, T. Freund, R. Baker, S. Agarwal, M. Godycki-Cwirko, A. Kowalczyk, E. Aakhus, I. Granlund, and J. van Lieshout. 2015. "Process evaluation of five tailored programs to improve the implementation of evidence-based recommendations for chronic conditions in primary care." *Implementation Science* 11 (1):123.

Kislov, R., C. Pope, G. P. Martin, and P. M. Wilson. 2019. "Harnessing the power of theorising in implementation science." *Implementation Science* 14 (1):103.

Moore, G. F., S. Audrey, M. Barker, L. Bond, C. Bonell, W. Hardeman, L. Moore, A. O'Cathain, T. Tinati, and D. Wight. 2015. "Process evaluation of complex interventions: Medical Research Council guidance." *BMJ* 350.

Rehfuess, E. A., A. Booth, L. Brereton, J. Burns, A. Gerhardus, K. Mozygemba, W. Oortwijn, L. M. Pfadenhauer, M. Tummers, and G. J. van der Wilt. 2018. "Towards a taxonomy of logic models in systematic reviews and health technology assessments: A priori, staged, and iterative approaches." *Research Synthesis Methods* 9 (1):13–24.

Slaughter, S. E., J. N. Hill, and E. Snelgrove-Clarke. 2015. "What is the extent and quality of documentation and reporting of fidelity to implementation strategies: A scoping review." *Implementation Science* 10 (1):129.

45 Dissemination

David Chambers

An old adage popularized in a 1910 book states, "If a tree falls in the woods and no one is around to hear it, does it make a sound?" (Mann and Ransom Twiss 1910). In the field of implementation science, we might modify this as follows: "If an evidence-based intervention fails to be disseminated, does it make a difference? Key to all efforts to integrate research into healthcare practice, we define dissemination as 'the targeted distribution of information and intervention materials to a specific public health or clinical practice audience'. The intent is to spread ('scale up') and sustain knowledge and the associated evidence-based interventions" (2020 PAR 13–055). Fifteen years ago, as the National Institutes of Health was soliciting applications for studies that would build knowledge on how best to improve the uptake of health interventions into clinical and community settings, a decision was made to include dissemination research as a core part of that effort. Why?

We recognized that the scientific community traditionally viewed dissemination as that to remain within academic circles. The primary method through which dissemination was expected to influence practice was the publication, and while some high-impact publication could directly influence guideline development and by extension, clinical practice, the vast majority of science (estimated by Balas and Boren (2000) as 86%) never made it into practising decision-making. Indeed, the need to advance our understanding of dissemination continues to cover all aspects of the process, from the creation of the evidence, to its packaging, transmission, reception, and how it is incorporated into actions by patients, providers, organizations, communities, and systems (Glasgow et al. 2012). We must also remember that dissemination channels vary by target audience, and the need for information (and in specific forms) will similarly vary.

In recent years, the complexity of dissemination has outpaced the research base. Innovations in technology have brought infinite sources of information to our handheld devices; new forms of media have arisen that have changed where, how, and why we seek information and how that information is provided. Even the journal publication process has significantly changed, with electronic publication of articles shortening the time from acceptance to access and new platforms streamlining the way in which investigators share their work.

The democratization of evidence has had clear benefits, as it has both expanded the ability for research findings to be disseminated and the capacity for target audiences to more easily find relevant information that can inform health decision-making. At the same time, it has enabled the spread of misinformation that can have adverse consequences for the health and healthcare of the population (Chou, Oh, and Klein 2018). With the dynamism of the evidence base (Chambers, Glasgow, and Stange 2013), and continuous innovation of communication technologies, dissemination has grown ever more complex. As a consequence, there are several things that the implementation science community can do to improve dissemination

DOI: 10.4324/9781003109945-49

as a necessary step toward integration of evidence-based interventions into clinical and community practice.

First, we should increase our focus on dissemination research questions within all portfolios of implementation science. A recent analysis of National Cancer Institute–funded grants has echoed prior studies, showing a relative paucity of dissemination trials (Neta, Clyne, and Chambers 2020, In Press). Second, the scientific community should practise what we know to be effective dissemination methods (e.g., active dissemination methods are far more effective than passive ones) and tailoring dissemination to the needs of heterogeneous stakeholders. Third, our evidence syntheses must uniformly provide better guidance around the evidence base for our existing interventions, as well as where the remaining knowledge gaps are. Finally, we should improve our understanding of how misinformation spreads and, analogous to the growing focus on de-implementation (Norton, Chambers, and Kramer 2019), focus on the development of strategies to disseminate evidence in the context of misleading or harmful information.

The research and practice of dissemination, like many things, is a work in progress. Vital to the ultimate benefit of our scientific discoveries on the health and healthcare of our people, dissemination can increase knowledge and awareness and, when effective, improve health behavior and health and healthcare outcomes. With greater emphasis on developing and utilizing its underlying knowledge base, we can ensure that our trees of evidence will always be heard.

References

2020 PAR 13–055: Dissemination and Implementation Research in Health (R01). National Institutes of Health.

Balas, E., and S. Boren. 2000. "Managing Clinical Knowledge for Health Care Improvement." *Yearbook of Medical Informatics* 1:65–70.

Chambers, D. A., R. E. Glasgow, and K. C. Stange. 2013. "The dynamic sustainability framework: Addressing the paradox of sustainment amid ongoing change." *Implementation Science* 8 (1):117.

Chou, W.-Y. S., A. Oh, and W. M. P. Klein. 2018. "Addressing health-related misinformation on social media." *JAMA* 320 (23):2417–2418.

Glasgow, R. E., C. Vinson, D. Chambers, M. J. Khoury, R. M. Kaplan, and C. Hunter. 2012. "National Institutes of Health approaches to dissemination and implementation science: Current and future directions." *American Journal of Public Health* 102 (7):1274–1281.

Mann, C. R., and G. Ransom Twiss. 1910. *Physics.* Chicago, IL: Scott, Foresman and Co.

Neta, Clyne, and D. Chambers. 2020, In Press. "Dissemination and implementation research at the National Cancer Institute: A review of funded studies (2006–2019) and opportunities to advance the field." *Cancer Epidemiology, Biomarkers & Prevention.*

Norton, W. E., D. A. Chambers, and B. S. Kramer. 2019. "Conceptualizing de-implementation in cancer care delivery." *Journal of Clinical Oncology* 37 (2):93–96.

46 A learning perspective on implementation

Per Nilsen, Margit Neher, Per-Erik Ellström, and Benjamin Gardner

Implementing evidence-based practice (EBP) in healthcare and other settings presents two interlinked challenges: adoption of evidence-based interventions (methods, programs, etc.) and abandonment of ingrained non-evidence-based interventions. We propose that two learning modes – adaptive and developmental learning – can enhance understanding of the challenges of achieving EBP.

Adaptive learning involves a gradual shift from slower, deliberate behaviours to faster and more efficient behaviours, yielding increasingly efficient and reliable task performances (Ellström 2001, 2006). This process occurs through habit formation. Habits form when a behaviour is repeated in a specific context. This reinforces associations between the behaviour and features of the performance context (e.g., an environment), to the extent that perceiving the context cues automatically activates an impulse to act, without prior forethought or conscious control (Gardner 2015b, Neal, Wood, and Quinn 2006). Over time, control over behaviour is delegated from effortful deliberative processes to contextual cues. Habits play an important role in instigating various healthcare practices (e.g., taking dental radiographs, placing fissure sealants, and managing low back pain (Eccles et al. 2012, Grimshaw et al. 2011, Presseau et al. 2014)).

Whereas adaptive learning involves a progression from deliberate to more automatically enacted behaviours, developmental learning is conceptualized as a process in the "opposite" direction, whereby automatically enacted behaviours become deliberate and conscious (Ellström 2001, 2006). Developmental learning may occur when an individual critically reflects on previously implicit assumptions and unconscious thought and action patterns. Many well-rehearsed tasks can be expected to depend on instigation of habits (Nilsen et al. 2012, Presseau et al. 2014, Rochette, Korner-Bitensky, and Thomas 2009). However, when unfamiliar problems or new situations arise, for example, a patient presenting with symptoms unknown to the physician, habitual responses built through experience may not suffice and deliberative processes must be engaged to find solutions.

Shifting from automatic to deliberate action necessitates overruling or breaking habits. The occurrence of unexpected problems offers an opportunity to inhibit activated habit impulses before their translation into behaviour (Gardner 2015a). This requires willpower or self-control, made more difficult when a person is stressed or distracted by cognitively effortful tasks (Neal, Wood, and Drolet 2013). Contextual changes also offer a possibility of limiting habitual responses. Discontinued exposure to habit cues can enable practitioners to bring behavioural decision-making under conscious control (Verplanken et al. 2008). For instance, reminders of appropriate indications and computerized decision support can decrease the number of routine chest X-rays in intensive care units (Sy et al. 2016).

DOI: 10.4324/9781003109945-50

Ultimately, achieving a more EBP depends on both adaptive and developmental learning, which involves both forming EBP-conducive habits and breaking habits that do not contribute to realizing the goals of EBP. From a learning perspective, EBP will be best facilitated by developing habitual practice of EBP such that it becomes natural to strive for an EBP in appropriate contexts by means of learning new interventions supported by empirical evidence. However, contexts must also facilitate disruption of existing habits, to ensure that use of evidence-based interventions in routine practice is consciously considered to arrive at the most appropriate response.

References

Eccles, M. P., J. M. Grimshaw, G. MacLennan, D. Bonetti, L. Glidewell, N. B. Pitts, N. Steen, R. Thomas, A. Walker, and M. Johnston. 2012. "Explaining clinical behaviors using multiple theoretical models." *Implementation Science* 7 (1):1–13.

Ellström, P.-E. 2001. "Integrating learning and work: Conceptual issues and critical conditions." *Human Resource Development Quarterly* 12 (4):421–435.

Ellström, P.-E. 2006. "The meaning and role of reflection in informal learning at work." *Productive Reflection at Work*:43–53.

Gardner, B. 2015a. "Defining and measuring the habit impulse: Response to commentaries." *Health Psychology Review* 9 (3):318–322.

Gardner, B. 2015b. "A review and analysis of the use of 'habit' in understanding, predicting and influencing health-related behaviour." *Health Psychology Review* 9 (3):277–295.

Grimshaw, J. M., M. P. Eccles, N. Steen, M. Johnston, N. B. Pitts, L. Glidewell, G. Maclennan, R. Thomas, D. Bonetti, and A. Walker. 2011. "Applying psychological theories to evidence-based clinical practice: Identifying factors predictive of lumbar spine x-ray for low back pain in UK primary care practice." *Implementation Science* 6 (1):1–13.

Neal, D. T., W. Wood, and A. Drolet. 2013. "How do people adhere to goals when willpower is low? The profits (and pitfalls) of strong habits." *Journal of Personality and Social Psychology* 104 (6):959.

Neal, D. T., W. Wood, and J. M. Quinn. 2006. "Habits – A repeat performance." *Current Directions in Psychological Science* 15 (4):198–202.

Nilsen, P., K. Roback, A. Broström, and P.-E. Ellström. 2012. "Creatures of habit: Accounting for the role of habit in implementation research on clinical behaviour change." *Implementation Science* 7 (1):1–6.

Presseau, J., M. Johnston, T. Heponiemi, M. Elovainio, J. J. Francis, M. P. Eccles, N. Steen, S. Hrisos, E. Stamp, and J. M. Grimshaw. 2014. "Reflective and automatic processes in health care professional behaviour: A dual process model tested across multiple behaviours." *Annals of Behavioral Medicine* 48 (3):347–358.

Rochette, A., N. Korner-Bitensky, and A. Thomas. 2009. "Changing clinicians' habits: Is this the hidden challenge to increasing best practices?" *Disability and Rehabilitation* 31 (21):1790–1794.

Sy, E., M. Luong, M. Quon, Y. Kim, S. Sharifi, M. Norena, H. Wong, N. Ayas, J. Leipsic, and P. Dodek. 2016. "Implementation of a quality improvement initiative to reduce daily chest radiographs in the intensive care unit." *BMJ Quality & Safety* 25 (5):379–385.

47 Alignment

Impact on implementation processes and outcomes

Mark G. Ehrhart and Gregory A. Aarons

How different forms of alignment within organizations influence implementation processes and outcomes

The concept of alignment arises in a number of forms throughout the implementation literature as being a critical element for implementation success although sometimes with different labels such as "fit" or "congruence". In this essay, we define alignment as the extent to which various elements internal to the organization or between the organization and external entities are congruent, consistent, and/or coordinated. We draw heavily from the literature on organizational climate and culture (Ehrhart, Schneider, and Macey 2013, Schein and Schein 2010) and describe five types of alignment that are critical for implementation effectiveness: internal systems alignment, horizontal unit alignment, vertical alignment, innovation–client alignment, and innovation–provider alignment.

Internal systems alignment

The degree to which organizational policies, practices, procedures, and systems are aligned has consequences for how employees perceive the organization's values and strategic priorities. In the implementation literature, internal systems alignment is perhaps best exemplified by the concept of implementation climate (Ehrhart, Aarons, and Farahnak 2014, Klein, Conn, and Sorra 2001, Weiner et al. 2011). Implementation climate is defined as "employees shared perceptions of the importance of innovation implementation within the organization" (Klein, Conn, and Sorra 2001). As providers experience the policies, practices, procedures, and systems in their organization related to implementation, they form shared perceptions of the extent to which implementation is indeed a priority in the organization. When these various structures and processes are aligned, it is clear to employees that implementation is a top priority (i.e., implementation climate levels are high), and they are more likely to act in support of the organization's implementation efforts (Williams et al. 2020). For example, internal systems alignment for evidence-based practice (EBP) implementation is evident when an organization adopts a mission statement explicitly mentioning the value of EBPs, hires providers specifically for their EBP expertise and experience, offers training to its providers on EBPs, reviews data on the fidelity with which providers are delivering EBPs as part of quality assurance practices, and formally recognizes staff who champion EBPs. However, when there is a lack of alignment, the messages employees receive are inconsistent, decreasing the likelihood that employees will prioritize implementation efforts.

DOI: 10.4324/9781003109945-51

Horizontal unit alignment

The organizational culture literature has discussed how organizations vary in the extent to which culture is shared across organizational units or subcultures (Louis 1985). Applied to implementation, this type of alignment captures the extent to which the various organizational units or subcultures support the implementation efforts and contribute to its success (Ravishankar, Pan, and Leidner 2011). For instance, poor horizontal unit alignment would occur if the clinical services department supports an EBP implementation effort because they believe that the EBP will improve service quality and client outcomes, but the accounting department opposes implementation because they are concerned about losing billable time while providers attend trainings to learn the new EBP. Conflicting perspectives on the prioritization of the implementation effort suggest horizontal unit misalignment and may result in challenges in securing the resources and infrastructure needed to effectively implement and sustain the practice (Stewart et al. 2016).

Vertical alignment

In contrast to alignment of horizontal units in the organization, the organizational culture literature also discussed whether the culture is shared across levels of the organization hierarchy (Louis 1985, O'Reilly et al. 2010). When applied to implementation, this type of alignment captures the extent to which leaders and staff at various levels are aligned in their support of implementation efforts (Aarons et al. 2014, Birken et al. 2015). For instance, vertical alignment for EBP implementation would emerge when a clinical director's decision to implement an EBP is supported by executive leaders doing such things as highlighting the importance of the EBP in organization-wide communication or coming to program meetings to discuss how the new practice aligns with the mission of the organization. Vertical alignment also captures the alignment between system-level leadership in the organization's external context and organizational leadership in the inner context (Aarons et al. 2014). For example, state mental health department leaders may request organizations' engagement in EBP fidelity monitoring procedures, but organization leaders may feel ill-equipped to implement fidelity monitoring procedures across their organizations without additional resources, technical assistance, and support from the state.

Innovation–client alignment

The extent to which the organization's culture or strategy aligns with the external environment has been referred to as external alignment or strategic fit in the organizational culture literature (Saffold III 1988, Schein and Schein 2010). One application of this type of fit related to implementation is the fit between the innovation or EBP that is being implemented and the needs or values of clients, or innovation–client alignment. For example, if a particular EBP is inappropriate for the organization's client base, then there is likely to be resistance from clients and/or reduced client engagement, which could ultimately lead to implementation failure. Critical to this type of alignment is the fact that the organization's external environment can change (Kotter and Heskett 1992). Practices that were implemented and sustained in the past may no longer be appropriate if, for example, the organization's client base has changed or if new practices with superior outcomes have emerged. Thus, leadership must maintain a firm grasp on shifts to the external environment to ensure that the practices that the organization adopts and implements are appropriate and will be sustained (Chambers, Glasgow, and Stange 2013).

Innovation–provider alignment

The final type of alignment described here is the alignment between the innovation and the users of that innovation, or innovation–provider alignment. This type of alignment has been referred to as innovation-values fit and defined as "the extent to which targeted users perceive that use of the innovation will foster (or, conversely, inhibit) the fulfillment of their values" (Klein and Sorra 1996). Using an example from mental health, if an organization's implementation effort targets a practice that is not aligned with the therapeutic philosophy (e.g., medication-assisted treatment versus psychosocial approaches) of many of its providers, the implementation effort is unlikely to succeed. Finally, this alignment can go beyond the values of the organization to include the skill and ability of its providers. If a new practice has requirements that are outside of the expertise or comfort zone of current providers, the implementation effort is unlikely to succeed without additional supports to strengthen the skill and ability of its providers.

We have enumerated and described five different types or aspects of alignment, although there are certainly others that we did not consider. Alignment can occur within outer context, inner context, and be implicated in bridging of outer and inner contexts (Moullin et al. 2019). The challenge is that alignment is usually the subtext of implementation. We recommend that alignment both within and across levels of context be elevated to a key consideration in implementation theories and strategies. Doing so will promote a greater understanding of the complex implementation environment and should lead to more nuanced and effective implementation strategies.

References

Aarons, G. A., M. G. Ehrhart, L. R. Farahnak, and M. Sklar. 2014. "Aligning leadership across systems and organizations to develop a strategic climate for evidence-based practice implementation." *Annual Review of Public Health* 35:255–274.

Birken, S. A., S.-Y. D. Lee, B. J. Weiner, M. H. Chin, M. Chiu, and C. T. Schaefer. 2015. "From strategy to action: How top managers' support increases middle managers' commitment to innovation implementation in healthcare organizations." *Health Care Management Review* 40 (2):159.

Chambers, D. A., R. E. Glasgow, and K. C. Stange. 2013. "The dynamic sustainability framework: Addressing the paradox of sustainment amid ongoing change." *Implementation Science* 8 (1):1–11.

Ehrhart, M. G., G. A. Aarons, and L. R. Farahnak. 2014. "Assessing the organizational context for EBP implementation: The development and validity testing of the Implementation Climate Scale (ICS)." *Implementation Science* 9 (1):1–11.

Ehrhart, M. G., B. Schneider, and W. H. Macey. 2013. *Organizational Climate and Culture: An Introduction to Theory, Research, and Practice*. New York: Routledge.

Klein, K. J., A. B. Conn, and J. S. Sorra. 2001. "Implementing computerized technology: An organizational analysis." *Journal of Applied Psychology* 86 (5):811.

Klein, K. J., and J. S. Sorra. 1996. "The challenge of innovation implementation." *Academy of Management Review* 21 (4):1055–1080.

Kotter, J., and J. Heskett. 1992. *Corporate Culture and Performance*. New York: Free Press.

Louis, M. R. 1985. "An investigator's guide to workplace culture." *Organizational Culture*:73–93.

Moullin, J. C., K. S. Dickson, N. A. Stadnick, B. Rabin, and G. A. Aarons. 2019. "Systematic review of the exploration, preparation, implementation, sustainment (EPIS) framework." *Implementation Science* 14 (1):1–16.

O'Reilly, C. A., D. F. Caldwell, J. A. Chatman, M. Lapiz, and W. Self. 2010. "How leadership matters: The effects of leaders' alignment on strategy implementation." *The Leadership Quarterly* 21 (1):104–113.

Ravishankar, M., S. L. Pan, and D. E. Leidner. 2011. "Examining the strategic alignment and implementation success of a KMS: A subculture-based multilevel analysis." *Information Systems Research* 22 (1):39–59.

Saffold III, G. S. 1988. "Culture traits, strength, and organizational performance: Moving beyond 'strong' culture." *Academy of Management Review* 13 (4):546–558.

Schein, E. H., and P. Schein. 2010. *Organizational Culture and Leadership*. Hoboken, NJ: Jossey-Bass.

Schweizer, K. 2011. "On the changing role of Cronbachs in the evaluation of the quality of a measure." *European Journal of Psychological Assessment* 27 (3):143–144.

Stewart, R. E., D. R. Adams, D. S. Mandell, T. R. Hadley, A. C. Evans, R. Rubin, J. Erney, G. Neimark, M. O. Hurford, and R. S. Beidas. 2016. "The perfect storm: Collision of the business of mental health and the implementation of evidence-based practices." *Psychiatric Services* 67 (2):159–161.

Weiner, B. J., C. M. Belden, D. M. Bergmire, and M. Johnston. 2011. "The meaning and measurement of implementation climate." *Implementation Science* 6 (1):1–12.

Williams, N. J., C. B. Wolk, E. M. Becker-Haimes, and R. S. Beidas. 2020. "Testing a theory of strategic implementation leadership, implementation climate, and clinicians' use of evidence-based practice: A 5-year panel analysis." *Implementation Science* 15 (1):10.

48 Work-as-Imagined and Work-as-Done

Erik Hollnagel and Robyn Clay-Williams

Resilient healthcare often uses two concepts borrowed from ergonomics, namely, Work-as-Imagined (WAI) and Work-as-Done (WAD). They make it possible to consider the difference between what people are expected to do and what they actually do without insisting that one is right and the other is wrong. The recognition of this difference is essential both for how work is managed and for how changes are planned and implemented. This essay will look at a specific use of the two concepts; a more detailed account has been given by Hollnagel (2015).

The need of Work-as-Imagined (WAI)

WAI represents how we think work should be done in order to bring about the intended outcomes. WAI covers our ideas about how others do, or should do, their work and, of course, also how we prepare our own work. Everyone naturally has ideas about how others do their work, but the WAI–WAD distinction is especially important where people are responsible for managing the work of others. Using the convenient but oversimplified description of an organization on three levels – macro, meso, and micro – the meso level manages the micro level, while the macro level manages the meso level and therefore indirectly also the micro level (Figure 48.1).

WAI is a composite of facts, experiences, and assumptions – and sometimes more the latter than the former. WAI will necessarily be incomplete and possibly also incorrect, for example, due to differences in experience, concerns, priorities, and so forth. A failure to recognize this may jeopardize how well changes can be planned and managed.

The reality of Work-as-Done (WAD)

When people carry out their work, they directly experience what happens. Their understanding is detailed and precise, and their priorities are directly related to the work at hand, first and foremost to meet the goals of the activities for which they are responsible. The plentiful feedback they receive is not limited to specific measurements or indicators and arrives with little or no delay.

Conversely, people who are not actually present where work takes place can only experience it indirectly via reports and indicators and from what others tell them about it. Their feedback is usually simplified and lagging and provides information that often has been filtered or interpreted several times. Managing work is usually done from a distance – often with the absence of precise knowledge or even a reasonable understanding of what goes on.

DOI: 10.4324/9781003109945-52

The larger that distance is – in time or proximity – the greater the gap between WAI and WAD will be.

It is both theoretically and practically impossible to describe work situations or activities so precisely that they completely match real situation so that any uncertainty or variability is eliminated. When work is done, some details will always be unknown, and some things may happen unexpectedly. Examples include interruptions, changes in priority, new demands, temporary unavailability of resources (colleagues, materials, time), and so forth. This kind of under-specification is inevitable in relation to how working conditions are described and contributes to WAD always being different from WAI.

Overcoming the WAI–WAD gap

The relative roles of WAI and WAD in management are shown in Figure 48.1. Although WAD obviously always is Work-as-Done regardless of the level on which it takes place, the term has traditionally been used to denote how people who are in charge of others think about what these others do. Thus, in Figure 48.1, what happens at the micro level is WAD relative to how people at the meso level think about it, which is the meso-level WAI. The same goes for the relation between the meso and macro levels.

For each level, information about what happens on the level below will be summarized, simplified, and delayed. Thus, reports used by the meso level are condensed and simplified descriptions of what happened on the micro level. The contents of, for example, quality surveys used by the macro level are even further simplified – and usually also further delayed. In the same way, the controlling interventions – targets, rules, procedures – can rarely be applied directly but require some kind of interpretation or "translation" to fill in the details. It is, therefore, hardly surprising that the actual outcomes of interventions always differ somewhat from the expected outcomes.

When considering the gap between WAI and WAD, the problem is not whether one is correct and the other is wrong, and the solution should never be to make WAD comply with WAI. The problem is rather to acknowledge the gap and to find ways to overcome it. WAD is, by definition, a function of the actual conditions – people, information, demands, resources, work environment – when it happens and can therefore only be changed by changing the conditions. But for WAI, the situation is different. To change WAI first of all requires that

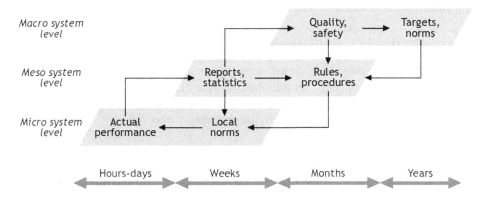

Figure 48.1 Differences between the blunt and the sharp end

Source: Created by authors

the delays in getting information about actual work practices, about WAD, are reduced. But it also requires that the information is more detailed and accurate and that it goes beyond condensed summaries, standardized measures, and indicators. At the very least, indicators should be chosen because they are meaningful rather than because they are convenient. The focus should also be on all operations and not just things that have gone wrong. This will eventually lead to a better understanding of WAD, which is the necessary condition for making successful changes. Managing work and changes to work must be grounded in a solid understanding of what actually goes on. Assumptions, even when they are widely shared, should never replace facts.

Reference

Hollnagel, E. (2015). Why is work-as-imagined different from work-as-done? In R. L. Wears, E., Hollnagel & J. Braithwaite (Eds). *Resilient health care, Volume 2: The resilience of everyday clinical work*. Farnham, UK: Ashgate.

49 Leading implementation by focusing on strategic implementation leadership

Gregory A. Aarons and Mark G. Ehrhart

Leaders in health systems and organizations are in a position of influence that can support or sabotage implementation efforts. Leadership is an important implementation determinant in multiple frameworks and is important across system and organizational levels (Moullin et al. 2019, Nilsen 2015). Leadership is also important for implementation in diverse healthcare and allied healthcare settings such as health (Richter et al. 2016, Gifford et al. 2007), behavioural health (Ingebrigtsen et al. 2014, Aarons et al. 2014, Aarons, Farahnak, and Ehrhart 2014), education (Lyon et al. 2018), and with both well-established and emergent interventions and technologies (Best et al. 2020). Despite recognition of the importance of leadership for implementation effectiveness, research has just begun to scratch the surface of the qualities and behaviours of leaders who are able to effectively lead evidence-based practice implementation and increased use of research evidence.

Leadership has been of interest to researchers and organizational change agents for many years (Lord et al. 2017), and the field has grown and evolved over time. More current studies of leadership address or integrate, among others, executive leadership, team leadership, follower-based approaches, ethical leadership, and gender (Avolio, Walumbwa, and Weber 2009). Research on transformational leadership has been most influential in health, behavioural health, and implementation science because of the substantial research base across settings and countries, with studies showing its associations with implementation climate, implementation attitudes, and implementation-related behaviours (e.g., Aarons et al. 2016, Michaelis, Stegmaier, and Sonntag 2010).

Recent leadership research has begun to address focused or strategic leadership that identifies characteristics and behaviours of leaders that support a particular objective (Aarons, Ehrhart, and Farahnak 2014). For example, past research has addressed the actions leaders take to support safety in organizations (i.e., safety leadership (Zohar 2002)) and leadership to support high levels of customer service (i.e., service leadership (Schneider et al. 2005)). When applied to implementation, this approach captures the characteristics and behaviours of leaders most influential in creating system or organizational context that clearly communicates to providers that evidence-based practice and use of research evidence are expected, supported, and rewarded by health systems and organizations (Aarons et al. 2014).

The Implementation Leadership Scale (Aarons, Ehrhart, and Farahnak 2014) assesses key dimensions of implementation leadership: 1) being knowledgeable about practices being implemented, their fit in routine practice, and nuances of application with diverse clients/patients; 2) being proactive in anticipating and addressing implementation challenges; 3) supporting clinicians in their efforts to use evidence-based practices; and 4) persevering through challenges in the implementation process (Aarons, Ehrhart, and Farahnak 2014). Similarly, a recent systematic review identified behaviours that leaders perform to facilitate

DOI: 10.4324/9781003109945-53

evidence-based practice implementation: 1) obtaining and diffusing information, 2) adapting information and the innovation, 3) mediating between strategy and day-to-day activities, and 4) selling innovation implementation (Birken et al. 2018). Finally, the Ottawa Model of Implementation Leadership (Gifford et al. 2017) identifies implementation-related behaviours within the broad categories of relation behaviours (e.g., recognizes efforts to change), change behaviours (e.g., demonstrates commitment to change), and task behaviours (e.g., clarifies roles and responsibilities).

Beyond identifying leader behaviours that impact implementation outcomes, it is critical to determine how to develop interventions to help leaders to become more effective implementation leaders. Progress has been made on this front, including the Leadership and Organizational Change for Implementation intervention (Aarons et al. 2015) and the iLead leadership intervention (Richter et al. 2016). Considering that almost all of the things that happen in systems and organizations are a result of leader actions or inactions, comprehensive approaches to further develop and test leadership-focused implementation strategies are needed. Interventions that support leaders in developing and enacting implementation-related policies and supports, engaging with implementation stakeholders, and setting a mission and vision related to implementation should increase the use of research evidence and evidence-based practice in their organizations.

By way of concluding, we must go beyond thinking of leadership as an abstract construct and instead focus on specific actions, activities, knowledge, skills, and abilities that help to create a conceptual and operational context that supports evidence-based care. There are many opportunities for doing just that through researchers partnering and collaborating with health systems and organizations to bring the best leadership-focused implementation science to develop leader-focused implementation strategies. A broader and more inclusive approach to understanding how leaders enact implementation-related change can advance implementation science and improve healthcare practices and outcomes.

References

Aarons, G. A., M. G. Ehrhart, and L. R. Farahnak. 2014. "The implementation leadership scale (ILS): Development of a brief measure of unit level implementation leadership." *Implementation Science* 9 (1):45.

Aarons, G. A., M. G. Ehrhart, L. R. Farahnak, and M. S. Hurlburt. 2015. "Leadership and organizational change for implementation (LOCI): A randomized mixed method pilot study of a leadership and organization development intervention for evidence-based practice implementation." *Implementation Science* 10 (1):11.

Aarons, G. A., M. G. Ehrhart, L. R. Farahnak, and M. Sklar. 2014. "Aligning leadership across systems and organizations to develop a strategic climate for evidence-based practice implementation." *Annual Review of Public Health* 35:255–274.

Aarons, G. A., L. R. Farahnak, and M. G. Ehrhart. 2014. "Leadership and strategic organizational climate to support evidence-based practice implementation." In *Dissemination and Implementation of Evidence-based Practices in Child and Adolescent Mental Health*, edited by R. S. Beidas and P. C. Kendall, 82–97. New York, NY: Guilford Press.

Aarons, G. A., A. E. Green, E. Trott, C. Willging, E. M. Torres, M. Ehrhart, and S. C. Roesch. 2016. "The roles of system and organizational leadership in system-wide evidence-based intervention sustainment: A mixed-method study." *Administration and Policy in Mental Health and Mental Health Services Research* 43 (6):991–1008.

Avolio, B. J., F. O. Walumbwa, and T. J. Weber. 2009. "Leadership: Current theories, research, and future directions." *Annual Review of Psychology* 60:421–449.

Best, Stephanie, Zornitza Stark, Helen Brown, Janet C Long, Kushani Hewage, Clara Gaff, Jeffrey Braithwaite, and Natalie Taylor. 2020. "The leadership behaviors needed to implement clinical genomics at scale: A qualitative study." *Genetics in Medicine*:1–7.

Birken, Sarah, Alecia Clary, Amir Alishahi Tabriz, Kea Turner, Rosemary Meza, Alexandra Zizzi, Madeline Larson, Jennifer Walker, and Martin Charns. 2018. "Middle managers' role in implementing evidence-based practices in healthcare: A systematic review." *Implementation Science* 13 (1):149.

Gifford, W., B. Davies, N. Edwards, P. Griffin, and V. Lybanon. 2007. "Managerial leadership for nurses' use of research evidence: An integrative review of the literature." *Worldviews on Evidence-Based Nursing* 4 (3):126–145.

Gifford, W. A., I. D. Graham, M. G. Ehrhart, B. L. Davies, and G. A. Aarons. 2017. "Ottawa model of implementation leadership and implementation leadership scale: Mapping concepts for developing and evaluating theory-based leadership interventions." *Journal of Healthcare Leadership* 9:15–23.

Ingebrigtsen, Tor, Andrew Georgiou, Robyn Clay-Williams, Farah Magrabi, Antonia Hordern, Mirela Prgomet, Julie Li, Johanna Westbrook, and Jeffrey Braithwaite. 2014. "The impact of clinical leadership on health information technology adoption: Systematic review." *International Journal of Medical Informatics* 83 (6):393–405.

Lord, R. G., D. V. Day, S. J. Zaccaro, B. J. Avolio, and A. H. Eagly. 2017. "Leadership in applied psychology: Three waves of theory and research." *Journal of Applied Psychology* 102 (3):434.

Lyon, A. R., C. R. Cook, E. C. Brown, J. Locke, C. Davis, M. Ehrhart, and G. A. Aarons. 2018. "Assessing organizational implementation context in the education sector: Confirmatory factor analysis of measures of implementation leadership, climate, and citizenship." *Implementation Science* 13 (1):5. doi: 10.1186/s13012-017-0705-6.

Michaelis, B., R. Stegmaier, and K. Sonntag. 2010. "Shedding light on followers' innovation implementation behavior: The role of transformational leadership, commitment to change, and climate for initiative." *Journal of Managerial Psychology* 25 (4):408–429.

Moullin, J. C., K. S. Dickson, N. A. Stadnick, B. Rabin, and G. A. Aarons. 2019. "Systematic review of the Exploration, Preparation, Implementation, Sustainment (EPIS) framework." *Implementation Science* 14 (1):1. doi: 10.1186/s13012-018-0842-6.

Nilsen, P. 2015. "Making sense of implementation theories, models and frameworks." *Implementation Science* 10:53.

Richter, A., U. von Thiele Schwarz, C. Lornudd, R. Lundmark, R. Mosson, and H. Hasson. 2016. "iLead – a transformational leadership intervention to train healthcare managers' implementation leadership." *Implementation Science* 11 (1):108. doi: 10.1186/s13012-016-0475-6.

Schneider, B., M. G. Ehrhart, D. M. Mayer, J. L. Saltz, and K. Niles-Jolly. 2005. "Understanding organization-customer links in service settings." *Academy of Management Journal* 48 (6):1017–1032.

Zohar, D. 2002. "Modifying supervisory practices to improve subunit safety: A leadership-based intervention model." *Journal of Applied Psychology* 87 (1):156–163.

50 Agents of change

The example of an allied health professional

Kate Laver

Although there is an increasing volume of research relevant to allied health professionals, gaps between evidence and practice remain.

Allied health professionals work with a degree of autonomy in many health settings. They have some degree of control over how much time they spend with each client and which treatments and interventions they offer. This autonomy is important when applying evidence-based practice which considers the best research evidence as well as the clinician's expertise and the client's values (Sackett et al. 1996). Autonomy can be conducive to knowledge translation activities as it means that allied health professionals can quickly and easily change practice.

Enlisting allied health professionals to act as "agents of change" in an organization can be an effective and rapid way to bridge the gap between research and practice. Allied health professionals employed in clinical positions are often those who are "doing the work" of the organization. They know the client group, are aware of their resources (and resource constraints), and understand the organizational culture and appetite for change. Supporting allied health professionals to become "agents of change" involves arming them with knowledge about the latest research evidence and the skills to translate this into practice.

The case

Our research team recruited allied health professionals working in dementia care across Australia to become "agents of change" as part of a quality improvement collaborative to improve adherence to guideline recommendations for dementia care (Cations et al. 2018). We built on their knowledge about the latest high-quality evidence through a start-up meeting, online learning modules, and webinars. We supported them to develop skills in knowledge translation through online learning modules and activities. We provided one-on-one advice, practice feedback, and access to tools to help support them through the process of identifying a quality improvement activity, conducting the activity (using Plan, Do, Study, Act cycles), and evaluating the outcomes.

We found that there was great interest in becoming an "agent of change"; allied health professionals wanted to collaborate across settings and workplaces, wanted to learn more about the evidence in dementia care, wanted to connect with academics and people with lived experience of dementia, and wanted to improve their practice and offer good quality care for people with dementia and their care partners. The "agents of change" reported high levels of satisfaction with participating in the collaborative at the end of the project.

DOI: 10.4324/9781003109945-54

The case indicated three key lessons around selection, flexibility, and diversity

In this study, selection of "agents" is important. We found that the agent should have clinical responsibilities (i.e., be at the coalface) and have some level of seniority in the organization. For example, he or she may be employed as a senior clinician or team leader. An opt-in approach ensures that clinicians choose to become "agents of change" rather than being asked or told to take on this role.

Flexibility was also noted to be important. "Agents" will have different learning styles, and it is useful to offer a range of different tools and activities to account for this. It is perennially seen to be hard to find mutually convenient times for busy clinicians, so taking advantage of online learning and communication platforms enhances accessibility.

Another key learning is to allow and encourage diversity. Allied health professionals work across different settings with a wide range of client groups and have pluralist workplace cultures. Creating a learning environment where diversity is acknowledged offers the opportunity for different professionals to learn from each other.

In summary, identifying, supporting, and empowering "agents of change" are likely to be more acceptable and positively embraced by allied health professionals than efforts which attempt to restrict autonomy or control practice.

References

Cations, M., M. Crotty, J. A. Fitzgerald, S. Kurrle, I. D. Cameron, C. Whitehead, J. Thompson, B. Kaambwa, K. Hayes, L. de la Perrelle, G. Radisic, and K. E. Laver. 2018. "Agents of change: Establishing quality improvement collaboratives to improve adherence to Australian clinical guidelines for dementia care." *Implementation Science* 13 (1):123–123. doi: 10.1186/s13012-018-0820-z.

Sackett, D. L., W. M. Rosenberg, M. J. Gray, B. R. Haynes, and S. W. Richardson. 1996. "Evidence based medicine: What it is and what it isn't." *BMJ* 312 (7023):71–72. doi: 10.1136/bmj.312.7023.71.

51 Clinical decision support

David W. Bates

Clinical decision support (CDS) is used to make suggestions to clinicians about what they should do when providing care. It is in this book because CDS delivers much of the value from the electronic health record in terms of improving quality, safety, and value, but to get benefit from it, it is essential to do it well. Simply delivering decision support does not necessarily deliver any benefit.

The key issues in decision support can be divided into two broad areas, getting the content right, and getting the delivery correct. Both are essential for securing care improvement. The content refers to the rules and underlying knowledge base. This means, for example, for drug–drug interactions, which interactions result in an alert to a clinician. If they are routinely warned about unimportant interactions, they will ignore the warnings. The second relates to how the warnings are delivered – whether they follow human factors principles in terms of how they appear and whether they are integrated into the user workflow.

One summary of the principles involved comes from one of our publications, in which our group summarized what we had learned over years of delivering CDS (Bates et al. 2003). Most of these are very important from the implementation science perspective. For example, "speed is everything" relates to delivering quickly from the electronic perspective – this is a need. In addition, anticipating needs and fitting into workflow also relate closely to implementation science, which argues that whether something will be accepted is closely related to the extent to which it fits the user's needs.

Two of the key issues in implementing are monitor, get feedback, and respond and have a management and maintenance plan. With respect to monitoring, organizations should be tracking the rates alerts and reminders are going off and how providers are responding to them. If a reminder is being routinely ignored, it should be turned off. There should also be easy ability to deliver feedback in applications and from decision support screens, and all the feedback that comes in should be assessed. When bugs or real issues are identified, they should be addressed, ideally quickly.

There are other issues which are more "meta" in nature, for example, whether decision support should be tailored to the individual clinicians who use the system, like doctors, nurses, and pharmacists. While many users argue for this, our experience has been that it is better not to do this, at least for a core of decision support. Experts make the argument that they know their area so well that they no longer need decision support in it; the data on the other hand suggest (Nanji et al. 2018) that many errors are caused by physicians going too quickly and that even experts should be receiving suggestions in their area. For areas outside this core, organizations might want to allow individuals to turn off or on certain functions to enable acceptance. A more critical issue today, however, is that most systems are delivering far too many "false positive" warnings (Edrees et al. 2020, Nanji et al. 2018), and it is

DOI: 10.4324/9781003109945-55

incumbent on organizations to systematically minimize the number of these warnings to minimize alert fatigue.

Another area which is important for user acceptance is making it easy for the interested user to get to information about why individual suggestions are being given. This can be done by linking monographs to individual warnings, for example, or providing the details around calculations. Soon, artificial intelligence will regularly be used to make recommendations, and it is likely to be more challenging to explain the underpinnings of these suggestions, but it will be important to attempt to do so.

Overall, today, decision support is delivering a modest benefit in terms of the percent of patients who received desired care – some 5.8 per cent based on a recent meta-analysis, but this benefit could be much greater (Kwan et al. 2020). If implementation science techniques are routinely applied when it is being implemented, it will be.

References

Bates, D. W., G. J. Kuperman, S. Wang, T. Gandhi, A. Kittler, L. Volk, C. Spurr, R. Khorasani, M. Tanasijevic, and B. Middleton. 2003. "Ten commandments for effective clinical decision support: Making the practice of evidence-based medicine a reality." *Journal of the American Medical Informatics Association* 10 (6):523–530.

Edrees, H., M. G. Amato, A. Wong, D. L. Seger, and D. W. Bates. 2020. "High-priority drug-drug interaction clinical decision support overrides in a newly implemented commercial computerized provider order-entry system: Override appropriateness and adverse drug events." *Journal of the American Medical Informatics Association* 27 (6):893–900.

Kwan, J. L., L. Lo, J. Ferguson, H. Goldberg, J. P. Diaz-Martinez, G. Tomlinson, J. M. Grimshaw, and K. G. Shojania. 2020. "Computerised clinical decision support systems and absolute improvements in care: Meta-analysis of controlled clinical trials." *BMJ* 370.

Nanji, K. C., D. L. Seger, S. P. Slight, M. G. Amato, P. E. Beeler, Q. L. Her, O. Dalleur, T. Eguale, A. Wong, and E. R. Silvers. 2018. "Medication-related clinical decision support alert overrides in inpatients." *Journal of the American Medical Informatics Association* 25 (5):476–481.

52 Interprofessional team working

The case of care pathways

Kris Vanhaecht and Ellen Coeckelberghs

We often hear from healthcare professionals: "Of course we work as a team!" "Yes, we follow our guidelines." "Sure we are accredited." "Yes, there is a good atmosphere and culture." But do we really track our performance as a team and follow our guidelines, or is it wishful thinking?

Optimizing interprofessional team working is a complex intervention. It is both complex in terms of difficulty and complex as defined by the UK's Medical Research Council (MRC) (Moore et al. 2015). MRC defines complex as multicomponent interventions (Moore et al. 2015). One of the methods and pragmatic approaches to enhance collaboration within and between teams, by making the care process transparent and standardized, is the development, implementation, and evaluation of care pathways. Care pathways, also known as clinical pathways or critical pathways, were first introduced in healthcare in the late 1980s and are now used worldwide to standardize care processes and align the roles of the multidisciplinary team members (Pearson, Goulart-Fisher, and Lee 1995, Deneckere et al. 2013). Care pathways are defined as "a complex intervention for the mutual decision-making and organization of care processes for a well-defined group of patients during a well-defined period" (Vanhaecht et al. 2010, 118). The ultimate goal is to improve outcomes by providing a mechanism to better coordinate care and reduce fragmentation and ultimately costs (Panella, Marchisio, and Di 2003). Based on research of the European Pathway Association, we know that, although teams think that they provide optimal and standardized care, unwarranted variation within and between teams persists (van Zelm et al. 2017, Seys et al. 2017).

Pathways can have a positive impact on teamwork and the organization of care processes (Seys et al. 2019, Panella et al. 2012, Deneckere et al. 2013). Generalizing the results must be done with caution, as several "active components", for example, preoperative examinations, induce change at different levels of the organization and the team (Rotter et al. 2008, Vanhaecht, Ovretveit, et al. 2012). Translating the implementation strategy from one organization to another, with a different context, could be inappropriate. Both the context and the intervention should be described in detail as the result is more than the sum of the different "active components", and each "active component" should be reported (Van Zelm et al. 2019–12). These "active components" include information on evidence-based key interventions, information on organization and design of the actual care process, and the phase-by-phase approach to develop, implement, evaluate, and follow up the care pathway. The European Pathway Association developed and published a seven-phase method to develop, implement, evaluate, and continuously follow up this structured care methodology (see Figure 52.1) (Vanhaecht, Gerven, et al. 2012).

But care pathway development and implementation is more than just following these seven phases; it is a complex process that is continuously influenced by individuals, teams,

DOI: 10.4324/9781003109945-56

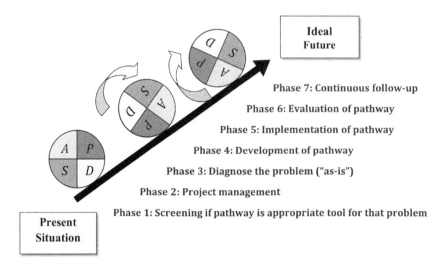

Figure 52.1 Care pathway, seven-phase development methodology (E-P-A.org)

Source: Author

organizations, and contexts. Van Zelm and colleagues analysed this challenge in an international multicentre study on pathways for colorectal surgery (Van Zelm et al. 2019–12). They found that the outcome of a pathway depends on a complex triad: 1) the perfect alignment of the intervention (e.g., the integration into daily management processes), 2) the implementation and use of the pathway (e.g., the fidelity to the key interventions and the continuous learning), and 3) the impact of the context (e.g., the internal and external incentives for standardization and optimal teamwork). A care pathway can only be successful when it introduces the appropriate "active components" in the appropriate social and cultural conditions (Vanhaecht, De Witte, and Sermeus 2007).

Care pathways are neither the Walhalla, nor the chicken with the golden eggs. But when team members are highly involved in the development, implementation, evaluation, and continuous follow-up, it gives them joy in work as it enhances their capacity to show their mastery and their purpose; they can have a positive influence on their autonomy and improve the relationships within their work environment (Vanhaecht 2020).

Acknowledgement: We thank Dr Deborah Seys, Prof Massimiliano Panella, Prof Dr Walter Sermeus, and Dr Ruben Van Zelm for their collaboration. Without their academic research, the content of this essay would not be available.

References

Deneckere, S., M. Euwema, C. Lodewijckx, M. Panella, T. Mutsvari, W. Sermeus, and K. Vanhaecht. 2013. "Better interprofessional teamwork, higher level of organized care, and lower risk of burnout in acute health care teams using care pathways: A cluster randomized controlled trial." *Medical Care* 51 (1):99–107. doi: 10.1097/MLR.0b013e3182763312.

Moore, G. F., S. Audrey, M. Barker, L. Bond, C. Bonell, W. Hardeman, L. Moore, A. O'Cathain, T. Tinati, D. Wight, and J. Baird. 2015. "Process evaluation of complex interventions: Medical Research Council guidance." *BMJ* 350:h1258. doi: 10.1136/bmj.h1258.

Panella, M., S. Marchisio, R. Brambilla, K. Vanhaecht, and F. Di Stanislao. 2012. "A cluster randomized trial to assess the effect of clinical pathways for patients with stroke: Results of the clinical pathways for effective and appropriate care study." *BMC Med* 10:71. doi: 10.1186/1741-7015-10-71.

Panella, M., S. Marchisio, and S. F. Di. 2003. "Reducing clinical variations with clinical pathways: Do pathways work?" *International Journal for Quality in Health Care* 15 (6):509–521.

Pearson, S. D., D. Goulart-Fisher, and T. H. Lee. 1995. "Critical pathways as a strategy for improving care: Problems and potential." *Annals of Internal Medicine* 123 (12):941–948. doi: 10.7326/0003-4819-123-12-199512150-00008.

Rotter, T., J. Kugler, R. Koch, H. Gothe, S. Twork, J. M. van Oostrum, and E. W. Steyerberg. 2008. "A systematic review and meta-analysis of the effects of clinical pathways on length of stay, hospital costs and patient outcomes." *BMC Health Services Research* 8:265. doi: 10.1186/1472-6963-8-265.

Seys, D., L. Bruyneel, M. Decramer, C. Lodewijckx, M. Panella, W. Sermeus, P. Boto, and K. Vanhaecht. 2017. "An international study of adherence to guidelines for patients hospitalised with a COPD exacerbation." *COPD* 14 (2):156–163. doi: 10.1080/15412555.2016.1257599.

Seys, D., S. Deneckere, C. Lodewijckx, L. Bruyneel, W. Sermeus, P. Boto, M. Panella, and K. Vanhaecht. 2019. "Impact of care pathway implementation on interprofessional teamwork: An international cluster randomized controlled trial." *Journal of Interprofessional Care*:1–9. doi: 10.1080/13561820.2019.1634016.

Vanhaecht, K., K. De Witte, and W. Sermeus. 2007. "The care process organisation triangle: A framework to better understand how clinical pathways work." *Journal of Integrated Care Pathways* 11:1–8.

Vanhaecht, K., E. V. Gerven, S. Deneckere, C. Lodewijckx, I. Janssen, R. V. Zelm, P. Boto, R. Mendes, M. Panella, E. Biringer, and W. Sermeus. 2012. "The 7-phase method to design, implement and evaluate care pathways." *The International Journal of Person Centered Medicine* 2 (3):341–351.

Vanhaecht, K., J. Ovretveit, M. J. Elliott, W. Sermeus, J. Ellershaw, and M. Panella. 2012. "Have we drawn the wrong conclusions about the value of care pathways? Is a Cochrane review appropriate?" *Evaluation & the Health Professions* 35 (1):28–42. doi: 10.1177/0163278711408293.

Vanhaecht, K., W. Sermeus, R. Van Zelm, and M. Panella. 2010. "An overview on the history and concept of care pathways as complex interventions." *International Journal of Care Pathways* 14 (3):31–31.

Vanhaecht, K., E. Van Bael, D. Seys, E. Coeckelberghs, C. Van der Auwera, E. M. Castro, and F. Decruynaere. 2020. *Mangomoment, a Small Act of Kindness & Leadership*. Leuven: ACCO. ISBN: 9789463440219.

van Zelm, R., E. Coeckelberghs, W. Sermeus, A. De Buck van Overstraeten, A. Weimann, D. Seys, M. Panella, and K. Vanhaecht. 2017. "Variation in care for surgical patients with colorectal cancer: Protocol adherence in 12 European hospitals." *International Journal of Colorectal Disease* 32 (10):1471–1478. doi: 10.1007/s00384-017-2863-z.

Van Zelm, Ruben, Walter Sermeus (Supervisor), Luk Bruyneel (Co supervisor), and Kris Vanhaecht (Co supervisor). 2019–12. *Understanding the Implementation of Care Pathways. Process Evaluation of the Implementation of an Evidence-Based Care Pathway for Colorectal Cancer Surgery in a Multicenter Setting*. Leuven, Belgium: KU Leuven.

53 Older people's care

Jackie Bridges

Just tell us what we need to be doing differently and we'll do it.

– Quote from a participant from fieldnotes

So said the emergency department (ED) clinical lead whom I was running an action research study with at the beginning of my research career. All were agreed that ED care for older people needed improvement, but the care failures weren't because staff didn't know better. In fact, the organization and delivery of care were expressions of a top-down organizational culture and a singular focus by managers on patient flow at the expense of supporting ED staff to deliver the support that older patients needed while they were in the department. As a result, staff felt highly stressed, under-resourced, and undervalued and unable to claim responsibility for the care of (often many) older people waiting in the ED corridors for a bed. These "trolley waits" and the efficiency of patient discharges or transfers to an in-patient bed had attracted close national government and media scrutiny. But sorting out patient flow was not an easy fix, and in the meantime, older people continued to wait in the corridors for an inpatient bed, sometimes for 24 hours, sometimes longer. Older patients in this transitory state received woeful medical and nursing care, worsening their conditions and their outcomes. As a "change agent", I found it a deeply unpleasant situation to work in, but, as set out below, focusing my efforts on training staff was not the answer.

This study was an important lesson for me in the influence of the context on the nature and delivery of care received by patients. Older people's care needs can be diverse and dynamic, requiring the provision of tailored care that can respond to individual needs and changes over time. This responsiveness is dependent not just on the skills, knowledge, and values of the healthcare worker at the point of care but also on a range of other factors that shape how the worker is able to act and the extent to which they can respond to what that individual patient needs in that moment. These factors centre on clinicians having the resources, authority, and flexibility to do what is required for an individual patient (Bridges, Pope, and Braithwaite 2019). Available resources are shaped by the extent to which wider society and hence policymakers value older people and the legitimacy of their healthcare needs. Taking a dynamic, ecological systems viewpoint encourages us to think about interventions as events in complex systems (Hawe, Shiell, and Riley 2009). Effective and sustainable interventions to improve care, therefore, identify and, where possible, harness or modify these conditions for action. Intervening to improve older people's care requires an analysis of the conditions in which staff at the point of care are able to act, and planning using a systems approach to optimize these conditions (Hawe, Shiell, and Riley 2009, Bridges et al. 2017). There are few

DOI: 10.4324/9781003109945-57

circumstances in which effective and lasting change will be achieved by merely telling staff at the point of care what care to deliver.

References

Bridges, J., C. R. May, A. Fuller, P. Griffiths, W. Wigley, L. Gould, H. Barker, and P. Libberton. 2017. "Optimising impact and sustainability: A qualitative process evaluation of a complex intervention targeted at compassionate care." *BMJ Quality & Safety* 26 (12):970–977.

Bridges, J., C. Pope, and J. Braithwaite. 2019. "Making health care responsive to the needs of older people." *Age and Ageing* 48 (6):785–788.

Hawe, P., A. Shiell, and T. Riley. 2009. "Theorising interventions as events in systems." *American Journal of Community Psychology* 43 (3–4):267–276.

54 Implementation interventions to enhance patient self-management

Michel Wensing

For planning the implementation of interventions to enhance patients' self-management, it is relevant to consider what these interventions are and what characteristics they have. From an implementation science perspective, the likelihood of implementation depends on characteristics such as the visibility of intervention effects and compatibility of interventions with prevailing ideas and practices. In addition, characteristics of the targeted users (patients) and mediators (healthcare professionals) and the organizational, physical, and cultural settings may influence the uptake of self-management support interventions. Barriers for implementation may be overcome by implementation strategies, such as information and education, engagement of patients, organizational change, financial incentives and resources, and regulatory changes.

Individualistic self-management interventions

Living with a chronic disease requires individuals' capacities to enact self-care and use healthcare, while the individuals are carrying on with their lives. A comprehensive review of qualitative research identified several types of activities, including rewriting of individual biographies and making meaningful lives in the face of chronic conditions, mobilization of resources for support, use of healthcare and self-care tasks, using individual social networks as social capital, and using the wider social environment for support (Boehmer et al. 2016). Despite the multifaceted character of self-management, it has frequently been conceptualized in terms of specific individual behaviours, such as taking medications and maintaining a healthy lifestyle, for which individuals need motivation and self-efficacy (Holman and Lorig 2004). Related interventions to support self-management comprise activities such as providing education, counselling, and training to individual patients. Depending on the available workforce and infrastructure, implementation may require additional training, resources, and infrastructure for health professionals and patients.

An example of this can be provided: take a randomized trial of individual counselling to enhance patients' self-management, which found changes in specific behaviours, such as clinical self-monitoring and elaboration of individual care plans, but no change in patient activation in engagement with disease (Eikelenboom et al. 2016). The intervention comprised personalized risk assessment, supported by a software tool, followed by counselling by trained nurses. It was likely that the implementation of this self-management support intervention was facilitated by the workforce and infrastructure of primary care (across the south of The Netherlands and locally), including the presence of trained nurses, routine use of information technology in patient care, a local support structure for practice organization, additional reimbursement by health insurers, collaboration with a commercial software

DOI: 10.4324/9781003109945-58

developer, and a local clinical opinion leader to push the implementation. These are personal assessments, because implementation was not formally evaluated. This seems typical for many studies of self-management support interventions. This poses challenges for the assessment of the transferability of interventions to other settings and target groups. Nevertheless, it seems unlikely that the described intervention could be implemented without strongly developed primary healthcare.

Alternative self-management support interventions

Some conceptualizations of self-management emphasize the role of social systems of support (Rogers et al. 2011). Associated interventions involved social networks and community support, for instance, through primary care or community organizations. Many self-management support interventions are currently delivered as information technology applications on smartphones or other devices. These alternative conceptualizations of self-management support may require different implementation strategies, such as changes in support networks or community organizations. A systematic review of studies (Harvey et al. 2015) categorized factors associated with the implementation of self-management interventions in terms of cost, morality, expectations of patients and healthcare professionals, individual motivations, and cultural ideas on learning and integration of new skills.

Need for theorizing

Much research on the implementation of self-management support interventions provides lists of factors associated with implementation, clustered in various domains. A major challenge of implementation science is to go beyond descriptive listing of factors and provide insight into the mechanisms of implementation. Focusing on telehealth interventions for self-management support specifically, a systematic review of research suggested three types of such mechanisms (Vassilev et al. 2015). First, these interventions can change relationships between patients and healthcare professionals (e.g., partially substitute them) and peers. Such changes influence the likely uptake of interventions. Second, telehealth interventions may fit well or less well into the everyday lives of people and their routines of healthcare use, resulting in various degrees of integration or disruption. Third, these interventions may or may not result in visible changes in knowledge, motivation, and sense of empowerment; engage network members; and provide monitoring and reinforcement of behaviours. The role of these concepts (relationships, fit, and visibility) needs testing and elaboration in future research on the implementation of self-management interventions.

Self-management support interventions fail to have impact if they are not effectively implemented into routine practice and embedded in individuals' lives. The implementation of these interventions in routine settings is an important area of implementation research.

References

Boehmer, K. R., M. R. Gionfriddo, R. Rodriguez-Gutierrez, A. L. Leppin, I. Hargraves, C. R. May, N. D. Shippee, A. Castaneda-Guarderas, C. Z. Palacios, and P. Bora. 2016. "Patient capacity and constraints in the experience of chronic disease: A qualitative systematic review and thematic synthesis." *BMC Family Practice* 17 (1):127.

Eikelenboom, N., J. van Lieshout, A. Jacobs, F. Verhulst, J. Lacroix, A. van Halteren, M. Klomp, I. Smeele, and M. Wensing. 2016. "Effectiveness of personalised support for self-management in primary care: A cluster randomised controlled trial." *British Journal of General Practice* 66 (646):e354–e361.

Harvey, J., S. Dopson, R. J. McManus, and J. Powell. 2015. "Factors influencing the adoption of self-management solutions: An interpretive synthesis of the literature on stakeholder experiences." *Implementation Science* 10 (1):159.

Holman, H., and K. Lorig. 2004. "Patient self-management: A key to effectiveness and efficiency in care of chronic disease." *Public Health Reports* 119 (3):239–243.

Rogers, A., I. Vassilev, C. Sanders, S. Kirk, C. Chew-Graham, A. Kennedy, J. Protheroe, P. Bower, C. Blickem, and D. Reeves. 2011. "Social networks, work and network-based resources for the management of long-term conditions: A framework and study protocol for developing self-care support." *Implementation Science* 6 (1):1–7.

Vassilev, I., A. Rowsell, C. Pope, A. Kennedy, A. O'Cathain, C. Salisbury, and A. Rogers. 2015. "Assessing the implementability of telehealth interventions for self-management support: A realist review." *Implementation Science* 10 (1):59.

55 Complex systems and unintended consequences

Robyn Clay-Williams

"[The road to] hell is paved with good intentions"

Henry G. Bohn, *A Handbook of Proverbs*, London, UK: 1855, p.10

Cane toads (Figure 55.1) were introduced into Australia from South America in 1935, to control a beetle that ate the sugarcane crops (Sutherst, Floyd, and Maywald 1996). The intervention not only failed to control the beetle but the cane toads were also large and poisonous and had no natural predators in Australia. The toad population spread invasively and now inhabits most of the Australian tropics and sub-tropics, reducing biodiversity and causing severe environmental impact (Shanmuganathan et al. 2010). What happened here? Those who introduced the cane toads did not consider interactions with other parts of the ecosystem or how that ecosystem would change over time (Urban et al. 2008). Unintended consequences, as in this example, are the outcomes of a purposeful action that are not foreseen.

Unintended consequences can be positive. In 1928, a messy Alexander Fleming returned to his laboratory after the holidays to find an unusual mould in one of his petri dishes. This "happy accident", the discovery of penicillin, was one of the most important medical findings of the twentieth century (Ligon 2004). The law of unintended [positive] consequences is a cornerstone of modern economics. An example is the trickle-down effect (Aghion and Bolton 1997) whereby reducing taxes and other financial burdens will allow businesses to flourish, increasing jobs and other investments. These advantages will "trickle down" to benefit the rest of society. While the validity of the trickle-down effect is highly debatable (Arndt 1983), we are usually delighted to accept any unexpected positive consequences of our actions.

We are less enamoured with consequences of the negative variety. We typically bring a positive intent to designing a change or improvement, and it is natural to focus on the change we are trying to make to the exclusion of peripheral concerns. Like figure and ground in a painting, however, where it is the ground that shapes the image (Figure 55.2), the context of the intervention can be critical, and often what we are *not* focusing on can have a great effect on the outcomes.

While nothing exists in isolation, and there are consequential effects in everything we do, often rippling out from the original action, some outcomes can be anticipated if a system view is adopted. Often, unexpected outcomes result from a mismatch between Work-as-Imagined (WAI) and Work-as-Done (WAD; refer to Essay 48), where the change has been designed with WAI in mind. Unintended consequences are more likely as system complexity increases, however, and these may be less predictable, as outcomes can be emergent and seemingly unrelated to action or input.

Health systems are dynamic, and it is important to recognize that consequences may be immediate, or delayed, as further flow on effects comes into play. Impacts on safety culture in healthcare organizations, for example, can sometimes take many years to be felt

DOI: 10.4324/9781003109945-59

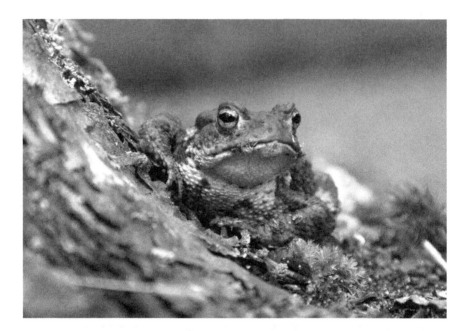

Figure 55.1 Cane toad
Source: Reprinted from Pexels

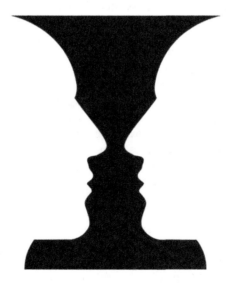

Figure 55.2 Figure and ground – a vase or two faces?
Source: Reprinted from Pexels

(Clay-Williams 2013). Unintended consequences may also be *noticed* now or not noticed until later. Having resilient systems in place, such as a capability for anticipating and monitoring (Hollnagel 2009), may enable countermeasures to be deployed early and thereby mitigate these effects. For example, during the COVID-19 pandemic in Australia, sewage systems were monitored for presence of the virus (Ahmed et al. 2020). This enabled small outbreaks to be detected early, and the source pinpointed to specific suburbs. Residents in those suburbs were then targeted through government messaging and encouraged to seek a test even if suffering only mild symptoms. This system of monitoring and anticipating may have contributed to the ability to curb outbreaks quickly and to the low overall incidence of COVID-19 in Australia in the latter half of 2020.

A system approach to the problem provides the best chance of characterizing (and thereby preventing) unintended consequences. Considering the whole picture, rather than just the "figure" or the "ground", designing an intervention or implementing change will help to protect us from introducing healthcare "cane toads" in our efforts to improve patient care.

References

Aghion, P., and P. Bolton. 1997. "A theory of trickle-down growth and development." *The Review of Economic Studies* 64 (2):151–172.

Ahmed, W., N. Angel, J. Edson, K. Bibby, A. Bivins, J. W. O'Brien, P. M. Choi, M. Kitajima, S. L. Simpson, and J. Li. 2020. "First confirmed detection of SARS-CoV-2 in untreated wastewater in Australia: A proof of concept for the wastewater surveillance of COVID-19 in the community." *Science of the Total Environment* 728:138764.

Arndt, H. W. 1983. "The 'trickle-down' myth." *Economic Development and Cultural Change* 32 (1):1–10.

Clay-Williams, R. 2013. "Restructuring and the resilient organisation: Implications for health care." In *Resilient Health Care*, edited by E. Hollnagel, J. Braithwaite and R. Wears. Surrey, UK: Ashgate Publishing Limited.

Hollnagel, E. 2009. "The four cornerstones of resilience engineering." In *Resilience Engineering Perspectives: Preparation and Restoration*, edited by C. P. Nemeth, E. Hollnagel and S. Dekker, 117–133. Surrey, UK: Ashgate Publishing Limited.

Ligon, B. L. 2004. "Penicillin: Its discovery and early development." Seminars in pediatric infectious diseases.

Shanmuganathan, T., J. Pallister, S. Doody, H. McCallum, T. Robinson, A. Sheppard, C. Hardy, D. Halliday, D. Venables, and R. Voysey. 2010. "Biological control of the cane toad in Australia: A review." *Animal Conservation* 13:16–23.

Sutherst, R. W., R. B. Floyd, and G. F. Maywald. 1996. "The potential geographical distribution of the cane toad, Bufo marinus L. in Australia." *Conservation Biology* 10 (1):294–299.

Urban, M. C., B. L. Phillips, D. K. Skelly, and R. Shine. 2008. "A toad more traveled: The heterogeneous invasion dynamics of cane toads in Australia." *The American Naturalist* 171 (3):E134–E148.

56 The nature and need for slack in healthcare services

Tarcisio A. Saurin

Slack is a cushion of actual or potential resources which allows an organization to adapt successfully to internal or external pressures (Bourgeois III 1981), contributing to the reduction of interdependencies and slowing down the propagation of variability (Safayeni and Purdy 1991). In turn, variability is the range of values or outcomes around the average, as well as all possible results of a given outcome (Story 2010). For example, medications may not be administered at the exact prescribed dosage and time on every occasion, and not all patients respond the same way to the same treatment. Occasionally, slack can also be useful to exploit opportunities arising from variability – for example, a surge in the demand for new treatments. Furthermore, slack is widely regarded as an asset for innovation, as it allows a forgiving environment for trial and error through experimentation (Kim et al. 2017).

Healthcare services offer plenty of examples of slack. An everyday instance refers to professionals on standby in emergency departments (EDs). In fact, EDs as a whole play a role as slack as they shield other hospital's units, such as in-patient wards and intensive care units (ICUs), from variations in demand from the external environment. The COVID-19 pandemic made the need for slack in healthcare services dramatically visible (Saurin 2021). From the perspective of built-in slack, the need for extra ICU capacity and extra supplies stands out. In turn, examples of opportunistic slack (i.e., repurposing and reallocation of resources) abound in the pandemic, such as the adaptation of factories to the production of hand sanitizer and respiratory ventilators, the use of hotel rooms for quarantining international travellers, and the installation of makeshift hospitals. Opportunistic slack also resulted from the mixed effects of the pandemic in the occupation of healthcare facilities, as demand for some services plummeted – for example, suspended elective surgeries freed up operating rooms. Thus, space and staff were reallocated to meet demands from COVID-19 patients. The pandemic also made it clear that slack is finite and that its provision must go hand-in-hand with the control of variability propagation – this lies at the heart of the widely discussed need for flattening the curve of infections and hospitalizations.

Slack also has drawbacks. First, slack formed by resources such as staff, equipment, and materials adds elements and therefore complexity to systems. This poses the risk of unintended consequences – for example, there may be complacency with hazards due to an over-reliance on redundancies. Second, there is a possibility that slack grows disorderly over time, to the point of being randomly distributed across the system, and thus not matching the variabilities (Saurin and Werle 2017).

Third, slack implies a cost, thus creating the problem of balancing costs against benefits. Too much slack can equate to waste, which corresponds to the use of more resources than what would be reasonably accepted to produce a desired outcome (Shingo 1981). Too little slack can make the system vulnerable even to everyday variability. Figure 56.1 represents

DOI: 10.4324/9781003109945-60

the range of possibilities involving the relationship between slack and their benefits. Benefits are conveyed in terms of resilient performance, which is the "ability of healthcare services to adjust their functioning prior to, during, or following changes and disturbances, so that they can sustain required performance under both expected and unexpected conditions" (2013). The inverted U-curve suggests that an optimal amount of slack is most beneficial. Based on Perrow (2011), it is hypothesized that slack in tightly coupled[1] systems is mostly built-in and offline (e.g., spare haemodialysis machine, to which there may be no other realistic alternative), while slack in loosely coupled[2] systems is mostly opportunistic and intrinsic to the system nature (e.g., nursing staff helping each other to mobilize a patient in a ward).

Despite these insights, Figure 56.1 is an oversimplification as it conveys resilient performance as a function only of the amount of slack. There may be situations where that amount is appropriate, but resilience is still low. Saurin and Ferreira (Saurin and Ferreira 2021) report one such situation in a hospital's pharmacy, in which physicians could order drugs at any time (i.e., out of the predefined window of time for regular orders) if the request was tagged as urgent. However, urgent ordering of drugs occurred in almost 40 per cent of cases rather than as a last resort, implying undesired safety and efficiency implications. In this case, the amount of slack, at least in terms of time, was reasonable. Shortcomings could be elsewhere, such as physicians' lack of awareness of the unintended consequences of their actions.

In addition, Figure 56.1 begs the question of how to determine the optimal amount of slack. This is essentially a matter of risk assessment and risk tolerance, therefore requiring the consideration of the likelihood and severity of known variabilities. These two criteria are associated with certain anticipated risk scenarios, which vary according to contextual factors and time horizon and, of course, according to the imagination of the analysts. Based on risk assessments, built-in slack might be defined and have its costs assessed. Depending on the nature of the slack, its amount can be determined more or less objectively and, in many instances, constrained by regulatory requirements (e.g., number of staff on duty in an ED). However, despite systematic approaches for defining the amount of slack, non-technical factors are likely to play a role on that decision-making. For example, political pressures and bargaining power of some social groups may be decisive for defining what counts as necessary slack and what counts as waste. In fact, the process of providing and adjusting slack is never ending in health services, as variabilities are ever changing, and new or revised forms of slack emerge from technological advancements and creative solutions from professionals.

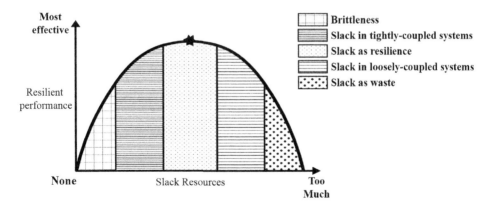

Figure 56.1 Relationship between slack and resilient performance
Source: Created by author

Notes

1 Tightly coupled systems have more time-dependent processes; they cannot wait or stand by until attended to. Sequences are more invariant (Perrow 1984).
2 In loosely coupled systems, expedient, spur-of-the-moment redundancies and substitutions can be found, even though they were not planned ahead of time.

References

Bourgeois III, L. J. 1981. "On the measurement of organizational slack." *Academy of Management Review* 6 (1):29–39. Hollnagel, E., Braithwaite, J, and Wears, R. 2013. *Resilient Health Care*. Surrey, UK: Ashgate.

Hollnagel, E., Braithwaite, J, and Wears, R. 2013. *Resilient Health Care*. Surrey, UK: Ashgate.

Kim, B.-N., N. S. Lee, J.-H. Wi, and J.-K. Lee. 2017. "The effects of slack resources on firm performance and innovation in the Korean pharmaceutical industry." *Asian Journal of Technology Innovation* 25 (3):387–406.

Perrow, C. 2011. *Normal Accidents: Living with High Risk Technologies-Updated edition*. Princeton, NJ: Princeton University Press.

Safayeni, F., and L. Purdy. 1991. "A behavioral case study of just-in-time implementation." *Journal of Operations Management* 10 (2):213–228.

Saurin, T. A. F. 2021. "A complexity thinking account of the COVID-19 pandemic: Implications for systems-oriented safety management." *Safety Science* 134:105087.

Saurin, T. A. F., and D. M. C. Ferreira. 2021. "Slack resources in healthcare systems: Resilience or waste?" In *Transforming Healthcare with Qualitative Research*, edited by F. Braithwaite and J. Rapport. Oxon: Routledge.

Saurin, T. A. F., and N. J. B. Werle. 2017. "A framework for the analysis of slack in socio-technical systems." *Reliability Engineering and System Safety* 167:439–451.

Shingo, S. 1981. "Study of Toyota Production System from Industrial Engineering View-Point, 'Japan Management Association'." *Business & Economics*.

Story, P. 2010. *Dynamic Capacity Management for Healthcare: Advanced Methods and Tools for Optimization*. New York: CRC Press.

57 Diagnosis errors

Gordon D. Schiff

Diagnosis. Is it a noun (a label applied to a disease) or a verb (the process of providing an explanation for a patient's problem)? Although both, we need instead to conceptualize diagnosis as a system (Schiff 2014). Not fixed labels, not cognitive wizardry, but a set of structural conditions and constraints that facilitate or hinder making accurate and timely diagnoses of patients' medical problems. Seen through this lens, diagnostic errors are less random events or variations in clinician skills and carefulness and more predictable consequences of system design and flaws.

Of Avedis Donabedian's model, the classical structure-process-outcome triad model (Donabedian 2002), when it comes to diagnosis quality, the least attention has been paid to structure. Although quality metrics for all aspects of the diagnostic process are underdeveloped (Balogh, Miller, and Ball 2015), most attention has been focused on outcomes (measuring rates of missed/delayed diagnoses) or processes (ordering the correct test, cognitive biases). What are structural elements of high-quality diagnosis? While these will require considerable additional future research and evidence to define and validate, we can reasonably postulate that diagnostic errors can be minimized with markedly better systems needed to transform our current ad hoc, poorly designed systems in the following areas:

Adequate time. Flexibly calibrated to the type of diagnostic problem, patient factors, communication conditions (language, health literacy), support staff, and work conditions (that include a number of factors below). Given growing "production pressures" on clinicians to see and help as many patients as possible, realistic time allocation is a prerequisite for avoiding diagnostic errors.

Informatics infrastructure. Which nowadays necessarily means computer interfaces, workflows, and information availability. Being able to quickly and easily access patients' prior records (notes, test results) and online resources (articles, textbooks, websites) means the clinician is not relying on memory or instinct to recall and easily integrate key pieces of information.

Diagnostic safety culture. A particular set of qualities derivative from generic overall patient safety culture. These include 1) patient and staff comfort in speaking up to question diagnoses that seem to be or become questionable (based on patient's course over time, lack of excepted response to treatment), 2) a supportive non-punitive environment for learning about and from diagnostic errors, 3) respect for human limitations, and 4) deep appreciation of the bedeviling role of hindsight bias (tempering retrospective conclusions "that the diagnosis should have been obvious"). A new, barely explored element of diagnosis safety culture is understanding and application

DOI: 10.4324/9781003109945-61

of conservative diagnosis principles (Schiff et al. 2018) to balance underdiagnosis with overdiagnosis.

Situational awareness. A set of signals, cues, and forcing functions to alert clinicians about potential key diagnostic considerations (most likely diagnoses; "don't miss" diagnoses) and potential mis-steps (diagnostic pitfalls) (Schiff In Press). This applies a general resilience principle to clinical diagnosis and points to the need to worry about and recognize so-called red flags that may be clues to critical or alternate diagnoses.

Safety nets. Along with an awareness that diagnosis is an inherently uncertain endeavour comes the need to create safety nets to monitor patients' symptoms, test results, and referrals in a "closed-loop" fashion. Thus, there need to be systems to ensure that things do not fall through the cracks and patients are reassessed when symptoms evolve or fail to respond as expected. Since designing and implementing such closed-loop systems can entail enormous manual efforts (e.g., ensuring that abnormal tests are followed up, or calling patients to track whether their symptoms have improved or worsened), we need to develop automated systems to support these tasks. Such hard-wired follow-up and feedback are important for both the patient's safety to minimize and mitigate errors and delays, as well as for providing feedback to clinicians and organizations for learning and improvement.

These five intersecting elements are bound together with the glue of trusting, continuous, caring relationships; many diagnostic errors are rooted in their absence. Thus, diagnosis needs to be co-produced by clinicians working with empowered patients in well-designed, reliable system to reduce errors and improve care.

References

Balogh, E. P., B. T. Miller, and J. R. Ball. 2015. *Improving Diagnosis in Health Care*. Washington, DC: National Academies Press (US).

Donabedian, A. 2002. *An Introduction to Quality Assurance in Health Care*. Oxford: Oxford University Press.

Schiff, G. D. 2014. "Diagnosis and diagnostic errors: Time for a new paradigm." *BMJ Quality & Safety* 23 (1):1–3. doi: 10.1136/bmjqs-2013-002426. Epub 2013 Sep 19. PMID: 24050984.

Schiff, G. D. 2021. "Diagnosis: Reducing errors and improving quality." In *Harrison's Principles of Internal Medicine 21e*. McGraw-Hill. https://accessmedicine.mhmedical.com/content.aspx?bookid=3095&sectionid=261486991.

Schiff, G. D., S. A. Martin, D. H. Eidelman, L. A. Volk, E. Ruan, C. Cassel, W. Galanter, M. Johnson, A. Jutel, and K. Kroenke. 2018. "Ten principles for more conservative, care-full diagnosis." *Annals of Internal Medicine* 169 (9):643–645.

58 "Scaling-out" evidence-based practices

Marisa Sklar and Gregory A. Aarons

Introduction/background

Widespread implementation and sustainment of evidence-based practices (EBPs) have been difficult to achieve across a variety of contexts and interventions. Even when there is empirical support for an intervention, only a small minority of these EBPs reach full implementation. Balas and Boren (Balas and Boren 2000) reported an average of 17 years for research evidence to move into clinical practice; furthermore, this paper illustrates how only approximately 14.4 per cent of research results in implementation over the course of approximately 15–22 years. Implementation science aims to reduce this well-documented research-to-practice gap by expanding the use of EBPs with fidelity appropriately and as broadly as feasible to maximize public health impact (Department of Health and Human Services 2017).

In this essay, we describe "scaling-out", a strategy for accelerating and expanding the benefit of EBPs through innovative study designs. When an EBP is implemented with fidelity in a setting that is identical to, or very similar to, where it was previously tested and found to be effective, one can anticipate that the EBP would result in similar benefit. However, every EBP implementation raises at least two critical questions: 1) is there sufficient empirical evidence or justification from prior evidence that this EBP would impact health as expected? 2) Are system, organization, and/or EBP adaptations necessary, sufficient, and culturally and organizationally appropriate to make it feasible, practical, and acceptable in the new context? Scaling-out proposes that when EBPs are implemented in health or service delivery systems, or with population/community contexts that are moderately different from the setting wherein the EBP was originally tested, a shorter time frame for moving from research to practice is possible by "borrowing strength" from evidence of impact in prior effectiveness trials.

What is "scaling-out"?

Scaling-out is the "deliberate use of strategies to implement, test, improve, and sustain EBPs as they are delivered in novel circumstances distinct from, though closely related to, previous implementations" (Aarons et al. 2017). The motivating questions when scaling-out are whether similar effects as found in previous studies can be expected and what additional empirical evaluations would be necessary to test for this without going so far as an entirely new effectiveness trial. If testing of this new scale-out requires the full empirical evaluation that would be required for establishing an EBP, this would be exceptionally costly, time-consuming, and would delay implementation, especially to populations underrepresented in scientific trials or in settings where its delivery could reasonably produce benefit. If we can

DOI: 10.4324/9781003109945-62

legitimately borrow strength from previous studies, and combine these data with a modest amount of additional empirical evidence, this could improve efficiency and lower costs while accelerating and expanding benefits of the EBP.

Types of scaling-out

Three distinct types of scaling-out have been proposed and are identified by whether or not the population and/or delivery system within which the EBP is to be implemented remains the same as prior trials that have established the evidence for that EBP. These three types of scaling-out differ from a typical scaling-up approach. In a traditional scaling-up approach, an EBP designed for one setting is expanded to other health delivery units within the same or very similar settings under which it has been tested. For example, scaling-up approaches are often used to expand the number of intervention recipients with an expanded number of service delivery organizations. A beneficial impact when scaling-up is expected because a nearly identical intervention is delivered in the same way to a similar population. When scaling-up, there is a heavy reliance on previous tests of effectiveness, and consequently, evaluation of implementation outcomes may be prioritized over that of clinical outcomes. In contrast, scaling-out approaches aim to implement EBPs to novel populations and/or delivery systems. There is more concern about the impact on effectiveness during scaling-out. There is more uncertainty whether the empirically supported clinical outcomes of the intervention will hold when adapted and tested under yet-unstudied conditions. As such, with scaling-out, we are unable to completely rely on findings of previous studies. Rather, evaluation of additional empiral evidence is necessary.

Scaling-out Type I

The first scaling-out variant, Type I: population fixed, different delivery system, involves targeting the same population as previously tested but through a different delivery system. This type of scaling-out pursues an alternative avenue to reach its target population. An example of Type I scaling-out involves the delivery of the "Familias Unidas" intervention, a parenting program for Hispanic families with young adolescents, which was originally designed and tested for delivery in middle schools (Pantin et al. 2009, Prado et al. 2010, 2012). With policy mechanisms such as the US Patient Protection and Affordable Care Act (Patient Protection and Affordable Care Act of 2010 2011) expanding access to healthcare in the United States, opportunity presented for engaging this population in the "Familias Unidas" intervention through the primary care system (Prado et al. 2019). As such, healthcare system changes may provide opportunity for scaling-out Type I.

Scaling-out Type II

The second type of scaling-out, Type II: delivery system fixed, different population, involves targeting a different population than previously tested but through the same delivery system. When implementing an EBP to a novel population through the same delivery system, the core elements of the EBP to retain, and the elements of the EBP to adapt for this novel population, must be determined. A large literature exists on cultural adaptation of EBPs, and many of these are examples of Type II scaling-out as the EBP is implemented in the same delivery system as originally tested. An example of Type II scaling-out is the adaptation of SafeCare (Hurlburt et al. 2014) for Spanish-speaking immigrant families from Mexico

(Finno-Velasquez et al. 2014). SafeCare is an EBP widely used in child welfare services with demonstrated improvements in parental management of children's health, increased home safety, and more positive and sensitive parent–child interactions (Bigelow and Lutzker 1998, Chaffin et al. 2012, Gershater-Molko, Lutzker, and Wesch 2003, Lutzker et al. 1998). In tailoring SafeCare for delivery to this novel population through the child welfare system, adaptation to materials, content, training goals, and program structure was made while retaining the core elements of the SafeCare intervention.

Scaling-out Type III

The final variant of scaling-out, Type III: different population and delivery system, involves targeting a different population, through a different delivery system, as compared to the original EBP trial. An example of this type of scaling-out is evident when attempting to expand access to behavioural health services to primary care patients through integrated primary care settings. One innovative approach for integrated primary care is the Patient-Centered Medical Home (PCMH) (Jones et al. 2015, Robert Graham Center 2007). Individuals with behavioural healthcare needs often present in primary care, though historically these behavioural healthcare needs would go unnoticed and/or untreated in the primary care setting as physical healthcare needs were prioritized. Integrating behavioural and physical healthcare through the PCMH model is an optimal way of addressing such mental health concerns in primary care patients through emphasizing improved care access and comprehensive, coordinated care and often via warm handoff wherein physicians refer patients to on-site behavioural healthcare service professionals by means of a personal introduction (Pace et al. 2018).

Implications

Scaling-out offers a strategy for improving efficiency, reducing costs, and achieving more widespread implementation of EBPs while assessing and testing implementation determinants and mechanisms and their effect on outcomes. It offers an approach to improve the efficiency of translating an EBP from one setting to another and/or from one population to another. When scaling-out an EBP, it may be possible to borrow strength from evidence of impact in prior effectiveness trials. Supplementation of this evidence with additional empirical data when scaling-out to a novel setting and/or population is determined by the extent to which the novel setting and/or population differ from the prior effectiveness trial. In the Type III variant of scaling-out, wherein both the delivery system and population differ from that of the original effectiveness trial, the demand for new empirical evidence is greater than that for Type I or Type II scaling-out variants, wherein only the delivery system or population varies from the original trial. While at the heart of the scale-out approach is borrowing strength through the use of mediational modelling, the creation and explication of statistical methods for scaling-out remain in development (Aarons et al. 2017).

References

Aarons, G. A., M. Sklar, B. Mustanski, N. Benbow, and C. H. Brown. 2017. "'Scaling-out' evidence-based interventions to new populations or new health care delivery systems." *Implementation Science* 12 (1):111.

Balas, E. A., and S. A. Boren. 2000. "Managing clinical knowledge for health care improvement." *Yearbook of Medical Informatics*:65–70.

Bigelow, K. M., and J. R. Lutzker. 1998. "Using video to teach planned activities to parents reported for child abuse." *Child & Family Behavior Therapy* 20 (4):1–14.

Chaffin, M., D. Hecht, D. Bard, J. F. Silovsky, and W. H. Beasley. 2012. "A statewide trial of the SafeCare home-based services model with parents in Child Protective Services." *Pediatrics* 129 (3):509–515.

Department of Health and Human Services. 2017. *Dissemination and Implementation Research in Health (R01) NIH Funding Opportunity: PAR-16-238.* Edited by NIH Funding Opportunities. https://grants.nih.gov/grants/guide/pa-files/par-16-238.html.

Finno-Velasquez, M., D. L. Fettes, G. A. Aarons, and M. S. Hurlburt. 2014. "Cultural adaptation of an evidence-based home visitation programme: Latino clients' experiences of service delivery during implementation." *Journal of Children's Services* 9 (4):280–294.

Gershater-Molko, R. M., J. R. Lutzker, and D. Wesch. 2003. "Project SafeCare: Improving health, safety, and parenting skills in families reported for, and at-risk for child maltreatment." *Journal of Family Violence* 18 (6):377–386.

Hurlburt, M., G. A. Aarons, D. Fettes, C. Willging, L. Gunderson, and M. J. Chaffin. 2014. "Interagency collaborative team model for capacity building to scale-up evidence-based practice." *Children and Youth Services Review* 39:160–168.

Jones, A. L., S. D. Cochran, A. Leibowitz, K. B. Wells, G. Kominski, and V. M. Mays. 2015. "Usual primary care provider characteristics of a patient-centered medical home and mental health service use." *Journal of General Internal Medicine* 30 (12):1828–1836.

Lutzker, J. R., K. M. Bigelow, R. M. Doctor, and M. L. Kessler. 1998. "Safety, health care, and bonding within an ecobehavioral approach to treating and preventing child abuse and neglect." *Journal of Family Violence* 13 (2):163–185.

Pace, C. A., K. Gergen-Barnett, A. Veidis, J. D'Afflitti, J. Worcester, P. Fernandez, and K. E. Lasser. 2018. "Warm handoffs and attendance at initial integrated behavioral health appointments." *The Annals of Family Medicine* 16 (4):346–348.

Pantin, H., G. Prado, B. Lopez, S. Huang, M. I. Tapia, S. J. Schwartz, E. Sabillon, C. H. Brown, and J. Branchini. 2009. "A randomized controlled trial of Familias Unidas for Hispanic adolescents with behavior problems." *Psychosomatic Medicine* 71 (9):987.

Patient Protection and Affordable Care Act of 2010.2011. Pub. L. No. 111–148, 124 Stat. 119 (2010).

Prado, G., Y. Estrada, L. M. Rojas, M. Bahamon, H. Pantin, M. Nagarsheth, L. Gwynn, A. Y. Ofir, L. Q. Forster, and N. Torres. 2019. "Rationale and design for eHealth Familias Unidas Primary Care: A drug use, sexual risk behavior, and STI preventive intervention for Hispanic youth in pediatric primary care clinics." *Contemporary Clinical Trials* 76:64–71.

Prado, G., S. Huang, M. Maldonado-Molina, F. Bandiera, S. J. Schwartz, P. de la Vega, C. Hendricks Brown, and H. Pantin. 2010. "An empirical test of ecodevelopmental theory in predicting HIV risk behaviors among Hispanic youth." *Health Education & Behavior* 37 (1):97–114.

Prado, G., H. Pantin, S. Huang, D. Cordova, M. I. Tapia, M.-R. Velazquez, M. Calfee, S. Malcolm, M. Arzon, and J. Villamar. 2012. "Effects of a family intervention in reducing HIV risk behaviors among high-risk Hispanic adolescents: A randomized controlled trial." *Archives of Pediatrics & Adolescent Medicine* 166 (2):127–133.

Robert Graham Center. 2007. *The Patient Centered Medical Home: History, Seven Core Features, Evidence and Transformational Change.* Washington, DC: Robert Graham Center.

59 Implementation sustainability

Sharon E. Straus

While initiating behaviour change is challenging, sustaining it is even more so, as those who have tried to sustain an exercise or weight loss program can attest. Similarly, despite initial implementation success, we can see a return to old practices as attention turns to the next evidence-based intervention (Straus, Tetroe, and Graham 2013).

Why is sustainability important?

Failure to sustain a successful intervention, even if it has a small beneficial effect, can have substantial long-term adverse impact (Straus, Tetroe, and Graham 2013). Failed sustainability has implications for cost and patient care and diminishes trust and support for future implementation efforts. Specifically, if an implementation scientist walks away from an implementation project without considering sustainability, the stakeholders involved with implementation may be reluctant to engage in future implementation projects. Indeed, sustainability was identified one of the most significant implementation problems of our time (Proctor et al. 2015), and our failure to address it threatens healthcare globally and leads to research waste (Chalmers and Glasziou 2009, Glasziou et al. 2017).

What is sustainability?

What is it that we are trying to sustain? Are we sustaining the clinical intervention or program? The implementation strategy? The outcome? In addition, how do we balance sustainability with the need to adapt interventions to the changing healthcare context? Not surprisingly, given all of these questions, Proctor and colleagues reported a lack of a consistent definition for sustainability in implementation science (Proctor et al. 2015). In response to this gap, we conducted a review and concept mapping exercise to define sustainability (Moore et al. 2017). While other definitions exist (Proctor et al. 2015), we defined sustainability as:

- After a defined period of time, the clinical/program and implementation interventions continue to be delivered.
- Clinician, patient, public, organization behaviour change is maintained.
- Clinical and implementation interventions may adapt while continuing to produce benefits (Moore et al. 2017).

DOI: 10.4324/9781003109945-63

Is sustainability considered in implementation science and practice?

Several systematic reviews addressed implementation sustainability (Tricco et al. 2015, Hailemariam et al. 2019, Francis, Dunt, and Cadilhac 2016, Shelton, Cooper, and Stirman 2018). Together, these reviews identified that few studies used a theory, model, or framework to inform their work (Tricco et al. 2015); of those studies that did evaluate sustainability, most reported on implementation process outcomes rather than evidence-based intervention outcomes (Hailemariam et al. 2019), most studies assessed sustainability at a single time point (Francis, Dunt, and Cadilhac 2016), and few described specific sustainability strategies. A systematic review of sustainability approaches explored those studies that considered sustainability prospectively versus those that used a retrospective approach (Lennox, Maher, and Reed 2018). Prospective approaches focused on building relationships and stakeholder buy-in and highlighted intervention adaptation; moreover, these efforts focused on building the initiative into the organization from its conception. It is more likely that these prospective approaches increase the potential for sustainability because of stakeholder buy-in and the opportunity to embed the initiative into the organization or system (Lennox, Maher, and Reed 2018). In contrast, retrospective approaches to sustainability tended to focus on identifying ongoing funding for the initiative (Lennox, Maher, and Reed 2018).

What factors influence sustainability?

Developing a sustainability plan requires consideration of the factors that influence it (Moore et al. 2017); these factors can be at the level of the intervention (clinical/program and implementation), the implementation team, the implementation setting, and the system. Some specific considerations for each of these are provided in Box 59.1. Reflecting on these factors helps us to understand and assess the sustainability context. This understanding can then lead to development of sustainability strategies, which we need to implement and monitor over time.

Critical to this process is the need to use an intersectionality lens when doing any implementation work, including sustainability (Etherington et al. 2020). Individuals simultaneously occupy intersecting social categories (e.g., sex, gender, ethnicity, age), which in turn interact with systems and power structures (e.g., healthcare system) (Crenshaw 1990, McCall 2005, Hankivsky et al. 2014). Intersectionality provides a way to situate individual behaviours within the larger context and acknowledges the intersections and interactions that characterize lived experiences and influence behaviour change (Hankivsky et al. 2014). Without attention to these intersectional factors, implementation will likely not realize its full potential for sustainability given increasing evidence of how social-structural considerations influence social care, healthcare, and public health.

Box 59.1   Factors influencing sustainability (Proctor et al. 2015, Moore et al. 2017, Hailemariam et al. 2019)

Factors influencing sustainability at the clinical/program intervention *and* implementation interventions include the following:

- What is the effectiveness of the intervention(s)?
- How can we adapt the intervention(s)?

- How easy is it to evaluate the intervention(s)?
- How accessible are the intervention(s)?

Factors influencing sustainability at the implementation team level include the following:

- Are frontline stakeholders engaged?
- Is there openness across the team to sustain change?
- What training and coaching are required by the implementation team?
- What interdisciplinary collaborations are required on the team?
- What is the incentive for team members (e.g., frontline clinicians, policymakers) to participate in implementation and sustainability?

Factors influencing sustainability at the implementation setting/organization level include the following:

- What are the organization's characteristics that may affect sustainability?
- What is the culture for monitoring and evaluation?
- Is the leadership supportive of sustainability?
- What funding is available for sustainability?

Factors influencing sustainability at the system level include the following:

- What are the characteristics of the health, education, and social systems that may affect sustainability?
- Are there networks across organizations that may influence sustainability?
- What economic factors may influence sustainability?
- What are the population characteristics that may influence sustainability?

What implementation theories/models/frameworks consider sustainability?

Several theories/models/frameworks could be used to inform sustainability (Strifler et al. 2018), including those that consider implementation from knowledge creation through to its implementation and sustainability (e.g., Knowledge Action Cycle (Graham et al. 2006)). Similarly, there are theories/models/frameworks that focus exclusively on sustainability such as the Dynamic Sustainability Framework (Chambers, Glasgow, and Stange 2013). There is no evidence to provide guidance on how to select one for use.

What are the research gaps in implementation sustainability?

Implementation sustainability is in its infancy, and there are many research gaps that can be tackled; while not an exhaustive list, a few examples are provided here. First, we need to identify determinants of implementation intervention sustainability across settings and time. Second, we need to understand how to adapt interventions (both the evidence-based intervention and the implementation intervention) over time and what the impact of adaptation is on relevant outcomes. Third, we need to determine the return on investment of implementation intervention sustainability over different periods and stakeholder perspectives. Fourth, we should leverage existing and planned projects across settings and countries to create a platform for studying sustainability. Fifth, how artificial intelligence can be used to model sustainability.

References

Chalmers, I., and P. Glasziou. 2009. "Avoidable waste in the production and reporting of research evidence." *The Lancet* 374 (9683):86–89.

Chambers, D. A., R. E. Glasgow, and K. C. Stange. 2013. "The dynamic sustainability framework: Addressing the paradox of sustainment amid ongoing change." *Implementation Science* 8 (1):1–11.

Crenshaw, K. 1990. "Mapping the margins: Intersectionality, identity politics, and violence against women of color." *Stanford Law Review* 43:1241.

Etherington, N., I. B. Rodrigues, L. Giangregorio, I. D. Graham, A. M. Hoens, D. Kasperavicius, C. Kelly, J. E. Moore, M. Ponzano, and J. Presseau. 2020. "Applying an intersectionality lens to the theoretical domains framework: A tool for thinking about how intersecting social identities and structures of power influence behaviour." *BMC Medical Research Methodology* 20 (1):1–13.

Francis, L., D. Dunt, and D. A. Cadilhac. 2016. "How is the sustainability of chronic disease health programmes empirically measured in hospital and related healthcare services? – A scoping review." *BMJ Open* 6 (5).

Glasziou, P., S. Straus, S. Brownlee, L. Trevena, L. Dans, G. Guyatt, A. G. Elshaug, R. Janett, and V. Saini. 2017. "Evidence for underuse of effective medical services around the world." *The Lancet* 390 (10090):169–177.

Graham, I. D., J. Logan, M. B. Harrison, S. E. Straus, J. Tetroe, W. Caswell, and N. Robinson. 2006. "Lost in knowledge translation: Time for a map?" *Journal of Continuing Education in the Health Professions* 26 (1):13–24.

Hailemariam, M., T. Bustos, B. Montgomery, R. Barajas, L. B. Evans, and A. Drahota. 2019. "Evidence-based intervention sustainability strategies: A systematic review." *Implementation Science* 14 (1):1–12.

Hankivsky, O., D. Grace, G. Hunting, M. Giesbrecht, A. Fridkin, S. Rudrum, O. Ferlatte, and N. Clark. 2014. "An intersectionality-based policy analysis framework: Critical reflections on a methodology for advancing equity." *International Journal for Equity in Health* 13 (1):1–16.

Lennox, L., L. Maher, and J. Reed. 2018. "Navigating the sustainability landscape: A systematic review of sustainability approaches in healthcare." *Implementation Science* 13 (1):1–17.

McCall, L. 2005. "The complexity of intersectionality." *Signs: Journal of Women in Culture and Society* 30 (3):1771–1800.

Moore, J. E., A. Mascarenhas, J. Bain, and S. E. Straus. 2017. "Developing a comprehensive definition of sustainability." *Implementation Science* 12 (1):1–8.

Proctor, E., D. Luke, A. Calhoun, C. McMillen, R. Brownson, S. McCrary, and M. Padek. 2015. "Sustainability of evidence-based healthcare: Research agenda, methodological advances, and infrastructure support." *Implementation Science* 10 (1):1–13.

Shelton, R. C., B. R. Cooper, and S. W. Stirman. 2018. "The sustainability of evidence-based interventions and practices in public health and health care." *Annual Review of Public Health* 39:55–76.

Straus, S., J. Tetroe, and I. D. Graham. 2013. *Knowledge Translation in Health Care: Moving from Evidence to Practice*. Oxford: John Wiley & Sons.

Strifler, L., R. Cardoso, J. McGowan, E. Cogo, V. Nincic, P. A. Khan, A. Scott, M. Ghassemi, H. MacDonald, and Y. Lai. 2018. "Scoping review identifies significant number of knowledge translation theories, models, and frameworks with limited use." *Journal of Clinical Epidemiology* 100:92–102.

Tricco, A. C., H. M. Ashoor, R. Cardoso, H. MacDonald, E. Cogo, M. Kastner, L. Perrier, A. McKibbon, J. M. Grimshaw, and S. E. Straus. 2015. "Sustainability of knowledge translation interventions in healthcare decision-making: A scoping review." *Implementation Science* 11 (1):1–10.

60 De-implementation

Iestyn Williams and Russell Mannion

De-implementation may require a separate theorization and the development of distinctive practical approaches. For example, as de-implementation programs often draw disproportionate critical attention, it may be that interventions are better targeted at the social, political, and economic contexts rather than at the behaviours and attitudes of individual adopters. Furthermore, if improved quality and equity are our goals, we must find ways to prevent de-implementation disproportionately affecting politically vulnerable services.

Introduction

We have been researching and thinking about de-implementation in healthcare for nearly two decades and, over this time, have come to appreciate its complexity and how it can be differentiated from other areas of implementation science. We will attempt to convey these in this essay, but in order to do this, it is first necessary to spell out what exactly we mean by de-implementation and situate it within the "natural evolution" of implementation science (Upvall and Bourgault 2018).

Defining de-implementation

Key defining properties of de-implementation are that 1) it is a *process* rather than a decision, and 2) it results from *intentional* (rather than accidental) activities to remove, replace, reduce, and/or restrict healthcare provision (Norton and Chambers 2020, Williams et al. 2020). Many current definitions of de-implementation assume benign motivations – that is, removing waste, increasing benefits, and so on – when in reality a variety of factors may inform such processes. In this essay we therefore adopt a descriptive definition of de-implementation as *processes for the deliberate removal, reduction, restriction, and replacement of established interventions, programs, and services*.

Commonalities between implementation and de-implementation

Like many similar terms (such as de-adoption, un-diffusion, disinvestment, exnovation), de-implementation is an inversion of a more established concept within implementation science (Niven et al. 2015). But the actual relationship between de-implementation and its opposite processes is unclear. On the one hand, there is much that is apparently shared, including the primary rationale of following evidence of effectiveness, cost-effectiveness, available alternatives, equity, local context, service cultures, and so forth (McKay et al. 2018). Taxonomies of implementation outcomes, including concepts such as "acceptability", "appropriateness",

DOI: 10.4324/9781003109945-64

and "penetration", can also be mapped onto de-implementation activities (Proctor et al. 2011, Prusaczyk, Swindle, and Curran 2020).

Furthermore, it seems likely that multilevel contextual analysis is as relevant to an understanding of de-implementation as it is to implementation processes. As an example, we might consider plans to bring about removal of services currently delivered in a community hospital setting (e.g., rehabilitation, palliative care, diagnostics, day surgery) and to relocate these into a larger, specialist acute provider organization. When introducing *new* practices, we would expect implementation to be influenced by the following:

- Characteristics of the new practice/s: how easily they can be adopted, what resources do they require, and how strong is the evidence for their efficacy?
- Patients and professionals: what degree of upheaval and change is required of those affected by the new ways of working, and what are their experiences and preferences?
- Organizations: how receptive is the unit or organization to new ways of working in general, and what is the role of strategy, structure, leadership, incentives, culture, prior histories of change, and availability of resources in this?
- Wider factors: what system, governmental, market, media, or social factors may influence implementation of the new ways of working?

It's not difficult to imagine how each of these categories and tiers might also be applied to the process of *de-implementation* of services from the community hospital setting, with the motivations and intended outcomes of the two processes mutually constituted and interlinked.

Differences between implementation and de-implementation

However, the detail of how these two processes play out can be quite different. If implementation science focuses on understanding and improving the uptake of research evidence into routine practice (Eccles and Mittman 2006), it is with some irony that we note that there is a paucity of robust evidence to inform de-implementation (Sevick et al. 2020). Linked to this, it is often much harder to make the case for the *benefits* of service removal (unless there are direct harms associated with the current program or practice) as some losses will inevitably be experienced. This in turn increases the likelihood of 1) negative organizational impacts, as current interventions are often tightly woven into the fabric of healthcare delivery and 2) risk aversion, anxiety, and distrust among patients and professionals "on the ground" (Gupta, Boland, and Aron 2017, Robert, Harlock, and Williams 2014).

For these reasons, de-implementation plans typically experience heightened levels of resistance, and this is exacerbated in cases where – as with our example of community hospitals– the removal of services presents an existential threat to the host organization. Healthcare organizations often perform roles (both real and symbolic) beyond the tangible impacts they have on patients and budgets (Prusaczyk, Swindle, and Curran 2020). Returning to our example of community hospitals, these functions may include:

> The physical presence of a community hospital, which acts as a visible expression of both historic and contemporary collective care and identity, but also . . . the different forms of interaction with it and the sense of ownership that this inspires. It extends beyond individual patients and their families to staff and, significantly, to the communities in which

they are based, and it connects together the different forms of value that community hospitals represent to these different stakeholders.

(Davidson et al. 2019)

In this context, de-implementation can trigger adversarial community responses in which the motives for de-implementation are impugned and recast pejoratively as "cuts", "closure", and "abandonment".

De-implementation theories and strategies

Implementation science aims to provide "models, theories, and frameworks" to examine how implementation works (Ronquillo et al. 2018), and the need for such models, theories, and frameworks applies equally to understanding processes of de-implementation (Nilsen et al. 2020). As of yet, we don't fully understand whether they are fundamentally linked and can be studied in unison or whether they require separate theoretical exposition. It certainly appears that de-implementation in its various forms encounters greater levels of opposition, partisan interests, and entrenched professional cultures. This suggests the need for distinctive de-implementation strategies that address its specific characteristics (Burton et al. 2019). As de-implementation programs often draw disproportionate critical attention, it may be that interventions are better targeted at the social, political, and economic contexts rather than at the behaviours and attitudes of individual adopters (Ronquillo et al. 2018). Our research also suggests the importance of examining prior *vulnerability* as a predictor of de-implementation outcomes; for example, by gauging the popularity of specific services and the level of political capital available to those that might seek to preserve them. And – returning to our example – we might also consider how small provider organizations such as community hospitals may themselves be in a relatively more precarious position and, therefore, vulnerable to losing their services, than larger, higher-profile hospitals.

Conclusion

De-implementation clearly has much to borrow from and contribute towards implementation science. But there are also clear differences in terms of drivers, stakeholders, and contexts which underpin the two processes. Our view is that greater attention should be focused on the uncomfortable reality that vulnerability may be an important predictor of successful de-implementation.

References

Burton, C., L. Williams, T. Bucknall, S. Edwards, D. Fisher, B. Hall, G. Harris, P. Jones, M. Makin, A. McBride, R. Meacock, J. Parkinson, J. Rycroft-Malone, and J. Waring. 2019. "Understanding how and why de-implementation works in health and care: Research protocol for a realist synthesis of evidence." *Systematic Reviews* 8 (1):194. doi: 10.1186/s13643-019-1111-8.

Davidson, D., A. Ellis Paine, J. Glasby, I. Williams, H. Tucker, T. Crilly, J. Crilly, N. L. Mesurier, J. Mohan, D. Kamerade, D. Seamark, and J. Marriott. 2019. "Health Services and Delivery Research." In *Analysis of the Profile, Characteristics, Patient Experience and Community Value of Community Hospitals: A Multimethod Study*. Southampton, UK: NIHR Journals Library.

Eccles, M. P., and B. S. Mittman. 2006. "Welcome to implementation science." *Implementation Science* 1 (1):1. doi: 10.1186/1748-5908-1-1.

Gupta, D. M., R. J. Boland, and D. C. Aron. 2017. "The physician's experience of changing clinical practice: A struggle to unlearn." *Implementation Science* 12 (1):28. doi: 10.1186/s13012-017-0555-2.

McKay, V. R., A. B. Morshed, R. C. Brownson, E. K. Proctor, and B. Prusaczyk. 2018. "Letting go: Conceptualizing intervention de-implementation in public health and social service settings." *American Journal of Community Psychology* 62 (1–2):189–202. doi: 10.1002/ajcp.12258.

Nilsen, P., S. Ingvarsson, H. Hasson, U. von Thiele Schwarz, and H. Augustsson. 2020. "Theories, models, and frameworks for de-implementation of low-value care: A scoping review of the literature." *Implementation Research and Practice* 1:1–15. doi: 10.1177/2633489520953762.

Niven, D. J., K. J. Mrklas, J. K. Holodinsky, S. E. Straus, B. R. Hemmelgarn, L. P. Jeffs, and H. T. Stelfox. 2015. "Towards understanding the de-adoption of low-value clinical practices: A scoping review." *BMC Medicine* 13:255. doi: 10.1186/s12916-015-0488-z.

Norton, W. E., and D. A. Chambers. 2020. "Unpacking the complexities of de-implementing inappropriate health interventions." *Implementation Science* 15 (1):2. doi: 10.1186/s13012-019-0960-9.

Proctor, E., H. Silmere, R. Raghavan, P. Hovmand, G. Aarons, A. Bunger, R. Griffey, and M. Hensley. 2011. "Outcomes for implementation research: Conceptual distinctions, measurement challenges, and research agenda." *Administration and Policy in Mental Healt* 38 (2):65–76. doi: 10.1007/s10488-010-0319-7.

Prusaczyk, B., T. Swindle, and G. Curran. 2020. "Defining and conceptualizing outcomes for de-implementation: Key distinctions from implementation outcomes." *Implementation Science Communications* 1 (1):43. doi: 10.1186/s43058-020-00035-3.

Robert, G., J. Harlock, and I. Williams. 2014. "Disentangling rhetoric and reality: An international Delphi study of factors and processes that facilitate the successful implementation of decisions to decommission healthcare services." *Implementation Science* 9:123–123. doi: 10.1186/s13012-014-0123-y.

Ronquillo, C., J. Day, K. Warmoth, N. Britten, Stein, Ken, and I. Lang. 2018. "An implementation science perspective on deprescribing." *Public Policy and Aging Report* 28 (4):134–139. doi: 10.1093/ppar/pry032.

Sevick, K., L. J. Soril, G. MacKean, T. W. Noseworthy, and F. M. Clement. 2020. "Unpacking early experiences with health technology reassessment in a complex healthcare system." *International Journal of Healthcare Management* 13 (2):156–162.

Upvall, M. J., and A. M. Bourgault. 2018. "De-implementation: A concept analysis." *Nursing Forum*. doi: 10.1111/nuf.12256.

Williams, I., J. Harlock, G. Robert, J. Kimberly, and R. Mannion. 2020. "Is the end in sight? A study of how and why services are decommissioned in the English National Health Service." *Sociology of Health and Illness* 43 (2):441–458.

The long and winding road

Navigating the field of implementation science

Jeffrey Braithwaite, Frances Rapport, and Robyn Clay-Williams

What does it take to solve the Rubik's cube of implementation science? We use the metaphor of Rubik's cube because it evokes an image of what the essays in this book represent – a multidimensional, many-faceted depiction of the omni-sided nature of implementation science which we have portrayed in the sections and essays of the book.

At the core of solving the problems of both the cube and in implementation science is the "combinations" issue. Most exponents of Rubik's cube know that the number of permutations is the daunting aspect of tackling it and the joy inherent in manipulating and solving it. Similarly, addressing implementation science is a combinations problem. Just like Rubik's cube, there are many aspects to implementation science, and it is both formidable and joyful to constantly strive to choose a pathway to get evidence of what we know works into routine practice. The 3-D puzzle that forms the implementation science "cube" is created by the domains making up this endeavour – research evidence itself, theoretical paradigms that account for getting that research into practice, methodologies ranging from randomized controlled trials (RCTs) to social science methods and models by which to explain getting evidence into practice and their applications. We need to manipulate these different factors to "align the colours" and solve the particular implementation problem facing us.

While there are limits to the cube metaphor, let's stay with it for a little while longer. Six sides, each with nine squares totalling 54 panels, are not enough to show the plethora of domains that must be called upon to understand implementation science. And, despite the number of combinations to Rubik's puzzle – in a cube there are 43,252,003,274,489,856,000 combinations or, more simply put, 43 quintillion – and regardless of the sheer size of this number, solutions are finite. In implementation science this is not the case. The number of pathways to getting evidence into practice and the number of ideas that can be harnessed to achieve this goal in any particular setting or instance are effectively infinite. Added to that, Rubik's cube is a static piece of puzzle equipment. The cube itself is a defined, known entity, fixed in time and space. That is not the case for any one implementation challenge in a defined setting.

Rubik's cube is, in short, *complicated* but not *complex*. That is to say, it is hard to solve, but there are solutions, and the problem it poses is addressable. Implementation science, or more aptly the pursuit of it, is ongoing, dynamic, and intricate and manifests as a challenge in many different ways and uniquely in every health setting. Like other complex problems, there are many unknowns and a myriad of interrelated factors which combine and are not reduceable to solutions that can be readily found by following rules or algorithms.

Still, despite the mind-bending complexities of implementation science, we promised in the title a book that shared its key concepts, and that is what we have, in conjunction with our authors, attempted to produce. We may have omitted some things that other people would

DOI: 10.4324/9781003109945-65

judge to be key, and no book in a field such as implementation science can sustain a claim that it is definitive. But we do hope that we have captured many of the recurring and important ideas which make up the implementation science domain.

Leaving the Rubik's cube metaphor behind and turning to what it is that we have documented above in 60 essays, we provide a summary in the accompanying Table 61.1 of the book in its entirety – with the central information of the authors and the essay title, lessons learnt, the country from which the authorship of that essay hails, the empirical stance they've taken, and their implied or explicit theoretical approach.

Part I took us on a journey through many of the important principles and concepts used by and applied to implementation science. These are the fundamental building blocks to a good understanding of the tenets of the field and what the contributors to it hold to be essential. These include taking a complex, systems approach, looking at theories and lenses for seeing implementation science in different ways, through to key theoretical ideas such as the Consolidated Framework for Implementation Research (CFIR), the Theoretical Domains Framework (TDF), Normalization Process Theory, organizational theory of various kinds, Diffusion of Innovation theory, and the number of ways people can choose in organizing and evidence building. There are many lessons to take from this section, but one point that should be apparent to readers is that despite implementation science being a relatively new field (the journal *Implementation Science* only began in 2006), it has matured sufficiently so that people can write very good essays on topics such as the principles of implementation science, organizational theory for implementation science, and various aspects of the environment within which interventions must be implemented. A science worthy of the title must be able to express principles and concepts underpinning the works of its practitioners; this has largely been achieved in Part I.

With a good understanding of the foundation principles under our belt, Part II moves into real-world strategies, taking us through the design and application process of implementation with renderings on methods and methodology. It begins with essays underpinning the key methodologies used for implementing interventions and then moves on to practical advice on individual methodologies. Rather than a specific "how to" for each methodology, the assembled contributions present an overview and key cues to guide the reader in choosing an appropriate approach by which to tackle their implementation problem. The section concludes with essays on the planning process and how to initiate change, followed by sensemaking and adaptation to round off our thinking and inform our strategies.

Turning to Part III, and by way of bringing the compendium to a close, we present contributions that account for important aspects that need our attention once implementation is underway. How do we evaluate our efforts, for example, and how do we make our successes sustainable? A variety of perspectives are offered to help with the messy process of making change happen in complex healthcare systems, in ways that are methodologically rigorous and informed by evidence, yet practical, and achieve improvement. As a comprehensive compendium, the book hopes to have offered a palette of implementation science choices: it is now over to you, the reader, to integrate and manipulate the various facets both in your mind and in practice, to successfully grapple with the myriad of problems and puzzles arising in your own projects, evaluations, and assignments. The overarching goal, put simply, is better, more evidence-based care for every patient in every health system. What more noble and motivating pursuit can there be?

Table 61.1 A summary of the book – authors, lessons, country, empirical stance, and theoretical approach

Author/s, Essay	Selected Key Lessons	Country	Empirical Stance	Theoretical Approach
Part 1: Setting the Scene: Principles and Concepts of Implementation Science				
Braithwaite, Complexity Science	• A linear approach to getting evidence into practice only gets you so far • A complexity approach, while challenging, more closely mirrors the real world that implementation science seeks to tackle	Australia	Secondary sources	Systems dynamics and complexity science
Ellen and Perlman, Taking a Systems View	• A systems approach helps focus across the micro, meso, and macro levels to meet implementation challenges • It helps focus on important interconnections and relationships	Israel	Secondary analysis of systems literature	Systems theory and health services research
Woods and Rayo, Resilience Changes the Lens for Healthcare Implementation Systems	• Understanding adaptive capacity via a platform of resilience engineering • Draws attention to recurring patterns in adaptive systems, for example, decompensation, cross-disciplinary working, and outmoded behaviours	United States	Analysis of resilience engineering studies applied to implementation	Resilience engineering, systems theory, and adaptive behaviours
Rayo, Implementation Systems that Support Resilient Performance	• Examines how to detect early patient decompensation and shows how clinicians exhibit resilient performance in clinical practice • Clinicians provide resilient performance to work around systems' limitations and constraints, applying a wide range of resources and resourcefulness	United States	Case study and associated research on clinicians' resilient performance	Resilience engineering, decompensation theory, and systems theory
Kilbourne, Principles of Implementation Science	• Argues that implementation science needs to get back to its roots and focus on tackling challenges of evidence-based practice in the real world • Highlights the US Department of Veterans Affairs Quality Enhancement Research Initiative (QUERI) and its implementation roadmap • QUERI provides a model for applying principles of implementation science in clinical settings	United States	Studies by the Veteran Affairs in improving the take-up of treatments known to be effective in routine practice	Implementation science theory

(Continued)

Table 61.1 (Continued)

Author/s, Essay	Selected Key Lessons	Country	Empirical Stance	Theoretical Approach
Clark, Medical Humanism: The Role of Character in Implementation Science	• Adopts a humanistic approach to implementation science examining the narratives, rhetoric, and differing stakeholders' perspectives on implementation • Argues the case for the character of the clinician as an important determinant of effective implementation practice	United States	Reliance on studies of ethics, narrative, and the attributes of clinicians	Medical humanities; narrative and storytelling theories
Kislov and Wilson, Theorizing	• Calls for researchers to consider not only the theories they use but also the process of theorizing • Explicates the role of differing kinds of theories ranging from small to mid-range to grand theory • Suggests how rich theorizing might support fresh insights into implementation	United Kingdom	Knowledge translation	Theoretical pluralism and theory-in-use
Nilsen, Theories, Models, and Frameworks in Implementation Science: A Taxonomy	• Categorizes theories used in implementation science and examines the aims of different theoretical approaches • Differentiates process models from determinant frameworks, classic theories, specific implementation theories, and evaluation frameworks	Sweden	Draws on studies applying theories, frameworks, and models used in implementation science	Theoretical categorization and theoretical pluralism
Damschroder, The Consolidated Framework for Implementation Research (CFIR)	• Articulates the contours of the Consolidated Framework for Implementation Research (CFIR) • Demonstrates its wide adoption and use across many studies	United States	Drawing on studies analysing and applying the CFIR	Implementation science theory
Lorencatto, The Theoretical Domains Framework	• Showcases the value of the Theoretical Domains Framework (TDF) and its flexible use as a determinant framework	United Kingdom	Applications of the TDF across multiples domains and settings	Application of theoretical framework (the TDF) in the field

Birken and Haines, Organization Theory for Implementation Science	• It is useful for implementation science to draw on organization theories; many are quite mature and are helpful in apprehending the dimensions of activities within organizations seeking to get evidence into practice • Examples are provided, ranging across public welfare, safer care, and collaborative teamwork	United States	Case studies exemplifying the use of organization theory	Multidimensional approach to organization theory
Moullin and Aarons, Exploration, Preparation, Implementation, Sustainment (EPIS) Framework	• The EPIS (Exploration, Preparation, Implementation, Sustainment) framework is a useful device for understanding implementation and constructing evaluations • It is sufficiently flexible that it can be applied to a wide range of implementation problems	Australia	Case examples and studies using EPIS	Implementation theory
May, Implementation Science as Process Ecology: Normalization Process Theory	• Outlines Normalization Process Theory (NPT), drawing attention to embedded routing practices which are often deeply etched into activities • This is an important focus for implementation activists and implementation science	United Kingdom	Summary of tools, studies, and models in NPT	NPT and theories of implementation
Yu, Diffusion of Innovation Theory	• Articulates the application of Rogers' famous Diffusion of Innovation theory in healthcare and the S-curve of innovation • The theory has provided generalized guidance for many implementation studies	Australia	Draws on some seminal studies using the Diffusion of Innovation theory framework and S-curve	Diffusion of Innovation theory
Smith and Durcinoska, Health-related Quality of Life	• Health-related quality of life (HRQOL) is discussed: the way disease and treatment affect people's physical functioning and wellbeing • More recently Patient Reported Outcome Measures (PROMs) have been used as a way of understanding HRQOL	Australia	Empirical studies of Patient Reported Outcome Measures (PROMs) and HRQOL	Theories of the use of PROMs and HRQOL as they are applied in practice

(Continued)

Table 61.1 (Continued)

Author/s, Essay	Selected Key Lessons	Country	Empirical Stance	Theoretical Approach
Elwyn, Shared Decision-Making: Consider Context	• Shared decision-making is centrally concerned with collaborating over choices made about treatment and care in a health setting • Its application has been uneven, so perhaps it will be better to consider the context within which shared decision-making takes place, including considering the person's *lifeworld*	United States	Studies and articles articulating shared decision-making	Theories of collaboration, sharing decisions, and context
Lamprell, Core Aspects of Nudge as a Behaviour Change Paradigm in Implementation Science	• Analyses theories of nudge and choice architecture and applies them to healthcare • Nudging clinicians is a better way of influencing behaviour than more blunt change mechanisms often used	Australia	Empirical studies of nudge and influence	Theories of change and influence
Hill and Knox, Pipeline and Cyclical Models of Evidence Building: The Roles of Implementation Research	• An important distinction arises between a pipeline from an idea through research to implementation, through to scale-up and an approach which is more cyclical, building improvement over time • Taking a cyclical approach is more attuned to the real world of practice and can help build adaptive learning organizations	United States	Studies of different modes of getting evidence into practice	Pipeline theory and cyclical theories for evidence building and implementation
Part II: Methodology and Methods of Implementation Science				
Sevdalis and Hull, Application	• Is implementation science applied, or is it mainly studied by researchers with little connection to the real world of practice? • In the past the field may have been more ivory tower, but more recently, implementation scientists are engaging directly with in situ problems	United Kingdom	Studies and papers addressing the tensions between implementation science researchers and practitioners doing implementation	Theories of application; theories of implementation
Braithwaite, Plan, Do, Study, Act (PDSA)	• Emerging from original work in the 1920s by Shewhart, the Plan, Do, Study, Act (PDSA) cycle was an innovation designed to guide change and improvement activities • It proposes a relatively simple algorithm for change	Australia	Studies using PDSA	Historical theories of change; PDSA and control charts

Braithwaite, Formative Evaluation Feedback Loops	• The Formative Evaluation Feedback Loops (FEFLs) model brings the idea of feedback as a powerful mechanism for creating more change and improvement • It also involves conceptualizing change as a longitudinal problem and stresses the importance of regular evaluation to monitor progress	Australia	Studies using FEFLs	Theories of longitudinal change and its stages and operationalization
Carayon, Implementation or Continuous Design? The Contribution of Human Factors and Engineering to Healthcare Quality and Patient Safety	• The Human Factors Engineering (HFE) discipline focuses attention on human characteristics and the design of work systems • In promoting both human wellbeing and better performance, the Systems Engineering Initiative for Patient Safety (SEIPS) model is a key example	United States	Studies of human characteristics, workplace design, and patient safety	Human Factors and Ergonomics theory
Ogden, Core and Variation Components	• Any implementation or intervention can be separated into the key things that make it work (core components) and additional things that help make it work better (variation components) • An example is Multisystemic Therapy (MST) and the adolescent and family treatment program	Norway	Papers on core and variable implementation science components; research on MST	Theories of what works, change, and adolescent and family theories
Aron and Leykum, Sensemaking: Appreciating Patterns and Coherence in Complexity	• Humans spend much effort in making sense – giving meaning – to their experience and the events, contexts, and issues that they encounter • Its role in implementation is critical; different people in different circumstances in different settings will give meaning to an implementation or an intervention, and the differing stages and components of them, and these need to be woven together to good effect	United States	Selection of studies and perspectives on sensemaking	Sensemaking theory, theories of change, complexity, and implementation

(*Continued*)

Table 61.1 (Continued)

Author/s, Essay	Selected Key Lessons	Country	Empirical Stance	Theoretical Approach
Rapport and Zurynski, Methodological Diversity	• Pluralist methodologies are one of the hallmarks of contemporary implementation science • This should not be seen as a weakness but leads to more rich information which can be addressed by approaches such as triangulation or mixed methods synthesis	Australia	Research using a wide range of methods and evaluation techniques	Theories of diversity and mixed methodology
Lorencatto, Applying the Theoretical Domains Framework (TDF): Its Uses and Limitations	• The Theoretical Domains Framework (TDF) brings attention to the multiple categories of theory that can be used to illuminate implementation models • It suggests conceptualizing implementation problems and adequately framing them with an appropriate theory	United Kingdom	Studies applying the TDF in various circumstances	Multiple theoretical paradigms
Waring and Clarke, Ethnography	• Seeking first-hand experience with people within their ecosystem in order to arrive at an enriched description and understanding of their practices and activities is the domain of ethnography • It seeks to understand naturalistically what's going on in the field; thus, it is a highly beneficial but often underutilized method in implementation science	United Kingdom	Studies applying ethnographic approaches to illuminate social activities in situ	Ethnographic theory and theories of social observation and practices
Rapport, Walking Methods	• Walking around in a social setting, gaining information "on the hoof" is a novel research technique also known as mobile methods • It can be highly insightful and lead to interesting data not otherwise harvestable by traditional methods	Australia	Studies using direct information gathered in situ	Theories of information gathering directly from social settings and ecosystems of interest to implementation and implementation science

Hollnagel and Clay-Williams, Modelling Complex Socio-Technical Systems: The Functional Resonance Analysis Method (FRAM)	• The Functional Resonance Analysis Method (FRAM) is a method for describing functions to model how a system performs • A relatively simple example, drawing blood to prepare for a transfusion, is mapped using the functionality of FRAM to illuminate how it can derive useful insights into the functioning of the system	Sweden, Australia	Case study of a FRAM	Theories of social structure and the functioning and performance of a system
Long, Getting a Handle on the Social Processes of Implementation: Social network Research	• One way to understand the social processes in healthcare and the relationships between stakeholders is to conduct a Social Network Analysis (SNA) – a depiction of the way components (individuals or their artefacts) connect with each other • The example of a network of translational researchers and clinicians in cancer care is provided to exemplify and depict the social networks and how they changed over time	Australia	Longitudinal studies into social network changes over time	Social Network Theory
Smith, Sentiment Analysis for Use within Rapid Implementation Research: How Far and Fast Can We Go?	• The opinions people hold about implementation can be measured and factored in to implementation processes • It has not been used to the extent it might; it remains an underutilized technique with much potential	Australia	Studies using and applying sentiment analysis	Sentiment and opinion theories
Palinkas, Mixed Method Designs	• Combining and synthesizing qualitative and quantitative approaches can illuminate questions and generate a wider range of rich findings • This can increase the credibility and complementarity of data findings • Mixed methods are useful in implementation science due to the complexity of its subject matter and implementation processes	United States	Studies and evaluations using mixed methodology	Pluralist research design, concepts, and theories

(Continued)

Table 61.1 (Continued)

Author/s, Essay	Selected Key Lessons	Country	Empirical Stance	Theoretical Approach
Patterson and Deutsch, Simulation to Improve Patient Care	• Simulation, whereby skills and knowledge are practised outside of normal work settings with a view to improving care, is a useful approach • It can also be conducted in situ; both off-site and on-site simulation can support implementation activities	United States	Studies both off-site and in situ of simulation	Theories of simulation; implementation and improvement
Nakamura and Nakajima, In Situ Simulation	• In situ simulation can be more realistic for participants than laboratory or other external simulation activities • Case studies of in situ simulation can illuminate the propensity for results to feed in to implementation and improvement	United States	Cases of in situ simulation	Theories of simulation implementation and improvement
Øvretveit, Emergency Implementation Science	• The need for rapid change is becoming greater and becomes especially apparent during a pandemic • A case study of the Stockholm care response to the COVID-19 pandemic provides useful insight into the emerging field of Emergency Implementation Science	Sweden	Studies of rapid implementation science	Theories of emergencies; disasters and implementation
Smith and Hutchinson, Planning for Implementation: Why, Who, and How	• If implementation is to be effective in the real world, it requires adequate baseline preparation and planning • This in turn requires tools and frameworks to help support such preparation	Australia	Research on implementation planning	Implementation theory and planning theory
Susskind, Consensus Building: A Key Concept in Implementation Science	• An important component of implementation science is to build consensus for the targeted change • There are various structured steps that can be taken to enhance partnership collaboration and consensus	United States	Studies of consensus and consensus building	Theories of consensus; governance and negotiation

Lamprell, Nudge: Finding Clues and Using Cues to Shift Clinician Behaviour	• Implementation science has discovered that clinicians don't necessarily take up the best evidence, and practice varies across settings • Nudges, while an important and often effective technique for influencing clinician behaviour, can be effective in one setting but does not necessarily work in the same way in another setting	Australia	Cases and studies of nudging clinician behaviour	Nudge theory and choice architecture theory
Ludlow and Westbrook, Design and Implementation of Dashboards in Healthcare	• The large amounts of data collected by healthcare organizations can be brought together in an informative dashboard • They require thoughtful design and application so that they are user-friendly and useful	Australia	Studies of dashboard construction and use	Information technology theory and theories of dashboard use
Leykum and Aron, Sensemaking: Paying Attention to the Stories We Tell to Improve Our Ability to Act	• People are often not unified in their work; they practise differently and differ in their views about why they are being asked to implement something new • One approach to tackle these problematics is to understand the sense people make of that new intervention or practice and to pay attention to the stories they tell each other	United States	Studies of physician sensemaking	Sensemaking theory and organizational theory
von Thiele Schwarz, Hasson, and Aarons, Adaptations	• Fidelity of implementation and adaptations are important and can be seen as oppositional forces • We can bring those two ideas together via a value equation, whereby value is created through an intervention in a context and resolving the tension between these via implementation strategies	Sweden	Studies of fidelity and adaptation	Theories of fidelity, value, interventions, context, and adaptation

Part III: Challenges with Evidence into Practice: Translation, Evaluation, Sustainability

Rycroft-Malone, Evidence Synthesis: Maximizing the Potential	• A key task to implementation science is bringing together findings as a platform for improvement • Realist synthesis is one approach to achieving this; whichever evidence synthesis approach is taken, there is an argument for greater multidisciplinary and collaborative efforts	United Kingdom	Studies of collaboration, multidisciplinary implementation science, and evidence synthesis	Theories of synthesis, context, and pluralism

(Continued)

Table 61.1 (Continued)

Author/s, Essay	Selected Key Lessons	Country	Empirical Stance	Theoretical Approach
Chen, Theory-driven Evaluation	• To achieve effective evaluation of an evidence-based intervention requires understanding of action and change • Various models have been proposed, and one crucial axis is to balance bottom-up and top-down approaches to implementation and dissemination	United States	Studies and evaluations of implementation science	Theories of evaluation, change, action, implementation, and adaption
Wensing, Process Evaluation of Implementation Strategies	• Of the many approaches to assessing implementation strategies, process evaluation focuses on implementation along its journey in contrast to the outcomes that it produces • Some key aspects of process evaluation are to consider implementation strategies, fidelity, end results, and transferability, and the evaluation should be adequately theorized	Germany	Studies and evaluations of the topics covered by process evaluation	Theories of evaluation, change, complex interventions, fidelity, and context
Chambers, Dissemination	• All the efforts of implementation need ultimately to make a difference in the world – this is where uptake, adoption, and scaling come in • Dissemination is highly complex and challenging to achieve, and the research and practice of dissemination is itself both a work in progress and worthy focus of study	United States	Dissemination case studies and research	Theories of adoption, take-up, scale, and communication channels
Nilsen, Neher, Ellström, and Gardner, A Learning Perspective on Implementation	• Getting evidence into practice requires adoption of new interventions and abandonment of non-evidence-based interventions • Adaptive (progressive, more incremental) learning and developmental (more deliberative and conscious) learning can support adoption	Sweden	Studies of learning and implementation	Theories of learning; adoption and de-adoption of new practices; theories of context
Ehrhart and Aarons, Alignment: Impact on Implementation Processes and Outcomes	• Organizational alignment (or fit or congruence) is an important factor in implementation success • Five types of alignment are stressed: internal systems, horizontal units, vertical, innovation–client alignment, and innovation–provider alignment	United States	Studies of fit, congruence, alignment, and sustainment	Theories of impact, institutionalization, and organizational theory

Hollnagel and Clay-Williams, Work-as-Imagined and Work-as-Done	• Work-as-Imagined (WAI), or a focus on ideas about how work should be done, and Work-as-Done (WAD), or actual performance, are different aspects of how people may do implementation • It is useful when doing implementation or an intervention to consider the gaps between WAI and WAD and find ways to reconcile them	Denmark, Australia	Studies of WAI and WAD	Theories of resilient healthcare; workplace theories; sociological constructs
Aarons and Ehrhart, Leading Implementation by Focusing on Strategic Implementation Leadership	• Leaders can make or break implementation efforts, but little research on leadership of implementation and getting evidence into practice has taken place • The Implementation Leadership scale examines multiple aspects, including leaders' knowledge, activities, support for interventions, and persistence through the implementation process, helping making concrete otherwise abstract ideas about leadership	United States	Studies of leadership behaviours pertaining to implementation	Leadership theory; theories of organizational change and improvement
Laver, Agents of Change: The Example of an Allied Health Professional	• Agents of change are those who provide leverage and actions to institute new ways of changing things • Allied health professionals can be key catalysts for productive change	Australia	Case study of allied health professionals as change agents	Change; agency; improvement; sustainment
Bates, Clinical Decision Support	• Simply delivering decision support to clinicians in the workplace is insufficient to improve care • Implementation science is needed to embrace a clinical decision support vehicle and leverage the benefits and potential of effective clinical decision support	United States	Studies of clinical decision support and adoption	Theories of take-up, change, benefits realization, and socio-technical theories
Vanhaecht and Coeckelberghs, Interprofessional Team Working: The Case of Care Pathways	• Interprofessional team working should not be taken for granted but is itself a complex, multifaceted intervention • If interprofessional teams collaborate along care pathways, there can be beneficial outcomes for both the teams themselves and patient care	Belgium	Studies of interprofessional care; research on clinical pathways	Theories of inter-professionalism, pathway theory, and theories of multidisciplinarity

(Continued)

Table 61.1 (Continued)

Author/s, Essay	Selected Key Lessons	Country	Empirical Stance	Theoretical Approach
Bridges, Older People's Care	• Almost everyone agrees that we can do better in providing care to older people, but a top-down focus on somethings such as patient flow often leaves carers feeling dissatisfied and demotivated • The influence of context and culture and the support of clinicians so that they can provide improved care are crucial determinants of better care to the elderly	United Kingdom	Case study of aged care provision in an emergency department	Theories of change, improvement, and older people's care
Wensing, Implementation Interventions to Enhance Patient Self-management	• Much care can be delivered by patients themselves; improving patients' self-management can be construed as an intervention • The different kinds of patients' self-management can be construed as those that are individualistic, or systems level – and much more research is needed in this area	Germany	Studies of self-management which have a positive effect on patients' lives	Theories of patient self-management, implementation, and adoption
Clay-Williams, Complex Systems and Unintended Consequences	• When we act in complex systems, despite efforts to make things better, there can be adverse or beneficial unintended consequences • Examples of the positive include Alexander Fleming discovering penicillin and examples of the negative are the introduction of cane toads in Australia; having resilient health systems can act to support positive consequences and mitigation strategies if things are going the wrong way	Australia	Studies and evaluations of systems and their outputs and outcomes	Complex systems theory and theories of adverse and beneficial effects
Saurin, The Nature and Need for Slack in Healthcare Services	• Slack in organizations provides the place to allow for adaptability; such redundancy can be regarded as an asset and latent buffer when things get busy or go wrong • On the other hand, slack can be a signal of inefficiency, or lead to greater complexity in systems or more complacency, and therefore, there is often a search for the optimal amount of slack	Brazil	Studies and evaluation of slack, redundancy, and organizational processes and outcomes	Theories of slack, waste, and unintended consequences

Schiff, Diagnosis Errors	• Reaching a diagnosis is a challenging clinical process • Providing better systems can help improve diagnosis but need to be better designed including providing adequate time, informatics infrastructure, diagnostic safety culture, support for situational awareness, and safety nets	United States	Studies of diagnostic safety and improving diagnosis	Theories of diagnosis, systems, change, and pitfalls
Sklar and Aarons, "Scaling-out" Evidence-based Practices	• Much new evidence does not get taken up into clinical practice, so we need ways to design strategies to get evidence into practice • Scaling-out is a conscious approach to doing this; there are various types depending on the target and the delivery system	United States	Studies and cases of scaling and getting evidence into practice	Implementation design theory, scale-up theory, and generalizability theory
Straus, Implementation Sustainability	• It is one thing to stimulate behaviour change and another to sustain it • Choices need to be made about what it is that needs to be sustained, and an examination of the multiple factors that influence or determine whether any new practice is sustained is critical	Canada	Studies of outcomes, adaptation, and anchoring sustainable change	Theories of sustainability, end results, and outcomes
Williams and Mannion, De-implementation	• A corollary of implementation is de-implementation – that is, the removal of a wasteful, non-beneficial, or non-evidence-based practice, program, or service • All in all, it is difficult to take something away that is already in place, and there is less research on de-implementation than there is on implementation	United Kingdom	Studies of de-implementation	Theories of de-implementation, de-adoption, un-diffusion, and clinical routines

Source: Created by author

Index

Printed in the United States
by Baker & Taylor Publisher Services